Body Moves

Body Moves

The Psychology of Exercise

James Gavin, Ph.D.

Stackpole Books

Published by
STACKPOLE BOOKS
Cameron and Kelker Streets
P.O. Box 1831
Harrisburg, PA 17105

Printed in the United States of America

10 9 8 7 6 5 4 3 2 1

Library of Congress Cataloging-in-Publication Data

Gavin, James, Ph.D.
   Body moves.

   Bibliography: p.
   Includes index.
   1. Exercise—Psychological aspects.   2. Personality.
I. Title.
RA781.G37   1988   616.89'13   87-18159
ISBN 0-8117-2272-4

To Mary and Paddy
   —for the lilt of Irish laughter,
Dick McDonald
   —for keeping the wind always at my back,
and Selina,
   —for stoking the fire within

Contents

1

Change Your Body—Change Your Mind

Have You Ever Noticed?

"I would never take up jogging! People who jog have to be crazy . . . they must like punishment." It's hard for some people to imagine engaging in certain exercise programs. It seems foreign to their makeups. No matter how popular an activity may be or how much social pressure they feel to go jogging, take aerobics, or start a Nautilus program, they will resist because "it's just not my kind of thing."

We can probably go a step further in saying that some people simply don't believe in exercise. As W. C. Fields once said, "Whenever I feel the urge to exercise, I just lie down and wait until it passes." It's clear that people have different attitudes toward physical activity—there are people who don't like to exercise, people who do it because it's good for them, and people who actually enjoy it. In fact, we can include another category for those who are hooked: the term *exercise addiction* has recently been added to the growing list of modern psychological problems.

We might wonder if some people are fitness fanatics because of a biological "exercise gene" that predisposes them to jog at lunchtime or

9

lift weights for fun. Of course, the heredity argument needs to be counterbalanced by the environment position, which suggests that if your parents and friends are jocks, then you will probably become a jock, too.

Without completely ignoring the heredity and environment positions, we should look at another possibility, which is that most people would enjoy, and indeed profit, from some form of exercise if they could find one that was right for them. Determining what is right for an individual is complicated. To get to the heart of the matter, we need a foundation that helps us understand why there is a right set of sports and exercises for us, as well as how some exercise programs can be psychologically damaging. For the moment, let's take a detour into today's fitness scene.

Commonsense Definitions

Everyday expressions reveal a commonsense understanding of exercise and personality. We hear remarks about body builders being overbearing, swimmers being introspective, ballet dancers being perfectionistic, football players being aggressive, and runners being compulsive. Are these just stereotypes — or is there some truth to these assertions?

Human beings defy simple categorization. Certainly, people who participate in a particular sport are not genetic clones. If they were, there would be very little difference between these athletes either in terms of physical or psychological makeup.

Why then do we agree with the stereotypes? Why is it that when we are told that someone looks like a swimmer, we concur so quickly? On a personal level, why do we feel attracted to some sports and not to others? Or, why is it that many of us prefer to associate with certain athletes and shun others? Honestly, who would want to admit that their ideal companion is a sumo wrestler — or a bowler?

A Grain of Truth

In studies of prejudice and stereotyping, psychologists have noted that we form stereotypes and find others to agree with these generalizations because there is a grain of truth in them. So, when your friend says that ballet dancers are perfectionists or that weight lifters are narcissists, you may agree. You may have read about a perfectionistic ballerina or you may know one. You may also have wandered through a Gold's Gym watching body builders strutting around the mirrored studio flexing their muscles and marveled at the looking-glass love affair.

At the same time, you may know of individuals who don't fit the stereotype. You may recognize the tendency to overgeneralize. Nonetheless, you are clearly aware that in your social network—at the office or in the community—there are the racquetballers, the noontime aerobics fanatics, the runners, the body shapers, the golfers, and even the bowlers. And to some degree, you may feel more identification with one of these cliques than with any other—you may even belong to one.

If you participate in a fitness activity, you would be hard pressed to identify one trait that somehow characterized all its participants. But then, you have to ask, "Why did we choose this exercise and not some other?"

Many answers are possible: I take aerobics classes because they fit my schedule; My boss plays racquetball, so I thought I would give it a try; My husband has been running for years and I decided to join him; I always wanted to have a body like Arnold Schwarzenegger. In spite of these rationales, the grain of truth about each stereotype persists with a nagging simplicity that clusters all runners, weightlifters, racquetball players, dancers, and bowlers into the same mold.

Birds of a Feather . . .

There is another revered psychological principle that helps justify the stereotypes we have about athletes and exercise buffs. Simply put, it asserts that similarity attracts or, in popular parlance, "birds of a feather flock together." This tells us that people who share personality characteristics find satisfaction in one another's company.

It may not always be obvious how two individuals are alike. We know we are drawn to people who have similar interest patterns or even similar physical features, but on a deeper level we also find we are connected to our friends by psychological factors as well. This is not to deny another basis for forming friendships, namely, that "opposites attract." But the evidence strongly favors the similarity hypothesis. We are more drawn together by the ways we are alike than by our dissimilarities.

Taking our discussion back to the locker room, we may need a closer look to see how we resemble those around us. Certainly, there is a wide assortment of body types and personalities jogging the streets. And if you walk into an exercise class, you will find a full array of shapes and sizes. Even on tennis courts and in swimming pools, body dimensions and personal styles are quite diverse.

Variation in body types will decrease, however, as we move from novice to advanced levels. There aren't too many seriously obese runners in the Boston Marathon. And the "Dolly Parton" look is rarely found in a classical corps de ballet. This is not to say that short people don't play basketball or that ectomorphs (frail, thin types) steer clear of the football field, but it does suggest a self-selection process coupled with body changes produced by particular sports.

Two popular questions are raised by this discussion of similarity: why do people first get involved in a particular activity, and why do they continue? Attempts to answer these questions represent a major focus of the new field of sports and exercise psychology. Although they have relevance to the concerns of this book, a third question is far more critical: *How do sports change you?* We need to consider what kinds of changes you will experience if you are involved in a sport or exercise program over a long period of time.

This question of how we are affected by our athletic experiences has an important impact on the similiarity hypothesis. It implies that we become more similar *because of* our athletic pursuits—regardless of whether we intend such changes or whether these changes are entirely beneficial. How can this happen?

The Missing Link

At the very least, we know that rigorous exercise changes our physical shape. We lose weight, muscles become more defined, and body proportions change. But what if we also change our personalities through exercise? This would cause serious concern. After all, we can see what is happening to our bodies—but mental changes?

The changes discussed in this book go beyond what is typically sought in exercise programs. We only need look at the exercise charts to find that marathon runners have the lowest percentage of body fat of any athlete. Does this mean that if we want to have low body fat we should go in for marathon running? Some people might answer yes without ever stopping to consider what it does to one's psyche to train one hundred miles a week. (Of course, others might opt for liposuction surgery!)

What if we were interested in improving specific personality traits? Are there charts to tell us what effects exercise will have on personality? For example, if you wanted to become more assertive, could you find a list of recommended sports? Unfortunately, no. On the other hand, are such charts possible? Most definitely yes! By the time you have finished this book, you will have a chart on personality change through exercise, along with answers to many related questions.

For now, let us take a closer look at one athletic experience—the aerobic dance class—for some insight into personality change through exercise.

Just to Illustrate

If you walk into an aerobics class, you will note that body shapes, ages, and sexes of participants vary considerably. What is common to all is that they have made time for a certain kind of experience on a more or less regular basis. And since the experience can be dissected, we have our first technique for probing the fitness personality.

Aerobics classes differ widely in style. Some instructors are more into dance than calisthenics, and some like high impact while others prefer low impact. If you have taken a few of these classes or even watched televised aerobics, you will be able to imagine the following experience.

You walk into a large mirrored room that allows you to watch your-self—and anyone else you care to—as you exercise. You notice the loud speakers that within minutes will blare a nonstop pounding sequence of pop rock. Your fellow aerobics worshippers begin pouring in. Some are clad in stunning color-coordinated leotards, tights, leg warmers, and sweat bands. Others may be masked in loose-fitting workout suits. In walks the instructor. She is about 5' 3", medium build, not much more than twenty-three years old, and obviously in great shape. It begins to hurt already. The music starts and there is a mild warm-up that tells you how stiff and uncoordinated you are. Your body just doesn't work the way hers does. You try to keep up and for the moment you fear that everyone is looking at you as you clumsily move through the first set of exercises.

Soon you have advanced to the aerobics part of the class—jumping up and down, throwing your body back and forth, side to side, hoping you don't go crashing into someone or that no one is taking particular notice of your spastic movements. Some people in the class have stopped. In fact, one middle-aged lady is simply standing in front of you making it all the more difficult to see the instructor. Others are really getting into it. The instructor is cheerleading the class with shrieks and cries. Then the hand-clapping begins: syncopated movements with everyone clapping on beat—except for you, of course. Now it's time to check your pulse. You know you are alive—your face is flushed, you are perspiring profusely, and you are completely out of breath! Why do you need to check your pulse?

The cool-down begins just before you thought you were going to melt down. This is when you do fifteen variations on the standard sit-up, innumerable push-ups, leg lifts, doggies, and whatever. You notice that the floor around you resembles a small wading pool. You furtively mop your sweat with a towel.

There isn't much talk throughout the class, and by the end people are beginning to recover. Loud clapping and it's over. The class files out as the next group filters in. A social atmosphere is more prevalent now. It's a little like being with the survivors of some misadventure. You feel good—you made it through. You rush into the spa to see whether your body has changed substantially. Unfortunately, it hasn't, so you know you will need to come back again—and again—and again.

So much for the novice aerobic dancer. What about the pro? By the time you have earned the right to wear color-coordinated unitards and warmers the whole routine is all too predictable. You know the warm-up sequence by heart; the aerobics movements have become monotonous. And you almost fall asleep during the cool-down. But you keep coming. It is a unique social experience, even though everyone seems to be into their private worlds during the class itself. In spite of the cheerleader's bouncy style and enthusiastic voice, there is something lacking. Eyes dart across the room—furtive glances make cautious contact. For the most part, people are alone in a crowd. But the movement feels good and the class is visually pleasing, especially when everyone works together. The music helps distract you from life's concerns, and you have made a few friends among the regulars.

The Analysis

In analyzing aerobic dance, we need to go beyond the customary ways of looking at exercise. We can start with simple observations. For instance, we know that aerobics is a group activity, yet there is little interaction among participants. Think of basketball for contrast: there are active verbal and nonverbal exchanges between players throughout the game. In aerobics, the only one who speaks is the instructor and her communications are mostly commands and cries of encouragement. Yes, there are other exchanges (brief eye contact, occasional stumbling into another, shrieks of pain), but these are not part of the prescribed activity.

Aerobics is a leader-centered activity. Participants are passive followers. They don't have to make a lot of decisions other than one to stay. In this regard, aerobics is unlikely to foster leadership skills or decision-making abilities.

For the most part, one competes with oneself. There are no prizes for the highest kicks, the loudest groans, or the best color-coordinated outfit. This doesn't mean that people don't compete. Participants come to class with whatever personality style they possess. If you are competitive, you will find opportunities in this or any other encounter to compare yourself to others and to better them. However, aerobic dance classes don't feed the competitive urge. If anything, they require cooperation.

In what ways do aerobics classes involve you mentally? At the outset you need to concentrate on the movements; your attention is consumed. Movements change frequently, so you have to focus on the instructor. The nature of this focus is follower to leader, requiring passive acceptance of commands. As time goes on, the class may be more predictable, so your body may be engaged but little mental effort will be needed. Why is this important? If you are preoccupied at the beginning, your mind remains free to dwell on problems throughout class. As a result, your body may experience some escape from tension but your mind will remain captive.

We can clearly see this by comparing basketball and running. Imagine that Miss Jogger runs the same route every day. She merely puts her body in forward gear and lets her mind drift. She may use this time to think through problems or plan her evening. Now, Miss Basketball Player gets her exercise by working in a few friendly games each week. The game forces her to watch the ball and other players. Any lapse in attention may result in a poor game or, worse, getting hit in the head by a missed hook shot. Such attentional demands take the individual away from other thoughts or obsessive worry.

Aerobic dance classes may sound like fun, but they are anything but playful. You only have to look at the serious expressions on aerobic dancers' faces to know they are not engaged in a free, spontaneous movement experience. Imagine children running in a field, rolling and tumbling as they go, and then think of the programmed movements of the aerobics class. You would not use words like creative or expressive to describe this exercise form.

What about the style of movement? Aerobics requires flexibility and coordination. Movements may be more or less stylized as in jazz dance. You can't muscle your way through the class as you might in weight lifting. Rather, you may have to search for that quality of gracefulness you never thought you had.

While there are other dimensions along which this or any other exercise program could be analyzed, let us review what is most apparent: Aerobic dance classes are group activities, yet they are minimally social and require few interpersonal skills. You are not asked to act aggressively. In fact, we could almost describe them as emotionally passive engagements. Someone hoping to become more assertive in daily life would not gain much from aerobics. It falls more toward the cooperative end of the continuum than the competitive. Mental effort and concentration required by aerobics varies from a relatively high level at the outset to a rather minimal level after a few weeks or a month. As a routine program, aerobic dance classes become undemanding mentally and repetitive in body action. Movements require some flexibility and even grace. In this sense, aerobics could be described as more stereotypically feminine than masculine. Finally, these classes might be characterized as more serious and controlled than spontaneous and free.

It is hoped this brief analysis of one fitness option opens some windows to your perception of exercise—how it can be examined psychologically and how it holds the potential for personal development. There are yet other ways to assess the aerobic dance class, but these require some background that will be provided in upcoming chapters. Having demonstrated that exercise programs have psychological as well as physical dimensions, let us look at the question of change. That is, what can we expect from exercise?

What Has Changed?

The aerobic dancer, the runner, and other exercise devotees are prone to make periodic assessments of change. Usually these take the form of weight or body fat changes, increases in muscular definition, or gains in cardiorespiratory function. Rarely do people ask how their personalities may be undergoing transformation.

We know that aerobic exercise has positive effects on physical conditioning. But what is it that changes psychologically as a result of exercise? And do all exercise programs have the same effect on a person's sense of well being? These are question whose answers have been clouded by the tendency to express the simplified observation, "I just feel better when I exercise." What does this really mean? Will any exercise make us feel good? Will five miles of running produce the same euphoria as will a routine of weight lifting? Can a yoga class give you the same release of aggression as would a round of racquetball?

Is it what you do or the results you achieve that matters? Is it the enjoyment of movement or the weight loss that keeps you going? We can readily recall images of pain on athletes' faces. We can see weight lifters groaning and marathoners grimacing. We might even detect a strained expression on the ballerina's face as she glides across the studio. And we can remember people telling us, "I do it because I feel so good when I'm finished." But what about the experience itself?

Many sports enthusiasts like what they do. They enjoy the competition of a good tennis match. They like the release of adrenaline in a fast race. They are hooked on the freedom of movement in dance. They relish the feel of water as they swim laps. So it may not be all pain, sweat, and masochism — there may also be some real pleasure in the activity!

Yet it still comes down to feeling good — during or after the activity. And it is hard to compare my feeling good with your feeling good to know whether one sport will make us feel better than will another.

The problem is complicated because change comes slowly. Not only do pounds melt away ever so gradually, but the process of psychological change is such that by the time we have changed, we will have little conscious awareness of how we were before. It's like learning how to ride a bicycle. Once you've learned, it's difficult to remember how it was before you could ride.

Another problem with understanding change is that we may be looking in the wrong places. When we exercise, we expect to see changes in our bodies, not in our personalities. Unlike the physical realm, where we can hop on a bathroom scale, look in a mirror, or take our pulse, we don't usually have psychological measures readily available.

Of course, we can measure personality change without tests. We can ask friends, relatives, or work associates. Aside from the chance they will tell us more than we want to hear, or comment on topics we didn't ask about, most often our social network will only have noticed general changes like, "You seem calmer" or "You have a lot more energy." This isn't very useful when trying to identify specific changes.

But important psychological changes *are* taking place as you exercise. It is a matter of knowing where to look for them and what kinds of questions to ask.

The Causality Question

With all this talk about change, we have ignored a crucial issue. How do we know these elusive psychological changes are the result of exercise? Maybe athletes choose sports that suit their personalities. Surely, a tough, demanding businessman is not going to choose ballet. After all, let's be realistic!

Measuring psychological change is more involved than standing on the bathroom scale. People start exercise programs for different reasons and with different personalities. For example, one person could be very sociable and another very shy. If you take a cross section of people engaged in an activity, you can't be sure what belongs to the person and what is produced by the exercise. This is also why it is difficult to find "sports types." Giving out personality tests at Gold's Gym this afternoon won't tell you where the body builders were when they started and how much they have changed. To understand change, you have to look at it from an individual angle—where were you when you began and where are you now?

To illustrate the problem, imagine two individuals who take up karate. Bill is a quiet, almost timid, individual who lacks muscular strength and coordination, is very methodical and emotionally reserved. Vance, on the other hand, is overly aggressive, "muscle bound," unorganized, and emotionally explosive. What will karate do for them? Good karate training should emphasize muscular strength and flexibility, emotional control, assertiveness (rather than aggressiveness), a realistic level of self acceptance and self-esteem, and mental concentration.

Vance and Bill begin training with different personalities and for different reasons. While karate training is likely to have some impact on them, it is unrealistic to expect that their personalities will ever be identical. On the other hand, karate should help Bill become more assertive and self-confident, as well as stronger and more coordinated. In turn, Vance's ego might be reined in a bit and he might become less impulsive.

Such changes would not occur overnight. In fact, you might not see much change until Bill and Vance were well on the way to earning black belts.

Sports Types

Let us build on the points discussed thus far. Our attention has centered around such questions as, "What would you expect to change through physical activity" and "Why should one exercise program affect you differently than another?" We noted that a general feeling of well-being tends to accompany regular exercise, but we might want to think of other kinds of changes. As examples, consider the following areas:

social skills
assertiveness or aggressiveness
competitive and cooperative styles
dominance versus submissiveness
leadership skills
decision-making processes
problem-solving skills
creativity
drive or motivation
interpersonal awareness

flexibility versus rigidity
anxiety level
emotional control versus impulsivity

We have seen how some of these areas were used in the analysis of aerobic dance. There may even be other changes pertinent to sports and exercise, but the list above is more than a sufficient start.

What is so important about these areas? When we think about sports and exercise programs, most of us have a feeling of attraction to or repulsion from certain activities. The reason for our response to exercise is related to the areas just listed. Sometimes a sport is too aggressive or mentally demanding. Some sports, like water ballet, require coordination and control, whereas others are more impulsive. Or we may dislike competition, preferring activities where we go at our own paces.

The question is whether we can actually change our personalities through the way we move and exercise our bodies. We know, at least on a superficial level, that we can characterize sports along psychological lines, so why wouldn't it make sense for us to see these activities as strategies for self change much as we view education, drama, psychotherapy, and reading?

It might help us to think of types of *sports* rather than types of *sportsmen*. In the comments about aerobic dance and karate, we saw some of the activities' psychological workings. These influences would be fairly constant, even though the outcomes might vary. This is like saying that everyone in a nutrition course is exposed to the same material, but individual learning may vary greatly.

Arguing that there are types of sportsmen runs into the complications of human nature. Individual personalities result from many influences. To infer that exercise has a paramount effect is hardly supportable. But persistent involvement in exercise *will* modify your personality. And with a solid understanding of *sports types,* you will at least have an idea of the direction in which you are headed if you choose a new fitness program.

Body Types

Understanding the psychological implications of exercise comes not only from knowing whether the activity is aggressive, social, or competitive, but also from understanding how the activity engages us physically: how we have to move and what muscles are employed.

We have already observed that some people look like football players, swimmers, or perhaps couch potatoes. Why do we have these impressions? It isn't merely the squashed nose of the prizefighter or the turned-out legs of the ballerina that identifies them—it is also the muscular development that comes with practice. The massive thighs of the speed skater, the short, firm calves of the long-distance runner, or the muscular chest and arms of the gymnast are natural outgrowths. It doesn't happen by chance that competitive swimmers look a bit like inverted triangles or that weight lifters look like anatomical muscle charts.

Muscular development is based on the fact that each muscle has a particular function. Some muscles extend a limb, others flex it; some move the limb away from the body (*abduction*), others move it toward the body (*adduction*); some muscles flex the torso, others extend it. Muscles are also located in and around areas where vital organs reside.

Muscles allow us to move about with grace and facility. We may characterize musculature as being wiry, bulky, undefined, or weak. Depending on muscle strength and flexibility, interactions with the environment are partially determined. We wouldn't expect a person with weak, undefined leg muscles to leap into action at a moment's notice or to run a mile in an emergency. On the other hand, we might not ask an overdeveloped muscleman to dust our precious knickknacks. These characterizations may seem extreme or even prejudicial, but the simple point is that our muscles can either limit or empower us in carrying out certain actions.

If we consider what different muscles are used for—lifting, pushing, running, reaching, taking, or holding—we can begin to appreciate the "psychology" of muscle. Translating this to the field of exercise, what do you think happens when a particular sport only develops your capacity to move quickly in a forward direction (like running)? Could it be that the potential for certain psychological responses, such as self-assertion or aggression, may be strengthened, whereas others, such as staying put or withdrawing, become less likely?

If you think this is crazy, read the following report by a devoted runner:

> One day last spring I was having an exceptionally good run . . . I was around the 14 mile point and I was preparing to cross a one-lane bridge when all of a sudden a large cement mixer turned the corner . . . I never thought for a second about stopping and letting the truck pass. I simply continued and said to myself, "Come on you son-of-a-bitch and I'll split you right down the middle—there will be concrete all over this road!" The driver slammed on the brakes and swerved to the right as I sailed by. That was really scary afterward, but at the time

I really felt good. I have felt equally strong and indestructable many times since then, but I have never taken on a cement truck again.[1]

It is relatively easy to assess where we are strong, where we are inflexible, whether muscles on one side of the body are tighter or stronger than those on the other side. Knowing this not only tells us something about what exercises we might need in our quest for the ever-elusive perfect body, but it may also suggest *psychological* strengths—and weaknesses!

The notion of *body type* has a long history in psychology. You may be familiar with William Sheldon's personology, which describes three primary body types: the round, fat endomorphs; the lean, wiry ectomorphs; and the square, muscular mesomorphs.[2] However, this classification and its variants is less helpful than some others that correlate specific psychological functions with different muscles and regions of the body. For this reason, we will be more concerned with the psychology of muscle in this book than with the establishment of body types.

Movement Types

One other approach remains: the analysis of movement. Most of us are familiar with body language. Crossed arms are supposed to mean you are feeling defensive; head cocked to the right is interpreted as meaning you are listening critically, and cocked to the left suggests you are being coy. Depending on your mood of the moment, your relationships with those present, and the context, you may adjust your body one way or another, communicating various nonverbal messages. Sometimes, however, crossed arms may simply mean that you are cold—and a cocked head may signal a stiff neck more than an interpersonal attitude. This illustrates the limitations of body language and the error of assuming that the same movement conveys the same meaning for all of us. These shortcomings may make us a bit skeptical about movement analysis.

There are, however, some carefully developed theories that take us beyond superficial analysis of body language to a more careful evaluation of movement patterns. Rather than focus on momentary changes in movement, these theories enable us to examine more stable patterns. For example, we hear people say, "I could tell it was you by your walk." Each of us has a characteristic way of walking. Not only are we identified by our gait, but we also have habitual styles of gesturing, movement tempos and ways in which we use the space around us. Some people seem to fill a room, while others recede into the background. There are those who are always running and others who do the "Sunday shuffle" no matter what the occasion.

These habitual patterns are related to personality. To illustrate, using a much-publicized example, we know that the Type A, or so-called coronary-prone personality, has been identified in movement as one who is direct and abrupt, moves rapidly, uses short, staccato gestures, and has a forward-leaning stance.[3]

How does this relate to personality and exercise? Different exercise regimes or sports emphasize different styles of movement. An individual who has had fifteen years of classical ballet training will betray this conditioning in her everyday movements. Likewise, someone who has studied yoga for years will show an ease and flexibility in movement. In brief, sports and exercise alter our movements in a more or less predictable manner. At the very least, they allow us to move in certain ways. To the degree our movement patterns are changed by exercise, to that degree we are also likely to find correlated personality changes.

Consider this. Exercise has been used to treat psychological conditions, including depression and anxiety. Yet it may be ill-advised for individuals who are suicidal or suffering from agitated depression, to take up running.[4] Why? Quite simply, the movement patterns encouraged by running might serve to increase the individual's forward mobility so that a suicidal leap off a bridge would become more likely. Doubtful? Remember the runner and the cement truck?

This discussion highlights the importance of proper exercise prescription. An individual who is coronary prone or Type A could be engaging in sports that foster quick, abrupt movements and in this sense do little to modulate his aggressive and potentially self-destructive pattern. A compulsive, uncreative person would do well to stay away from such exercises as daily jogging because the inherent movement pattern might reinforce these psychological traits instead of develop other characteristics.

With the aid of movement analysis, not only can we diagnose our personalities, but we can also categorize the patterns of different sports and exercises. Then we will know to what extent our movements match those of our chosen activities and, more critically, whether we need to recondition our movement patterns through different exercise programs.

A New Perspective

The slogan for Nautilus Clubs, "Fitness is everything!" captures the spirit of the fitness boom. We have become a nation of runners, aerobic dancers, body shapers or, as some might say, fitness fanatics. Not only do we have marathons, biathlons, and Ironman triathlons, but we now have ultrasports like cross-continent bicycle races—the ultimate in fitness challenge.

We have emerged from a world where exercise was a natural by-product of work to one where exercise is something we do to ourselves in our leisure time to condition our muscles, trim our bodies, and remain ever-youthful. What is curious about this new devotion to fitness is that there is relatively little consciousness about the nonphysical effects of fitness programs. Exercise continues to be something we do to ourselves. Like applying some magic potion, we attempt to put on muscles and curves to match a fantasized ideal. And it doesn't much matter what we make ourselves endure as long as it has the desired result.

Exercise programs represent a vast, untapped resource for personal development. Although this has been partially recognized in such experiences as the "runner's high" and other reports of mood changes following exercise, the influence of exercise programs on our psychological condition has been vastly underestimated.

Consciously or not, we are changed by the exercise we do. The extent of change depends on the depth of involvement in an exercise program and its inherent potential for altering physical and psychological structures.

The inclination to choose exercise programs that match our personalities frequently prevents any change. Socially isolated individuals pick activities where they exercise alone. Aggressive people select aggressive sports. Compulsive people develop compulsive exercise regimes. If we end up in an activity that doesn't suit our personal style, we may become early dropouts.

Exercise should be viewed not only as a body-change strategy, but also as a means for altering our psyches. When we ask for professional advice about exercise, we seek out cardiologists, sports medicine experts, or health club trainers. The idea of discussing exercise with a psychologist or some other mind specialist sounds preposterous, even though the kind of advice we get from the body experts leaves us only partially satisfied. We may be told that our heart is in good enough shape for us to initiate a program or that we should choose exercises with certain levels of intensity. Beyond this we are given little guidance as to the kind of program that makes the most sense for us. Left to our personal wisdom, we yield to our inclinations; we choose what reinforces our personal habits.

Sometimes these selections are straightforward and uncomplicated. They neither aggravate our psyches nor worsen psychological conditions. On the other hand, they simply may not be as helpful as they could be. The right moves are those that not only condition our bodies but also help develop our personalities. We can expand our "psychophysical" functioning through new movements that enhance psychological flexibility and coordination, through interactions that widen our range of social behaviors, and through muscular development that enables us to better stand our ground or move through the world more efficiently.

By definition, if there are right moves, then there are wrong moves. There are exercise programs that will help us become more compulsive, more aggressive, or more introverted—and all of this will happen while we naively hold onto the belief that we are merely working on our bodies. The adage "Sports build character" is usually interpreted to mean sports foster good character. Unfortunately, this is not the case.

It is important that we discover what the right moves are for us. By honest self-examination and understanding the hidden psychological dimensions of different sport and exercise programs, we will find programs that are developmental, as well as identify those that are potentially damaging.

2

The Natural Choice

The Need for Consistency

Human beings strive for consistency. We do things that fit our self-images. An aggressive, super-macho businessman who played college football and who enjoys a few brews with the boys would feel pretty uncomfortable in leotard and tights doing *pliés* in a dance studio. This doesn't mean it hasn't happened—but we must admit it is rare.

Sports and exercise programs are not value-free. Each activity has an image that may appeal to us based on who we think we are and perhaps who we want to become. We see in them *means* that are more or less compatible with our *ends*. Culture tells us there are sports for men and sports for women. Even while the grounds for sexual stereotyping shift beneath our feet, many people argue that football is a man's sport while ballet is mostly for women. We also know that some sports are more prestigious or tougher or require greater skill. It doesn't take much training to tie on running shoes and pound the pavement. And bowling doesn't have the prestige associated with tennis.

Self-definitions are deeply ingrained and not easily altered. We guard against putting ourselves in situations where we might be out of our league or where our image will become vulnerable. Carried to an extreme, this can be a formula for personal rigidity—for becoming stuck. We may fail to adapt when adaptation is required. We may hold onto old patterns when new ones are called for. We may persist in protecting our egos, our archaic self-definitions, when it is time to change.

This may take the form of remaining in a job that has lost its meaning because we say, "I'm not a quitter!" Or we may hold onto outdated views of masculinity or femininity because that's the way the world "should be." In exercise we may unduly restrict ourselves to activities that are no longer practical ("Oh sure, I'm big on outdoor sports . . . I go hunting and fishing whenever I can"—which actually was three years ago!). Or worse, we may approach our fitness agenda with the same zeal that we apply to our careers and end up on another treadmill, with another kind of addiction. This is the negative view.

On the positive side, some of us may live in worlds requiring little modification. Our days have a comfortable security and we know reasonably well what we will be doing next week, next month, even next year. We may have found a lifestyle that suits us—an enjoyable occupation, a satisfying relationship, a pleasant locale, and perhaps a physical activity that is well integrated with our needs. In this scenario, our exercise program merely reinforces what is; it does not change our psychology, it simply increases physical strength and cardiorespiratory functioning while supporting our basic personality structure.

Sport Selection

Personal consistency is so paramount in our choices that we must recognize it as a major determining force in sport selection. This is not to deny the impact of other factors like cost, availability, and social networks in determining our activities. Yet, when left to ourselves, unguided by experts and professional wisdom, what "natural choice" do we make—and why? Why do some people become marathon runners or triathletes? Or how is it that some women choose weight lifting while others become ballerinas? Or what would cause a person to become a boxer versus a yoga master? These questions highlight the issue of selection: why do we choose certain sports or exercise programs over all others?

An important question asked in this book is whether these natural choices are always best for us. And for those who don't exercise, is there some fitness program that might actually be appealing if the right kind of match could be found?

We become involved in fitness activities for many reasons, but the satisfaction we derive depends largely on how well they meet our psychological needs. To understand the self-selection process, let's get acquainted with some people involved in movement, sport, or exercise. The cases you are about to read are based on real life, on athletes and exercise addicts who made unique adjustments to life's demands. They range from Olympic-level athletes to midlife converts to the fitness boom[1] *Do not interpret them as prototypes of their sport*. It would be an error to conclude that all runners will be more or less like the characters described. These portrayals are offered as individual studies highlighting personality traits of the athletes and suggesting how these traits affect not only their exercise choices but other areas in their lives as well.

Ten Case Studies

The Body Builders

Jan. Jan walked into the weight room as if she owned it. She made her way through the maze of benches, weights, and other paraphernalia, smiling and saying hello as she passed her buddies. There were subtle acknowledgments of her presence even from those who were in the midst of some herculean power lift. She had earned her place in the club. As she reached the mat where she would begin her warm-ups, one heavily muscled man turned to a much leaner individual and commented, "She's ranked second in the state and she only started a couple of years ago." The listener grunted as if to say how impressed he was, although in truth there wasn't much by which to judge: Jan's body was well hidden beneath layers of tee shirts and sweats.

It was 5:30 P.M. and she had just left the office. Her job offered little satisfaction, except to her tyrannical boss who delighted in squelching any sign of enjoyment employees might show. Since she had taken up body building three years ago, Jan's boss seemed to find particular pleasure in making remarks about how "butch" she looked and in keeping her overtime, knowing that she tried to stick to a rigid workout schedule each day. It was less than one month before the national body-building competition and this was the first day this week she had been able to get to the club on time. Jan wanted to quit her job and devote herself to body building fulltime, but she had to eat, and jobs were hard to come by—even the bad ones.

She felt like an addict. Her whole life was governed by body building. And it all began as a whim. She had been playing racquetball for about a year. She started because at the age of twenty-eight she was worried about her health and didn't want to end up with her mother's pear-shaped figure. Her brother had been a superb racquetball player and that helped her begin.

Even though she wasn't very good, her wiry muscular figure enabled her to pull off some surprising victories. Best of all, from her perspective, she was able to soundly trounce a few male partners. She had always seen herself as competitive, but winning against men accentuated the triumph. Her love life had been turbulent—relationships had started well, but all too soon they revealed the fatal flaws that lead to breakup. And shallow waters had little cushion for headlong romantic dives.

At the point when she first joined a health club, she had more or less sworn off men, or at least romantic entanglements. The club was a place to displace her energies. She was always available for a game when she wasn't working, and the more she played, the more competitive she felt. But something else was happening. She was beginning to bulge out with muscular development. It was less than a year into her fitness plunge when a friend jokingly told her she ought to become a "lady body builder." Something clicked.

In her school years Jan had always been a ham. She loved getting up in front of audiences and clowning. She relished attention, no matter what the arena. She liked to be good at things and the better she got the harder she tried. When she failed, however, that was the end. It was difficult for her to motivate herself when she thought of herself as mediocre. At one point in childhood she had taken a ballet class and felt so clumsy that she never returned. From that point on, she stuck to things she was sure of.

Body building was something she felt almost born to succeed at. It didn't take much for her to gain muscular definition. Within weeks her biceps made most men wish they were wearing long-sleeved shirts. She luxuriated in the expressions on men's faces when, at the end of a workout, she would pose in front of the mirror flexing one muscle group or another. Their mouths dropped in envy—or perhaps it was lust. That didn't matter; she had decided to remain celibate. She could be in control far better when she didn't complicate her life with love, and besides, she felt that body building was a more or less acceptable substitute for sex. There was something sensual and stimulating about watching her gleaming muscles ripple in the mirror, particularly when she oiled her body and dressed in her skimpy bikini. Call it narcissistic or egocentric, it was satisfying nonetheless, and it enabled her to call the shots. She could challenge herself as much as she wanted, there was no one else telling her what to do. And she was on her way. She had already won the regional championship this year, was ranked second in the state, and now had a good chance at being a finalist in the nationals.

Thirty-five hours a week, that's what it took, and she would gladly have spent more if she could afford to. It was beyond dedication. It was a substitute for so many things—for a satisfying job, for a relationship she could count on, and perhaps for an ingrained sense of self-worth that didn't require external validation. It worked for her and she was happy. It was hard to get motivated to lift some days, but for the most part, going to the club was like coming home.

Ted. Ted almost thought of himself as a caricature: the Charles Atlas hero who used to have sand kicked in his face but now had a bevy of beauties surrounding his muscular frame. He had been the typical small kid on the block who wasn't very athletic and who had trouble defending himself. He envied his friends who attracted attention with their athletic prowess, so he compensated by excelling academically. Although he was bright enough, he tended to be an overachiever, working extra hard to stay ahead of the pack.

At twenty-two he was just under 5' 5" and about 120 pounds. He had taken up jogging but didn't seem to have the stamina for it. A friend suggested that he build up strength with weights—and thus began his transformation.

He was in his second year of medical school when he became heavily involved in weight lifting. His body showed remarkable change that year. He gained over fifteen pound while losing more than an inch in his waistline. More impressively, Ted's popularity skyrocketed. He had always been perceived as a rather cautious, unidimensional guy, but now people began to notice him. His unimpressive stature had made it difficult for him to get dates, but what he lacked in height, he made up for in muscles.

After finishing medical school, Ted continued to body-build. It had served him well by providing an outlet for his energies, and it was an area where he had control. His workouts were precise and rigorous. He calculated his nutritional intake and knew exactly how much weight he could gain or lose, depending on the intensity of his workouts.

He thought of himself as being worse than a heroin addict. He needed to lift every day, otherwise he would feel depressed. It was his "fix." He spent five to six evenings a week working out. He tried to mix in some aerobic exercise because, as a cardiac specialist, he knew weight lifting's limitations. But he much preferred lifting to anything else. It gave him a high, and he liked what it did to his body. He enjoyed looking at himself in the mirror—at the spa, at home, or, in fact, anywhere.

His father had been a doctor and so Ted's career choice was a bit predetermined. What really interested him, though, was science: the rigor and control, the precision of the methodology. Medicine was too much of an art; there were too many unknowns. He directed his profession toward clinical research in cardiology, and by the age of thirty-two had achieved a moderate national reputation.

He was puzzled, however, by his lack of success romantically. This is not to say that his popularity had declined. Quite the contrary, women seemed to fall all over him. He had no trouble dating some of the most attractive women in town. He would walk into a singles bar and heads would turn. The problem wasn't dating—it was keeping up a relationship. He just couldn't seem to feel much for his dates. Oftentimes he thought he ought to love a current girlfriend because of the qualities she possessed, but it was as if the softer emotions couldn't penetrate his thick muscular armor.

Ted remembered one woman he had dated in medical school. She was head over heels in love with him, but he couldn't respond. He experienced himself as being blocked, and he seemed more interested in himself than in anyone else. There were too many beautiful women who were aching to get into bed with him; his ego simply could not ignore the attention. He dated this woman off and on for about two years after which she simply gave up. She told him it was like banging her head on a brick wall trying to get through to him. As time went on, Ted continued to be active on the dating scene but he also began to feel a sense of loss. More than three years after the breakup he finally admitted to himself that he had been in love but just had not realized it at the time.

Commentary. When Jan got hooked on body building, it seemed to suit her. It made sense psychologically and perhaps physically as well. But what did she avoid, and why? How did her body building serve to protect her ego and make her feel less vulnerable? She didn't want to be opened up. She feared situations she couldn't master immediately, such as love or dance.

Ted displayed his fear of relationships in another way: he dabbled, he gratified his ego, but he avoided involvement. From a psychological perspective, he was heavily defended against being hurt—even to the point of blunting genuine emotions for a woman. And coincidentally we find that Ted's body had a certain armored appearance, one that resulted from his self-described addiction to weight lifting.

These two individuals built their muscular defense systems for very personal reasons: they needed them to adapt, to function in a way that helped them feel safe, protected, and, to some degree, satisfied. It doesn't work this way for all body builders. A great deal depends on the psychological issues you bring to your fitness regime. And there is no intention of implying something is wrong. Jan and Ted did what they needed to in order to adjust to their unique situations. The question is whether there is a better way, one that would enable Jan to experience relationships in a less threatening way and Ted to know his inner emotional world before it is too late.

The Dancers

Pam. Pam remembered the first time she went to the ballet. She was only three, but the impression was permanent. She pestered her mother for weeks until she was allowed to enroll in a dance academy. Years went by and she ascended the ranks of the dance world, performing in numerous small productions and eventually being selected for apprenticeship in a national ballet company.

Pam was a "good" girl, well liked but consumed by dance. It was all she talked about, all she ever wanted to do. She was never any trouble to her family, and in a way, dance classes became a substitute for family life. Her parents thought she was being well taken care of while she was dancing and didn't feel the need to devote much time to her.

Classes were arduous. She had some bad teachers, those who pushed the students too hard, too fast. She learned how to dance on *pointe* at an early age, probably too early. She learned to be submissive, to bend her will to that of her instructor. She learned to tolerate pain, to deny the fierce resistance of her body as she strained for greater turnout, higher leaps, longer stretches—all the while smiling and looking unruffled by the agony of her art. She learned to be self-critical, to doubt herself, to strive for a level of perfection always beyond her grasp.

At seventeen she was dancing with the junior company. She was an A student, and she was in a lot of pain—emotional pain. She could never do enough, she could never be good enough. In a strange way her family colluded with her. She was so good that her parents became upset if her grades were less than perfect, if something she did wasn't the best possible. Of course, that was Pam—she never had any problems, she was always good at everything.

She crashed. After three weeks of not sleeping and working on one project after another in a frenzy to get it all done, to get it all perfect, she was hospitalized: nervous exhaustion.

Years later she would look back upon this period only to understand what she had become through dance, what it had done to her. She continued to dance after her breakdown but moved out of the professional program to take classes at a local studio. Her teacher was a sensitive woman, consistently warm and encouraging in manner. Even so, Pam knew what perfection was and by this time didn't need anyone else to criticize her—she did that well enough on her own. She majored in science and landed a good job in a research laboratory after college. She was a perfectionist and that was important for the kind of work she did. Years in psychotherapy enabled her to let go of some of the extreme edges of her perfectionism, but she continued to be highly self-critical.

She tended to stick to things, and to people. She had a deep sense of commitment and in that regard mourned the loss of her career in dance. She couldn't do anything partway and even though dance remained as her chosen form of movement and exercise, she would never perform again. In relationships, she favored monogamy. By twenty-seven she had been involved with only three men, not counting a few dates between long-term relationships. Her present relationship was a metaphor for her experience in dance. Infatuation, falling in love, and then a lot of hard work—reaching for the ideal and being disappointed when she couldn't achieve that elusive end point. But she was committed. She knew the meaning of adversity, and she believed with all she had learned that she could be more forgiving, more accepting—of herself, of those close to her, and of the fact that life is not perfect.

Holly. She moved like the wind on the prairie: sometimes soft, sometimes more powerful, always in motion, always an elemental force to be reckoned with. At twenty-six Holly had her own dance studio where she taught and choreographed. She admitted she didn't know how to manage it, but her husband had a good head for business and could take care of practical matters. She was most interested in dance. She had been interested in dance for as long as she could remember, but it wasn't until she was in her early teens that she actually began taking classes. At first, she enrolled in a ballet school, but that didn't last long. It was too rigid, too "constipated," and Holly was a free spirit. She imagined herself like the legendary Isadora Duncan: in endless romantic adventures, dancing around the globe.

She trained in modern dance. Graham, Cunningham, Limon all gave her roots, but she developed on her own, creating her own style and threading her emotional life in and out of her dance. She was not an easy student, but her teachers seemed to value her idiosyncrasies. She was tall, almost six feet, and when she moved across the floor, other dancers simply faded into the background. There was music and motion—and Holly. She seemed boundless—arms and legs extending infinitely through time and space. When she leaped into the air, one fully believed she would never land. She was everywhere and then at times she would almost disappear—much like an illusion, a dreamlike shadow on the stage.

How she got through college was one of life's great mysteries. She couldn't seem to pull it together. Books were always getting lost, class schedules slipped her memory and exams invariably conflicted with dance rehearsals. But she was a minor legend—the dance department had never had such good attendance at its performances. This was not simply because half the students were in love with her (the other half were too proud or too shy to admit to such feelings); it had a lot to do with what she created and how she danced.

After college Holly wanted to start her own company—she also wanted to go to New York or perhaps Paris or, who knows? At twenty-two, for her the world was wide open, and she was in love. Sam was handsome, ambitious, and mature. He was someone Holly could lean on for all those annoying little realities like rent for the studio and management for her productions.

But then the world closed around her: she became pregnant. She loved Sam and didn't want to have an abortion, and he said he would take care of the baby. She danced through most of her pregnancy, enjoying the exploration of balance with her constantly changing form. Within weeks of the baby's birth, she was back in the studio. Sam kept to his word, becoming the principal parent as Holly pursued her role as principal dancer in her company.

Her students loved her and the company grew in reputation. Her capacity for creation seemed infinite, and her romantic spirit would not be tamed. She loved wildly: Sam, her baby, her friends and students. She had no limits, but others did. Sam was not the jealous type—that would never do for Holly's mate—but he could only tolerate so much, and the arguments increased. For Holly this was too much like the real world. It was true that she was committed to dance, that she had to work hard on her technique, but it felt effortless for the most part and it didn't have all those nasty connotations of obligation and duty. Marriage and motherhood were beginning to feel that way.

Just when the pressures seemed to peak, the world reopened its doors: a call came from a company in New York. Sam would understand, and she would visit the baby whenever she could.

Commentary. The dancers, Pam and Holly, exhibit almost opposite characteristics, and when one considers the differences between ballet and modern dance, the contrast is not so surprising. The movements required in ballet tend to be very exact and repetitive. Training is demanding and even painful. The ballet dancer learns to be perfectionistic, to be self-denying, and to endure. Modern dance allows more creativity, more variety, more personal interpretation. Rules exist in order to be broken.

It is hard to say whether Pam's mental collapse was precipitated by her pattern of self-denial and perfectionism or how much her dance training reinforced these tendencies. We can only note the similarity between her lifestyle and her dance training.

So, too, when we think of Holly's exuberance, her unbounded nature, and free-spirited approach to life, we can see these same elements in the form of dance she preferred. A coincidence? It is hard to imagine Holly as a dedicated marathon runner, especially considering all of the pain such runners endure. What she did suited her—it captured the qualities she valued in living.

Did either Pam or Holly profit greatly or suffer unduly because of their movement expressions? It is hard to say, but at the very least we need to pay attention to the consistencies in their lives, in the choices they expressed and the outcomes they realized.

The Runners

Warren. Warren was a stickler for detail. He was well suited to his job as a financial executive. Everything had its place, its category. Things could be quantified and tabulated, and answers came in black and white, or sometimes red. He liked what he did and he did it well. When people met Warren, they saw a square peg in a square hole—everything seemed to fit.

Warren had always been lean and trim without having to work at it, but when he passed the thirty-year mark, his pants squeezed his waist—and he noticed. He was meticulous about his appearance, as about most other things, and he wasn't going to allow middle-age spread to creep up on him. It was time to get serious about fitness. He had never been very athletic, mostly because he was preoccupied with other things, but now fitness was his priority. He would tackle it the way he dealt with everything else—head-on, no nonsense, no halfhearted efforts.

He liked to be in charge and he didn't like depending on others. This is not to say he was a loner. Warren liked people—he just didn't want to get bogged down by them. Trying to schedule squash games seemed like a waste of time, even though a lot of his office mates were avid squash players. After careful consideration, he decided on running. He could set his schedule and his standards. He could clock himself, estimate his mileage, and chart his progress.

He researched footwear and bought the best running shoes for the money. He read all about warm-ups and cool-downs, as well as running schedules for novices. Warren studied the sports medicine articles on running injuries because he didn't want his program interrupted by something that was avoidable. Within six months he was running fifty miles a week. He supplemented his runs with muscle strengthening exercises and weight training.

His friends thought he was a bit fanatical. He became the local expert on exercise — which, in his mind, equated with running. His days revolved around his runs. His diet changed, reflecting his heightened attention to his body and its needs. He started running competitively. First it was the "Five Mile Fun Run," then the ten-milers, and on to the marathon. He was obsessed with running and what it did to his body. From the point where he began to notice his increased muscular definition, Warren systematically measured his percentage of body fat. He had always been clothes conscious, but now he wore clothes to accentuate his physique.

At home he became very critical of his wife, Jenny, and her lack of involvement in exercise. After three children, her body was less than perfect — and that annoyed him. He put her on a training program that she followed scrupulously, not because she wanted to, but because if she didn't, Warren would be angry. After a while they became like trains crossing in the night: she was on her schedule and he on his. Rarely did they run together because he was so much faster and he didn't want to downgrade his workouts. Running was serious business, as was everything else. Even parties at Warren's house tended to be serious affairs: planned games, scheduled events, and long-winded monologues by Warren on topics of his choosing.

Jenny tried to keep up with Warren but he outpaced and outdistanced her, and the gap kept growing. He was ever more talking about his body, his diet, his running, his races, with occasional pauses to criticize Jenny's lack of dedication. At poolside during the summer Warren could be seen strutting around, proudly displaying his gorgeous body. Jenny, who was in fact quite shapely, felt so inferior that she often hid beneath large towels or blankets.

The inevitable moved one step closer when Warren began running with a younger woman who had somehow beaten him in a marathon. They compared body fat and diet and schedules and running times — and then other performances. Soon Warren became remote and disinterested in Jenny. He even stopped criticizing her, which might have felt good had Jenny not realized its meaning.

It would not be quite accurate to say that Warren and his new romance ran off into the sunset one bright and beautiful day—that would not be characteristic. Warren had analyzed the situation, studied its pros and cons in minute detail, and logically concluded that Jenny would be better off without him. And certainly, it made more sense for him to be with someone more suited to his lifestyle. Like most things Warren decided on in life, once he had satisfied his own objections and concluded the rightness of his choice, he was unshakable—some might say rigid.

Phil.   Phil had his priorities straight. Whatever he did in life, there had to be time for running. He had been a sprinter in school—the 440 was his favorite race. He wasn't great, but he always placed in state meets. He studied physical education in college and afterward landed a job in teaching. Over the years he gravitated toward guidance and counseling because he felt he understood kids, and he liked working with them.

Through the years he kept up a respectable training program. He had other interests, but running was his passion. He especially liked "speed work"—short, compact, and efficient. He kept a notebook of his workouts, and at the age of thirty was consistently bettering his high school times.

His job, however, wasn't quite right. Administrative duties cluttered his days and his working hours increased with his age. Work began to infringe upon his running. He would not have quit for that reason alone, but other factors—location, job duties, limitations of the educational system—added to his malaise. He had gone back to school for a master's degree and thought he could move somewhere and open up a private practice. He also knew it wouldn't be that simple.

Everyone thought of Phil as a levelheaded guy. Even when he quit to go off into the unknown without a job, no one said he was crazy. They knew he had a plan and that it would work out for the best. The idea that his career took second place to his running seemed entirely consistent. He led an orderly life knowing his values and pursuing them carefully. He rarely did things on a whim or out of impulse.

Phil's new home was in the right location for running. The climate was dry and sunny most of the year. It took him a while to get his private practice together and in the interim he worked in a supermarket. He had enough to live on and a free rein to work out as much as he desired. That's what counted.

Ten years later his counseling practice was booming. He had earned a reputation for being quick and effective. As a therapist, he got right to the point, established realistic goals, and worked efficiently to reach them. He didn't muddy the waters with fancy theory. He was a common-sense person who was clear about what he could do and what he couldn't, whom he could help and whom he couldn't. He didn't waste your time and you didn't waste his.

One bright day, as he was doing some roadwork, a car hit him. He survived, but his left leg was smashed, broken in six places. The doctors gave him little hope of ever running again. The injured leg would be slightly shorter and, more critically, he had little range of movement in his knee. At first he was devastated. But he took his own medicine. Within weeks he had studied his situation well enough to direct his rehabilitation.

Phil made up a program. He consulted the best sports medicine people he could find. He codesigned physiotherapy sessions with the hospital staff. Soon it became evident that the worst forecasts would not be fulfilled. He had already regained more flexibility in his knee than had been predicted, and it was only six months postsurgery. Throughout he was practical and cautious. He worked within his limits but continually pushed the boundaries. He was no stranger to pain. Running had conditioned him to endure, to go beyond normal tolerance. He understood training and physiotherapy was just another training program. The doctors were impressed. He soon added a new component to his private practice—counseling injured athletes.

Five years hence Phil is running: speed work, distance, the full program. None of it was easy, but the recovery process was typical. It was a challenge, it could be structured, and he could measure progress. And he did it his way. He directed his rehabilitation the way he guided his life—deliberately, thoughtfully, and with commitment.

Commentary. The runners, Warren and Phil, share certain similarities—a kind of order and discipline along with perhaps a compulsive edge. They needed to have things a certain way, to have a well-organized and controllable routine. Life events and personal inclinations led them to different outcomes. Warren became more compulsive and obsessed with such things as his physical appearance and diet. Phil took his discipline and channeled it in a critical rehabilitation effort. Depending on circumstances and needs, personality traits reinforced by running may prove essential in making life adjustments, or they may aggravate situations that otherwise would be tolerable.

Warren was thorough and methodical. Under stress he became rigid. These are not inherently bad traits. It is only when carried to an extreme that perspective gets lost and decisions are less than optimal. Phil shared some of Warren's tendencies, but somehow the conclusion of his story was different. He obviously had other traits that enabled him to curb the extremes and to turn adversity into triumph.

Running was only part of their makeups. They molded their training as extensions of themselves, but there was more to them than just running. Yet, their running selectively reinforced certain traits and ignored other dimensions of their personalities—for better or for worse!

The Swimmers

Grey. Grey had tried a lot of sports in his adult years. He liked the idea of being in shape. For a while he had been a runner, long before it was fashionable to do so. And he did some cycling, but that was only seasonal. He had even lifted weights, kept to a Nautilus regime and occasionally practiced yoga. In spite of all this, he just seemed to have what he called "a swimmer's body"—long, relaxed muscles without much definition. He said it was due to all the years he labored in pools as a competitive athlete.

Grey didn't join a swim team until high school, although he swam every summer from a very early age. Once when he was eight, he almost drowned in the ocean after being caught in a riptide. He prided himself on having swum to safety while his friend had to be rescued by lifeguards. The experience didn't frighten him enough to keep him from swimming; he felt a special affinity for water. One of his favorite memories was swimming after the boat his father rowed across their lake. By the age of twelve he could swim the length of the lake, which was over two miles.

Grey had a few good friends but thought of himself as shy and socially awkward. In high school he had been recruited for the football team because of his size, but after a few practice sessions he quit. He didn't like all the aggression he had to muster in order to play. Swimming wasn't like that.

Grey was best in long-distance events but was only a mediocre sprinter. Although workouts were grueling, the real test came in getting psyched up for competition. He had to be mentally prepared and that was particularly hard when he knew the times of swimmers he was up against. It came down to believing in himself, but there was a lot of time to play mind games in a 1,500-meter race. And for whatever reason, his performance in meets was never as good as it was in practice.

He liked being on a swim team. For the most part, he thought the other guys were pretty much like him. They tended to be serious students and, except for a couple of the sprinters, they were relatively quiet and easygoing. There were no big egos and only a few personality clashes on the team.

Swimming was a good hideout for Grey; he had a hard time dealing with reality. He wasn't sure what he wanted to do when he grew up so he picked things he thought he ought to do without knowing whether they were right or not. He entered the novitiate after his sophomore year in college. He wasn't just going to be a priest; he was going to be a Jesuit — fourteen years in the making. He put forth his best but couldn't do it. He made it through seven years and then dropped out to become a poor poet living on New York's Lower East Side. Eventually he found himself in a doctoral program at the New School. His field was philosophy.

Even though he was persistent in what he tried, he just couldn't get his feet on the ground. He couldn't make sense out of life. In relationships it was the same. He would gravitate more and more toward a deep relationship with a woman, but his emotional uncertainties made him hard to live with. He felt too vulnerable. He needed a mother more than a wife.

At thirty-eight he had a job at what used to be a women's college. The student body was still predominantly female. He didn't feel settled, but then he thought he probably never would. A friend had coaxed him into Masters swimming. It was like a second chance. He loved the feel of water; he could lose himself swimming endless laps. It comforted him and gave him a sense of purpose, as if he were going somewhere, even though it was just to one end of the pool in order to turn around and do it all over again.

Beth.   Beth described herself as a "psych case." She had been a nationally ranked middle-distance swimmer, but was cut in the Olympic trials even though her personal bests would easily have placed her on the team. It made her mad. She felt she had talked herself out of winning, which is not so hard to do when there is just you, the water, and all those hard laps to go. It was a strange perception, particularly if you looked at Beth objectively. She was a straight A student, Phi Beta Kappa, a computer whiz, and an accomplished pianist. But she liked certainty and control. Not being able to perform the way she expected made her doubt herself.

In adolescence, she had hated her body. Her shoulders were too broad for a girl and she complained about being rounded forward from swimming. She never thought of herself as very attractive, and even at age twenty-five considered herself average. But in fact she was a knock-out, a real beauty who could turn heads when she walked into a room.

She was just too self-conscious and shy. She had lots of friends and publicly acted like a social butterfly. Privately, she hid. When her fears took hold, she couldn't face people. She had to withdraw with the phone off the hook and the curtains drawn. These feelings frightened her. She couldn't explain them and she certainly couldn't control them.

The Olympic trials marked the beginning of the end of Beth's swimming days. But she had to work out because it made her feel good and it kept her body trim. After college she took aerobics classes to stay in shape. They represented an acceptable mix — she didn't have to worry about the competition and it was great for muscular conditioning. Occasionally, she got frustrated by instructors who acted like dancers. Dance was a little too creative for her taste. It also threatened her.

For about three years she stuck with aerobics, eventually graduating to a part-time instructor's position. Her classes were the hardest workouts in town. But they were also highly repetitive, almost mechanical, in the way one muscle group was worked to exhaustion before she attacked another. The class format was always the same, only the intensity varied. Beth's class was popular with men. They felt more comfortable with simple, repetitive routines and were challenged by the endurance contests she created.

Around her twenty-fifth birthday, Beth got the whim to go back to swimming, but it was in the context of a triathlon. Once again she felt the charge of competition along with the agonies and ecstasies of training. The first time out she finished fifth in a field of 110. The second time, her performance remained about the same, but the third time it declined and she feared the reappearance of her old "psych out" syndrome. At the end of the season she hung up her gear, bathing suit included, and went back to aerobics. Here at least she could get the intensity of workout that she had become accustomed to in swimming — without all the competitive trappings. What surprised her was that she seemed more tuned into the social layer of her classes, something she had not given much thought to before, certainly not when she was swimming. She even noticed that she enjoyed it.

Commentary. What does the mind do when you are swimming those endless laps, when you are pushing hard and you can't even see the competition? Struggling through water when your arms feel like lead and your lungs are burning from lack of oxygen, you have to find something inside yourself to keep going, to kick faster, to pull harder — and to believe you haven't miscounted laps. That's competitive swimming: you against you. You get to know yourself in a different way. You play mind games to chase away the pain, to make you forget how much more you have to do. Sometimes you feel in harmony with the water, as if you are part of it, and sometimes you fight it.

It's not like that for most people who enjoy recreational swimming, but then people like Beth and Grey wouldn't call that swimming. For them it was an endurance contest with their psyches—pushing the limits, always asking for more—and trying not to get down on themselves. Swimming creates a very private world, one that is different from most other hours you spend. There's not much to see when you are swimming, so you end up looking inside.

Grey had a hard time coming to grips with reality. He had a persistent character, but he never learned how to weigh things. He couldn't figure out what he needed in life and how to get it. He lacked a feeling of support, a sense of being firmly rooted. He worked hard and was serious, but his vision seemed obscured. He didn't know where he was going.

Beth took her tumble from the Olympic trials pretty hard. She felt guilty, as if she should have perfect control over her performance at all times. Competition wore on her even though she was a great competitor. She didn't like looking inside and playing around in her murky psychology. But unwittingly, she trained her mind to focus inward throughout her years as a competitive swimmer. It came as a relief to find her social side emerging in aerobics. She was more comfortable and happier when she was dealing with the outside world. So, steering clear of those isolating periods in lap pools was a wise choice for her adult years.

What might have happened if Grey stuck with the football team in high school or if Beth had played basketball? Would they have ended up on the same paths, or would their experiences have rechanneled them? We raise the question not to say what they did was wrong, but to suggest an image of how they might have been had their athletic pursuits been different.

The Racquetball Players

Will. You knew immediately when Will arrived at the club. There would be a ripple effect as he walked down the corridor: quips, cackles, and guffaws echoed along the hall announcing the coming of the "King of Squash." In the locker room his partners—past, present, and future—would begin to flex their wit in the unspoken knowledge that the game was always in play; what happened on the court was only an extension of the competition.

Will was more than a successful stockbroker, he was the guy others would come to for advice. He had an edge, an uncanny insight that enabled him to pick the winners. It was always that way with Will. In college he was just an average student but that had little to do with his reputation. He always had a thousand things going, mostly business ventures or schemes to turn a dull event into a spectacle. He was fun to be with, but you had to be ready for rapid fire. His forte was keeping things light, keeping the action rolling, and creating a sense of adventure.

In sports he wasn't a team player as much as he was a star. He didn't belong to teams in school, but when someone was getting together a game of basketball or touch football, Will was always available—and usually one of the first to be picked. He never went in for "all this jogging stuff" and thought that aerobics was for "sissies." He liked to interact, to pit himself against others, and to come out on top. This is not to say that he was a sore loser; in fact, he was gracious in defeat, but the victor always knew it would just be a matter of time before the tables would be turned.

At the age of thirty-six Will was still single. He liked it that way. He wasn't really a ladies' man, just a guy who didn't want to be tied down. His life included work, squash, and social events—in that order of priority. When he dated, he was quite particular. It wasn't that he wanted to be seen with only the best-looking women in town. Appearances were far less important than the challenge of dating women known for their ability to bring something novel to the exchange. He was not a dull date and he expected reciprocity.

It was no surprise that squash was his game. It was fast and competitive. Winning was an individual achievement and Will didn't like having his personality submerged in a group. His racquet went where he did; he needed an outlet that was as flexible as he was.

Sean.   Sean was the last of five children in a close, nurturing family. At thirty-eight he was a well-respected director in a manufacturing company, traveling extensively and away from home for long periods. He had been romantically involved twice. It just didn't work out either time but the partings were friendly. He was the only bachelor in his family and he felt a bit overripe for the picking. He wanted to get married, but as with most other things in life, he was very cautious.

Sean was a hard worker. In school he was consistently in the top ten percent and, considering the schools he attended, that was no mean achievement. He recalled his years in college as some of the most trying of his life: long nights followed by full weekends in the library for months on end. When he was studying for his MBA, he found the program a holiday compared to his earlier studies. He completed his MBA while holding down a fulltime job. Sixteen years later he was working with the same firm.

Sean didn't expect he would ever be president of the company, but if it did happen, he wouldn't be surprised. He didn't play office politics, but preferred to put his energy into his job. He got along with most people, never being too pushy and, on the other hand, not being a pushover. He thought of himself as someone who was flexible to a degree. He had clear values about what was right and wrong, but when it was merely a choice between one good procedure and another, he didn't let his ego hang him up.

Studies took most of his time during his school years and that was his excuse for not becoming more involved in sports. At the age of thirty Sean joined a health club. It was close to home and he thought of it as a reward for his efforts. He also thought it might be a good place to meet women, since the bar scene was never to his liking. The club offered a range of athletic programs, but Sean immediately gravitated toward the racquetball courts. He was a tough competitor. Although his skill level was modest at the outset, he played a hard game, and as time went on he became one of the club's top-ranked players. Then he broke his hand on a camping trip.

While recuperating, he started taking aerobics. He had always enjoyed looking in on these classes and watching the women. Now that there were a few men in the classes, he felt less intimidated. He described aerobics as "a real turn-on." The classes suited his social nature and it was nice getting to know some of the women at the club. Racquetball had been mostly a male domain and competition seemed to complicate relationships.

In looking back over the four years since his accident, Sean saw a change in himself. He still played a lot of racquetball, but he mixed in a few aerobics classes each week. He didn't really understand the change until one day, when he played a much weaker partner. Normally he would have been bored or he would have trounced his opponent just to get on to a more challenging game. This day he remembered setting some goals in returning the ball, not so his partner could hit it, but more to create his own challenge. He didn't want to give away the game, instead he wanted a real contest for himself and his partner. In a sense they played by different rules, but in the end they both had a lot of fun. In reflecting on this experience, Sean became clearer about what he called "the social dimension of sports." The competitive part had always been there, but for Sean, people mattered a great deal. Winning was fun only if everyone could join in the victory.

He had enough confidence in himself to know he would do well in this world. Beyond a certain level of achievement, however, gains had to be weighed against the human costs. He would rather have a friend than have his ego boosted through hollow victory. It struck him that even his attitude about climbing the corporate ladder reflected this mix of social and competitive drives. He had a secure job that challenged him and provided ample rewards. He didn't need to become president of the company to satisfy himself. It was enough to know that he did a good job and had valued friends.

Commentary. Competition: the thrill of a good match, the joys of victory, the frustration of defeat. Racquet games can bring out the best and the worst, but bringing it out is what they are about. They don't just permit aggression and competitiveness, they require such expressions. And that's just fine for some people.

Will liked the challenge, the rush of competition. He enjoyed pitting his talent against someone else's. It was what he was used to, what he had come to expect in any encounter. He was sociable enough, but there was a certain edge to his relationships. The game was always in play.

Sean had another meaning for sociability; he needed to be liked, and people didn't always have friendly feelings after losing a game. He was also an achiever, a hard-working and serious-minded guy. But when he worked or when he played he was acutely aware of others, of the interpersonal world. This world was not, as with Will, a means to an end, it was important in itself. Sean's sensitivity would limit him—there were things he wouldn't do, there were prices he wouldn't pay—but that was all right. He bargained for a certain level of accomplishment and a degree of social comfort. Will struck a different kind of bargain: he was a "winner," a guy who, when he saw a pile, wanted to be on top of it. And that was just fine with him. He liked action and got bored when things were too predictable.

Choice—and Knowing What's Best

The ten cases are based on people who range in their level of involvement (some might say addiction) to movement and exercise. Most people don't exercise as much as the individuals portrayed in this chapter, and in that sense we are looking at more extreme variations. The value of examining this end of the exercise continuum is that it provides a more dramatic illustration of the interplay of exercise and personality—both how personality affects our choice and, in turn, how exercise shapes our personality.

The concept of "natural choice" implies we are drawn to certain exercise programs or sports and, conversely, repelled by others. What makes some activities attractive is perhaps the sense of fit not only on the physical plane but also in psychological terms. Needs for order, security, control, the release of aggression, for people, or for creative expression are just some of the reasons we find ourselves in one sport and not another. Each activity involves us in particular ways and requires certain behaviors in order to engage us. Whether it is height or weight or strength—or interactional demands, leadership skills, or creativity—we generally know what is called for, and we make our choices accordingly.

What we might consider for each of the ten cases is how well the activity suited the person. If, in general, we were aware of a congruence between the people and their activities, then we need to ask whether the choice was always the best or if there were any negative effects. Did it tend to draw out or overemphasize personality traits that should have been curbed? Such drawbacks may have been more evident in some cases than in others. It is important to bear in mind that this is not so much a function of the activity as it is a result of the match. That is, there are no bad sports, but there are bad matches between people and sports.

If we were to play an imaginary game and pretend that we could select exercise programs for these individuals, what would we choose, and why? In a way, this is what we will be doing in the upcoming chapters: trying to understand what we would change—and why—not for the case studies but for ourselves.

The approach that we have taken in this chapter is an intuitive one. We have examined sketches of individuals with significant investments in some sport or exercise and we have seen how their lives reflected these activities. These are normal people leading productive lives. Each person made a reasonable adjustment to life conditions, and so the question of what it is that might be changed is tricky. Even more complicated is how we would ever motivate these people to undertake other activities.

Our intuition may tell us that something is wrong or at least that something could be better, but it is only with the weight of solid evidence that we might be able to convince someone to try something new. And that is the task of this book: to provide the evidence, the arguments, and the means of knowing what will work better for us and for others.

3

Psychological Benefits of Exercise

> ... the fully functioning person must have a fully functioning body ... the self-actualizing individual must reside in a self-actualized body. — George Sheehan[1]

Psychologically Speaking

As we noted throughout the first two chapters, exercise is generally considered a body-change strategy. Other than the ancient wisdom that "sports build character," we didn't hear much about the psychology of exercise until recently, when mental health practitioners began exploring the benefits of fitness. As this mental health bandwagon got rolling, a lot of fitness converts jumped on to add their personal tales of how exercise had changed their lives.

A current survey found over eleven hundred articles proclaiming the psychological effects of exercise.[2] Of this number, *only twelve* met rigorous criteria for scientific research! This means that a lot of what we read — even in the more prestigious professional journals — about the positive or negative influences of exercise doesn't stack up scientifically.

In most cases we have little more than personal testimonials (like "Running made me a much happier person," or "I was an addict to Jane Fonda's aerobics"), or case studies involving one or two psychiatric patients who made it back from the depths of depression through exercise.

Some scientists scoff at the evidence on exercise, but we have to be careful not to throw out the baby with the bath water. There is a lot of evidence pointing in the same direction. Something is happening with high consistency, even though individual reports may not stand up to scientific scrutiny. As interest grows, more sophisticated studies are being conducted, providing a solid base for exercise effects.

What Are the Potential Effects of Exercise?

If we were to believe all that has been written about the psychological payoffs of exercise, we would enshrine exercise as the twentieth century panacea for humanity's mental ailments. Based on professional and popular accounts, benefits such as those listed below have been attributed to exercise:[3]

EXERCISE INCREASES:
academic performance
assertive behaviors
feelings of self-confidence
emotional stability
a sense of independence
feelings of control
positive moods
feelings of euphoria
the relaxation response
popularity
sexual satisfaction
a sense of well-being
adjustment to life
work efficiency
intelligence
memory
perceptual skills
body image
self-esteem
energy level

Not only have investigators reported how exercise accentuates the positive, but there have been numerous other studies or case histories attesting to exercise's effects on negative emotional conditions. As examples, we can find evidence of the following improvements:[4]

EXERCISE DECREASES:
alcohol abuse
drug abuse
anxiety
depression
dysmenorrhea
PMS (Premenstrual Syndrome)
headaches
emotional hostility
phobias
tension
psychotic behavior
insomnia
Type A or "coronary prone" behavior
stress reactions
mood swings
emotional fatigue

Now, if that isn't enough to justify buying a pair of running shoes or joining a health club, then you will never be convinced. Right? Well, it's not quite so simple.

Not only are there other ways to improve psychological functioning (for example, meditation, relaxation training, reading, psychotherapy), but this evidence is not definitive; exercise can be hazardous to your health. While you may immediately think about physical injuries, you shouldn't gloss over the potential for psychological injuries.

People who exercise regularly have been labeled narcissistic, neurotic, inhibited, egocentric, masochistic, addicted, compulsive, fanatical, hedonistic, and so on. They have been likened to anorexics with their obsessive worries about weight, body fat, and diet. Many exercise addicts are thought to suffer from poor self-image, emotional instability, and a lack of self-confidence. They are described as joyless and as having a low capacity for self-reflection.[5]

With all these conflicting findings, it's easy to defend any position you wish about fitness. Our position is that exercise has a lot to offer, but it does have potential for harm. It largely depends on what you do and how you do it.

Loopholes in Exercise Research

When researchers expect to find exercise benefits, why do some of their studies show no gain or even negative psychological effects? To answer this, we have to delve into the methods of exercise research. Aside from the standard scientific bugaboos of faulty measurements, lack of control groups, or inadequate sample sizes, there are some unique problems in fitness research that can create misleading results.

When research shows *unexpected* negative effects of exercise, we would say it is due to one or more of the following factors:

1. The exercise program doesn't match the research subjects' psychological needs, and as a result reinforces dysfunctional or negative traits.
2. Research subjects don't spend enough time in their exercise program to reap psychological rewards.
3. Research subjects are not coached properly, so that bad habits are reinforced instead of changed.

Probably the most critical of these three design flaws is the first. If the exercise program is not well suited to the individual's needs, then it has the potential for being harmful, or at the least ineffective. This is partly due to the prevailing model for exercise prescription. The American College of Sports Medicine's criteria for prescribing exercise are based purely on physiological, not psychological, considerations.[6] They include three factors: the *intensity* of the exercise, the *frequency* of exercise sessions, and the *duration* or length of each exercise session. As a result, a twenty-minute game of racquetball might be physiologically equated with thirty-minutes of aerobic dance. There is no evaluation of the activity itself, particularly along psychological lines.

As long as we look at exercise in an undifferentiated, might we say unsophisticated, way, we will continue to get conflicting reports about exercise benefits. We have to be more discriminating. We have to add questions like the following to the physiological evaluation of exercise: 1. What is the individual's personality? What are the personality traits emphasized by the exercise program? And how well does the program match the individual's personality (see Chapter 5)? 2. What does the exercise program do to develop the body? What psychological functions are emphasized through this body development? And how does this development match the individual's needs (see Chapter 6)? 3. What are the movement patterns emphasized by the exercise program? What psychological qualities do they reinforce? And how well matched are they with the person's movement profile (see Chapter 7)?

By asking questions like these we will begin to sort out the benefits from the liabilities of exercise, and to understand conditions under which an exercise program will be most effective.

Separating the Wheat from the Chaff

Despite all the research difficulties, there is good consensus about specific outcomes of exercise. If we take a conservative view, we may not have a list of exercise benefits nearly as long as those presented earlier, but we will have something we can trust. In the next section, we will review reliable trends on exercise benefits. We will describe qualifying conditions to achieve these benefits, and detail reasons these benefits occur. The final segment of the chapter will look at the liability side, the cautions about exercise.

Ridding Yourself of Tension and Anxiety — At Least for a While

What is anxiety? Perhaps the more common terms are tension and nervousness — an unpleasant experience signaled by uneasiness, apprehension, headaches, butterflies in the stomach, sweaty palms, or tingling sensations. Anxiety is distinguished from fear, which is an emotional response to something we consciously recognize as a real threat or danger.[7] Anxious feeling are not always easy to pin down to specific causes or origins. We just feel anxious sometimes with no apparent reason.

Psychologists distinguish between *state* and *trait* anxiety.[8] State anxiety is the anxiety you feel at a given point in time, whereas trait anxiety is a general characteristic. You might feel anxious right now (state anxiety), but if you feel anxious most of the time (trait anxiety), then anxiety is one of your personality traits. These two types of anxiety are not mutually exclusive. You can be both trait and state anxious, or trait anxious but not state anxious.

Another important distinction is between *cognitive* and *somatic* anxiety.[9] Cognitive anxiety is akin to worry or lack of concentration, whereas somatic anxiety refers to bodily sensations that occur in moments of anxiety (like physical tension, headache, sweating, rapid pulse).

Why make these distinctions? Research tells us that exercise is most beneficial for certain types of anxiety but may have little effect on others. We need to know where the payoff lies.

Anxiety has been shown to decrease for anywhere from thirty minutes to several hours after exercise. This means that exercise lessens state anxiety. Exercise is as effective as biofeedback and certain tranquilizing drugs in treating anxiety. Some reports document more long-range effects of exercise on trait anxiety, but, unfortunately, these results are not as reliable as those for the temporary effects of exercise.[10]

By examining the data more closely, we can tease out some of the special conditions for the anxiety-reducing effects of exercise: Intense exercises (running or racquetball, for example) offer a greater chance of anxiety reduction than do light to moderate exercises (walking or slow jogging, for example). Exercise intensity must be sufficient to produce sustained heavy breathing without exhaustion. A second condition for anxiety reduction is that the exercise period should be at least twenty minutes, although it could be as long as one to two hours. So, if you want tension relief or body relaxation, you have to work for it.[11]

Remember, most reports on exercise and anxiety tell us that effects are short-lived — from thirty minutes to six hours. This means you have to work up a sweat again tomorrow in order to reap the benefit. It's not a pill you take once to make your anxiety go away forever.

What happens in the long term? If you keep on exercising, you will continue to experience anxiety reduction. But if you stop, you may be back where you started. If you think of yourself as an anxious type, there is some real promise that a regular program of aerobic exercise will help you manage your tense and anxious feelings.

Is exercise any better than other anxiety-management procedures? Let's answer this first by ruling out medication or tranquilizing drugs. Drug treatment has its place, but it also has a number of drawbacks, including negative side effects, increased tolerance, and dependency.

Some research suggests that exercise is no more effective than rest breaks, quiet walks, listening to music, biofeedback, or meditation. The rationale is that exercise helps because it distracts us or takes us away from anxiety-provoking situations — it is another kind of "time-out" from our stress-filled days. This is neither bad news nor good news. It simply says that exercise helps reduce anxiety, as do a number of other pastimes, by taking us away from stress.[12]

At this point, the distinction between cognitive and somatic anxiety comes in handy. A unique benefit of intense aerobic exercise is that it works especially well to reduce anxiety's uncomfortable body sensations. You are less likely to reap these benefits from reading, walking, or even meditation!

However, some exercise programs may be less beneficial than activities like meditation for reducing cognitive anxiety or worry. For example, if you go for a run, you may spend the entire time worrying. When the run is over, your body will be relaxed, but your mind may still be stirred up. Of course, your upset mind will be housed in a quieter body, so you should feel somewhat better.

How can you reduce both cognitive and somatic anxiety? That's what we will be exploring in upcoming chapters. A brief answer is that you need to choose exercise programs that give you mental as well as physical relief. Sometimes this can happen by changing *how* you exercise; for example, concentrating on what you are doing, on the sensations in your body, in essence, making the exercise a moving meditation. An easier approach is to pick sports or fitness programs that make you shift gears. For example, you have to pay attention when you are playing racquetball. When you are running or sitting on a stationary cycle, your mind can worry all it wants.

Where you exercise can also be important. Running through midtown traffic is not going to produce nearly the level of benefit as running through a quiet park. Sitting on a stationary cycle at home may not be as relaxing as going to a health club.

Exercise can help you lead a more anxiety-free life, but there are some qualifications to this proposition. You have to keep at it, and you have to do more than light or even moderate levels of workouts in order to achieve somatic anxiety reduction. There is no permanency to the exercise payoff. Once you stop exercising you may lose that wonderful inner feeling of calm. And since exercise only reduces anxiety for a limited number of hours, each day needs to be an exercise day if you want that feeling of relaxation. In brief, lots of regular huffing and puffing is what you have to give in order to get temporary tension relief. While this may be heartening to anxiety sufferers, bear in mind that many exercise professionals would not recommend a daily regimen of aerobic exercise that can become addictive and increase chances of injury.

Fighting the Blues with Exercise

There is good news when it comes to the antidepressant effects of exercise, but first let's be clear about the term "depression." All of us go through ups and downs, through times of feeling sad and unhappy. These feelings may be brought on by specific events, such as the loss of a relative, relationship problems, financial difficulties, and other life changes.

When feelings of sadness and despair go on for a long time, or when they are exceptionally severe, depression becomes a clinical matter requiring professional help. At the clinical level, depression is marked by such symptoms are insomnia, chronic fatigue, appetite changes, low self-esteem, social withdrawal, irritability, pessimism, crying, decreased effectiveness, and even suicidal thoughts.

Exercise has a marked effect on moods. Dramatic inprovements occur not only for people suffering from temporary mood swings but also for more serious cases of clinical depression.[13]

One of the most important studies of exercise's antidepressant effects compared a running program to traditional time-limited psychotherapy. After twelve weeks of running, clinically depressed psychiatric outpatients showed as much relief from their depression as outpatients treated with psychotherapy. Something even more impressive was discovered twelve months later when, in a follow-up study, eleven of the twelve exercise outpatients remained free of symptoms while half of the psychotherapy outpatients had returned for treatment.[14]

There have been so many other reports on the antidepressant effects of exercise programs that we have high confidence in this exercise benefit. But how does exercise affect moods? Answers range from physiological to more psychological explanations.

On the physiological level, one theory is that increased blood flow and oxygenation of the blood influence the central nervous system, producing positive mood changes. Another theory tells us that positive mood changes result from exercise-induced increases in the hormone norepinephrine (depressed people are known to have low levels of norepinephrine). Since exercise increases norepinephrine levels, this hormone is believed to be a key to the antidepressant effect. Another hormone theory tells us that cortisol increases during vigorous exercise may be partly responsible for mood improvements.[15]

Aerobic exercise is also known for its positive effects on sleep patterns and thereby serves to alleviate one of the major symptoms of depression, insomnia. With better sleep, the depressed person is also likely to suffer less from chronic fatigue.[16]

One psychological theory is based on the development of mastery through exercise.[17] The idea is that people feel better because they are able to master an activity. They feel more competent and therefore less depressed. To ensure this psychological payoff, there are some important considerations to keep in mind when embarking on an exercise program. First, the exercise program should be developed slowly and in a carefully graduated manner. This way you won't get discouraged—or worse, injured. Second, the program should have reasonable goals so you feel a sense of accomplishment as you progress from one level of exertion to the next. Undertaken in this manner, an exercise program stands a high chance of improving your self-image and decreasing feelings of depression.

Another psychological theory is that exercise works on depression by providing opportunity for emotional release, for catharsis of negative emotions.[18] A good example of this comes from a runner who enjoyed nothing better than racing headlong into gale-force winds and yelling at the top of his lungs. No matter how badly he felt before such a run, he would end up experiencing the tranquility of a Buddhist monk.

However, there can be too much of a good thing. High-performance athletes, including professionals and highly ranked amateurs, sometimes develop a feeling of staleness that seems like depression.[19] Even habitual exercisers who, for example, run six to ten miles every day, have feelings of depression because progress is not perceived, improvement goals are not attained, or the routine becomes monotonous and unsatisfying. For these individuals, a suggested cure of time off has the potential for increasing depressed feelings due to the attendant loss of physiological benefits and the addictive aspects of exercise. A better solution is to change the exercise program from one activity to another, rather than merely take time off.

You can count on exercise as an effective antidepressant for symptoms ranging from normal mood swings to moderate levels of clinical depression *when* the exercise program is slowly developed according to a graduated plan that ensures mastery, and when it does not go to extremes (as in cases of exercise addiction). The antidepressant effect of exercise derives from physiological changes as well as from psychological feelings, including enhanced self-esteem, emotional relief, and mastery. Once again, it's something you have to work for. While the evidence doesn't say you have to do a lot of huffing and puffing, as was true for exercise-induced anxiety reduction, you do have to stick with it. So long as you exercise in a reasonable manner, you can count on buffering yourself against depressive symptoms. This doesn't mean you will never feel depressed. Rather, the severity of your depression will be reduced.

Exercising to Manage Stress

Hans Selye believed that stress was an integral part of human existence.[20] In his words, it was both the "spice" and the "wear and tear" of life. It could be positive (*eustress*) or negative (*distress*). He defined stress as the result of *any demand on the individual to cope*. Since we have to cope continually to survive, we experience stress throughout life. What makes the difference in terms of wear and tear are such factors as the intensity and frequency of demands to cope, the nature of these demands (positive or negative), and our resources and resilience—which brings us back to exercise.

More and more research points to the significance of exercise in the ongoing management of stress. In fact, according to some researchers it is one of the best stress-management tools available. Why?

There are physiological and psychological explanations of how exercise benefits stress management. When exercise is assessed physiologically, researchers are usually talking about aerobic or cardiorespiratory fitness programs (running, aerobic dance, racquetball) rather than anaerobic or isometric exercise regimes (weight lifting, Nautilus training).

Exercise is a preventative approach to stress management. It enhances body function, strengthens the heart, and generally buffers the individual from the physical ravages of stress. Muscles become more efficient, thereby reducing the load upon the heart. Under physical stress, the heart experiences less of a demand because of the body's increased efficiency and also because the training effect of exercise increases the efficiency of cardiac muscle. This allows the heart to return to a normal rhythm in a shorter period of time. More important, it allows the heart to meet the physical stress with a smaller increase in heart rate or work. At rest, the heart works less. Normal or resting heart rate may drop anywhere from ten to thirty beats per minute as a result of regular aerobic exercise.[21]

Harmful chemical byproducts of stress may be reduced through exercise training or they may be countered by the production of more beneficial ones. For example, blood (plasma) cholesterol levels have been associated with heart disease, but recent studies distinguish between "good" cholesterol (HDL, or high-density lipoprotein cholesterol fraction), and "bad" cholesterol (LDL, or low-density lipoprotein cholesterol fraction). Exercise is known to increase the production of good cholesterol and decrease the amount of bad cholesterol, thereby improving our resistance to heart disease.[22]

We might also recall that stress reactions are known as the *fight or flight response*. This refers to the evolutionary function of stress as an adaptive process whereby the body readies itself to deal with life-threatening situations. Even though many modern-day stressors are not life-threatening, we nonetheless respond with all the chemical, hormonal, and other physiological reactions that prepare us to fight or flee. Unfortunately, these modern stress situations don't allow us to fight or flee, so we have no immediate way of expressing the body's charge. We react with increased heart rate, but the body remains at rest; hormonal secretions take place throughout the body, and we end up feeling jittery and uncomfortable. What was once an adaptive mind-body reaction for our primitive ancestors has become like a dysfunctional pressure cooker linked to a host of psychosomatic disorders.

Exercise lessens these harmful reactions and allows a more natural expression of the byproducts of the fight or flight response. Even though a fitness activity may occur hours after the stressful situation has passed, it will use up chemical deposits and put our bodies back in balance. Moreover, exercise conditions our bodies to respond more efficiently to stress. The magnitude of our stress reaction is less extreme, and we bounce back faster from the stressful event.[23]

Exercise provides an escape, a diversionary time-out from stressful encounters. Going to an exercise class or taking a run in the park marks a transition from the daily routine. It is personal time, or, as some would argue, adult playtime.[24]

We can get more out of exercise by making a few changes. The unrealized potential of exercise is due to the way most people go about fitness. They separate mind and body, telling themselves that as long as they get their heart rates up and breathe heavily, they are doing as much as they can to capture the exercise benefit. The fault in this logic is that many people keep their minds tuned into stressful thoughts while exercising and perpetuate the wear and tear of worry. This is why many studies found exercise superior to most other stress-management methods for reducing somatic tension but not for easing cognitive tension. To capture the full benefits of this time-out, we need to refocus our minds as we are getting our hearts beating faster. The best exercises for achieving this added effect will be identified in Chapter 8.

Exercise is rated as one of the best stress-management approaches available. Despite the advances in relaxation training, biofeedback, and other mind-control methods, none of these approaches achieves the physiological benefits of exercise. On the psychological side, exercise is similar to a number of other time-outs or diversionary recreational activities that help us manage stress. Some of the untapped potential of exercise comes from learning how to shift mental gears while exercising. As we will see later on, some exercise programs are inherently better at making us shift. If our natural tendency is to dwell on stressful problems during exercise, we may need to choose an activity that more naturally helps us get out of our worry-filled heads.

Improving Self-Esteem

Probably the most important factor in our personal psychology is what we think about ourselves — our self-concepts. This is also referred to as self-image or self-esteem.

So much has been written about self-concept that it is hard to offer a concise definition. Self-concept refers to how we see ourselves and whether we like what we see. Liking, or self-valuing, has a number of parts. We hear people saying, "I feel good about my career, but socially I'm a mess" or "I like the way I look, but any time I open my mouth I feel like a fool." This tells us that self-image comes from different aspects of ourselves. Some psychologists say it results from ways we identify ourselves, such as spouse, lover, worker, friend, or athlete. Others say it is a general feeling of worth based on personal assets and liabilities, abilities and competencies, or successes and failures.

How does exercise fit into this picture? Your physical characteristics constitute one of three major components of self-concept, the other two being social identity and personal disposition.[25] Exercise is a *means to an end* where that end is a more positive feeling about your physical appearance.

For some people, body image plays a smaller role in overall feelings of self-esteem. Yet, with the fitness boom continuing through the 1980s, most people have at least had their body consciousness raised. Physical appearance is not solely a matter of aesthetics and beauty. It strongly reflects psychological and physical health. Medical practitioners are keen on advising patients to manage their weight and to engage in reasonable fitness programs as a preventive measure. And other health practitioners advocate weight control and physical fitness programs for reasons ranging from quality of life to promoting youthfulness and longevity. The good news in this current body focus is that efforts to enhance health and attractiveness through physical fitness will pay off in higher self-esteem.

A recent review concludes that exposure to physical fitness programs is associated with increases in self-esteem.[26] And an earlier review indicated that the personality variable with the highest payoff from fitness programs is self-concept.[27] This earlier review reasoned that body changes resulting from fitness training improve body image, which, in turn, builds self-concept. So, it's a safe bet to assume that a good exercise program is going to make you feel better about your body and that this will do a lot for your self-image.

Whether or not you subscribe to modern-day idolatry of the human body, you cannot help but be affected by this culture of body worship. Society places a high premium on physical appearance. Efforts to enhance appearance will be amply rewarded through positive payback to self-image. Even if you ignore this idolatry, you cannot escape the deluge of popular press releases on the medical importance of moderate exercise. And in a looking-glass world, if you exercise for either psychological or physical payoff, it must mean that you care about yourself—and if you care about yourself, you must like yourself. With this kind of logic, the inevitable consequences of exercise participation work their way to your psyche and soma, causing you to feel better, for at least as long as you exercise.

Joy, More Joy, and the Runner's High

Ask any marathon runner and the chances are she will tell you about some peak experience, a euphoric moment, or some other pleasant state of consciousness while running. Average mortals who simply exercise regularly are also likely to recall emotional highs during or after their fitness rituals.

What is this strange and wonderful experience? Is it really like nirvana? Do we get it every time we exercise? How much does it cost; that is, how far do we have to run, how much do we have to sweat? Answers vary and, in brief, the jury is out.

A recent explanation is based in neurochemistry. It implicates a chemical family known as beta-endorphins. Because these opiate-like chemicals increase with intense exercise and because they block pain sensations, acting like the body's own morphine, the "runner's high" has been attributed to increases in beta-endorphins. Elevated endorphin levels have also been measured for up to two hours after vigorous activity, suggesting they may be responsible for positive mood states following exercise.[28]

Scientific findings do not wholly support this theory. For example, in one study, beta-endorphin production was inhibited by injection of a chemical blocker, yet athletes still reported euphoric moods.[29] One study does not a theory break, but even so, other research brings into question the role of beta-endorphins as the sole explanation for mood lifts.

Other explanations of the runner's high argue for meditative states and corresponding brain-wave changes, body-temperature changes during intensive exercise, elevations in blood-plasma norepinephrine, cortisol increases, and so forth. None of these theories has come through the science gauntlet unscathed. This has caused some researchers to back off completely and others to drop back to simpler explanations.

Statistical estimates of the percentage of runners who experience a high range from ten percent to seventy-eight percent.[30] No doubt the truth lies somewhere in between. One study notes that the words runners use to describe these emotional highs include no less than twenty-seven variations, making it far less than uniform.[31] Words like "spirituality," "spin out," "a glimpse of perfection," or "moving without effort" typify the diversity of subjective experience in the exercise high. Even so, there is something here that requires examination.

Simpler theories revert to ideas previously discussed in this chapter—that is, anxiety reduction, decreases in depressive feelings, and increases in self-esteem—as accounted for on both physiological and psychological levels.

We need to find a way to unite these observations. No doubt neurochemical, hormonal changes, coupled with other physiological processes, contribute to the experience of mood euphoria. Also, the psychological benefits of increased competence in an activity, of having a time-out or playful period, and of increased self-esteem through creating a better body have to make us feel pretty good while we are exercising.

It's unlikely that we will feel euphoric every time we exercise, but as we know from psychology, an unpredictable payoff pattern, such as Las Vegas slot machines have, hooks us solidly. We may never be sure when we are going to get it, but we do know that sooner or later we are going to feel great during an exercise session, and that keeps us going, keeps us reaching for the brass ring.

Anything That Good Has Got to be Dangerous

Without considering precisely what a person does, the conservative picture is that regular exercise will make you feel less anxious, less depressed, more euphoric, more self-satisfied, and more effective in stress management.

Wait! There's got to be a catch!

You're right—there is. And that's why this book is so important.

Exercise critics have not been nearly as active in publicizing their opinions as have fitness advocates. Nonetheless, various studies of fitness participants have reported negative side effects of exercise. A partial list of these potential hazards is listed below:[32]

EXERCISE MIGHT INCREASE:
behavioral compulsivity
an escapist pattern or avoidance of problems
a tendency toward exercise addiction
feelings of fatigue
poor eating habits
preoccupation with fitness, diet, and body image
overcompetitiveness
overexertion
self-centeredness or narcissism
masochistic tendencies
violent behavior

EXERCISE MIGHT DECREASE:
involvement in career or job
marital stability and family involvement
social involvements
sexual interest
frequency of sexual activities

One can argue that not all of these potential harms are necessarily bad. For example, it may be beneficial to some individuals to decrease their career identification, particularly if they tend to be workaholics. And whoever said we should squarely confront all our problems? Even our primitive ancestors knew there was a time to stand one's ground and a time to run. Escape from a world that may be beyond our control is not a bad trait to nurture—as long as it is kept in perspective.

The issue is one of limits, knowing when enough is enough, when something is healthy and beneficial and when the solution itself has turned into the problem.

Addictions—Positive and Otherwise

A consistent complaint about our exercise-conscious society is that people get hooked. They become addicts, needing their daily fix of exercise. This is another one of those chicken-and-egg dilemmas where one cannot be certain which comes first, the addictive personality or the addictive exercise.

Whatever the answer, there is reason for concern. People who become addicted allow fitness to assume higher priority than most other things in life—family, friends, work, even personal health. Exercise addicts go through identifiable withdrawal symptoms when for some reason they are forced to stop exercising. They show signs of depression, irritability, and anxiety. Interpersonal relations begin to deteriorate. They may have disturbed sleep. Appetite may decrease. Muscle tension, tics, and general soreness may develop. In response, the addict will attempt to resume exercising even though it may be harmful emotionally, socially, or medically.[33]

The incidence of exercise addiction is not at all clear, but it is likely to be high among people who work out five or more times per week. If you exercise this frequently and you show any of the above symptoms when you miss a day or more of exercise, the possibility of addiction needs to be considered.

What confuses the issue is that addictions can be positive. In his book *Positive Addiction,* William Glasser popularized the idea that certain kinds of regular activity can be beneficial to health and well-being.[34]

What is a positive addiction and how does it differ from a negative one? Negative addictions are pretty clear, according to Glasser. Like addictions to alcohol and drugs, they can weaken and eventually destroy us. On the other hand, positive addictions "strengthen us and make our lives more satisfying." They allow us to live with "more confidence, more creativity, more happiness, and usually in much better health." Positive addiction provides enjoyment but does not dominate your life.

Glasser established six criteria to distinguish positive addictions from negative ones. Let us review these criteria to determine how your fitness activities match up.

Six Criteria for Positive Addiction

1. The activity is noncompetitive, freely chosen, and engaged in for about one hour daily.
2. It is something you can do easily and without a great deal of mental effort.
3. It doesn't require others' involvement — you can and often do engage in it alone.
4. You believe it has some physical, mental, or spiritual value for you.
5. You believe that if you persist, you will improve — but improvement must be based on your personal scale.
6. The activity is done without self-criticism.

How did you do? Did your fitness program pass the addiction test? Keep these points in mind as you read upcoming chapters on personality and fitness matching. For now, let's press forward in understanding the addictive process.

In the typical pattern of becoming addicted, an individual may initiate a program for health or personal reasons. Soon the psychological and physiological payoffs sink the hook deeper. The person feels better, looks better, and often experiences a gratifying sense of accomplishment.[35]

As the benefits increase, another transition may occur. The fitness novice becomes fearful that if he stops exercising, all will be lost. Fear fuels the addictive process, as well as marks the border between positive and negative addiction. The addict needs to increase the dosage. It becomes more and more difficult to keep the fitness regimen in check. His world revolves around exercise. Social and recreational patterns change. Time with the family is decreased. Eating habits become obsessive. The addict worries about weight and appearance. Eventually, performance in other areas of life begins to decline. Work and career concerns become subjugated to the tyranny of fitness. The person needs a daily fix to feel good, indeed, in order to function.

There is some speculation that the beta-endorphins may be involved in the addictive process.[36] If the endorphins act like morphine and if they require an ever-increasing intensity of exercise for their production, we can appreciate what might happen if the fitness fanatic doesn't go through his daily ritual.

Three signals of negative addiction have been identified. First, significant relationships with family and friends begin to suffer and eventually are ignored as exercise commitment increases to three or more hours per day. Second, the addict becomes self-absorbed while at the same time expressing less and less concern for external affairs, including job and even financial obligations. Third, as with drug and alcohol addictions, the exercise addict's highest priority is feeling good, even when the production of this feeling-state through exercise jeopardizes his mental and physical health.[37]

When the person is addicted, deprivation of the daily fix produces withdrawal symptoms. Feelings of increased anxiety, depression, and irritability may be accompanied by insomnia, muscle aches, and eating disorders. In the extreme, suicidal feelings may develop.[38]

As a practical benchmark of addiction, there is evidence to suggest that when fitness buffs are exercising the equivalent of running seventy or more miles per week, the likelihood of addiction is high.[39] In terms of hours, this would equate to about fourteen hours or more of exercise per week. Bear in mind that even Glasser's more appealing positive addiction, involving one or more hours per day, is likely to produce some unpleasant withdrawal symptoms.

We simply cannot ignore problems of exercise addiction. If you happen to be an ultramarathoner or triathlete whose life is sport and competition, it's hard to say how much this is different from the lifestyle of a career professional. But for the recreational athlete whose fitness pursuits are crowding out primary involvements in family and work, there is reason for concern. Exercise initiated as a solution to health or emotional concerns may have developed into a serious problem of its own. Why some people become addicted and others do not is no doubt related to personality makeup and the nature of the exercise program that is chosen. Diagnosing your personality and the psychological demands of different exercise programs will help you steer clear of this pitfall to fitness programs.

The Bottom Line

When we examine the publications of sports and fitness experts, the weight of evidence is substantial enough to say that if you exercise moderately, you will be amply rewarded. You can pretty well count on feeling less anxious for a period of some hours after a moderate-to-intense workout. You will experience a lift in spirits. Whether this means feeling less depressed or attaining a more positive state of euphoria will have a lot to do with where you are emotionally at the outset of your exercise session. You will become better at coping with stress, partly through having a more tuned body, and partly from giving yourself a stress break each day that you exercise. Your self-image is likely to get a substantial boost from regular exercise. This will come chiefly through a more positive body image, but will also derive from feelings of competence and mastery in your exercise program.

There are many other benefits that have been attributed to exercise. These include improved mental functioning, greater independence, better self-control, and more sexual satisfaction. How reliable these gains are is subject to debate. As a more conservative proposition, exercise promises better anxiety and stress management, relief from depression, euphoric feelings, and an enhanced self-image. These benefits seem considerable on top of all the physical health payoffs. Whatever other gains come your way from exercise are raisins in your granola.

4

The Traditional Approach to Exercise Prescription

Better to hunt in fields, for health unbought
Than fee the doctor for a nauseous draught.
The wise, for cure, on exercise depend;
God never made his work for man to mend.
                                        John Dryden

Why Bother?

The typical argument for exercise has more to do with physical well-being than with personality. Down through the ages, people have been advised to keep fit for health reasons. Of course, in earlier times there was hardly a need to convince people about the value of exercise. Lifestyles — even of the rich and famous — required a certain amount of physical effort for personal maintenance and worldly involvement. Today, people of all income levels have the dubious advantage of remaining relatively immobile for long periods of time while working or recreating. The consequences of our sedentary lifestyles have been the subject of some debate. While there is consensus that we need to move around a

bit to maintain healthy functioning of the body, the degree of movement—or might we say, exercise—is not at all agreed upon.

In fact, Dr. Henry Solomon, author of *The Exercise Myth*[1] and a
prominent New York cardiologist, argues that the case for exercise has
been grossly overstated. Not only does he believe that the minimal
efforts we make to get us from bed to breakfast to work and home again
are sufficient to maintain the human body, but, more critically, he asserts that the current advocacy of exercise may be hazardous to our
health. In his view, "Exercise will not make you healthy. It will not make
you live longer. Fitness and health are not the same thing."

One man's opinion? Well, not exactly.

Dr. Solomon's arguments are well supported by research. Unfortunately, the language of research ("perhaps"—"under certain circumstances"—"it might be the case that"—"some potential effect of") allows
for a variety of interpretations. The same publications, when reviewed
by other exercise specialists, end up as citations for preventive health
benefits of exercise.

One distinction Dr. Solomon makes that is well worth remembering
is that between fitness and health. Health has to do with the presence or
absence of disease entities or abnormal body conditions, whereas fitness
is a measure of ability to perform physical work. Health and fitness are
considered to be independent of one another. This means you can be fit
but unhealthy—or healthy but unfit.

The Health Argument

We know that if we exercise, we will become more fit, but will we
become healthier as well? The consensus seems to be yes, Dr. Solomon
and others notwithstanding. This does not mean that by becoming fit,
we will rid ourselves of all disease, but rather that exercise can help us
prevent certain diseases, and, if we are afflicted with particular diseases,
exercise can help alleviate some of their symptoms.

Dr. William Haskell of Stanford University School of Medicine
summarizes the evidence as follows:[2]

> Of the various claims made regarding the health benefits of exercise,
> those with the most substantial scientific basis appear to be the main-
> tenance of optimal body weight or composition, the prevention of
> coronary heart disease, and the normalization of carbohydrate metab-
> olism. Other areas in which benefits are likely but persuasive data are
> not so available include the prevention of elevated blood pressure or
> hypertension, the maintenance of bone density (the loss of which

occurs with aging), the prevention of lower back pain syndrome, and improved psychological status.

Haskell goes on to note that patients with certain diseases show clinical improvement with exercise. These diseases include chronic obstructive lung disease (emphysema or bronchitis), kidney failure, and arthritis. The evidence does not support the theory that exercise prevents these diseases from occurring.

Problems of Obesity and Weight Management

Statistical estimates tell us that out of 225 million Americans, about 50 million men and 60 million women between the ages of eighteen and seventy-nine are overly fat and need to reduce excess weight.[3] When we add to this an estimated 25 million youngsters[4] who have weight problems, we are looking at an astounding sixty percent of the U.S. population contending with problems of being overly fat.

The approach most frequently taken for weight loss is some extreme form of caloric restriction which, as numerous studies have demonstrated, creates problems of its own.[5] Not only are we likely to induce dangerous chemical, hormonal, and mineral imbalances, but the objectives of these programs are rarely achieved. By this we do not simply mean that the dieter doesn't lose the desired amount of weight, but that the goal of losing body fat while maintaining lean body tissue, including muscle and bone, is usually not attained.

While diets that involve moderate (as opposed to severe) caloric restriction are less harmful, evidence weighs strongly in favor of *exercise plus moderate caloric restriction* as the most effective weight loss plan.[6] The rule of thumb for weight loss is that you have to burn off more calories than you consume. There are three good reasons why exercise gives our weight management program that extra boost.[7]

First, exercise can have an "appetite suppressant effect," so the exercising dieter eats less at mealtimes. Usually this means exercising a short while before eating so that appetite is lower during mealtime.

A second reason is "energy expenditure." Most of us know that exercise really doesn't burn off that many calories. For example, jogging five miles in an hour uses up about 570 calories, compared to 100 calories that we use while sitting quietly. The net difference of 470 calories will help promote weight loss, but it will be slow. (One pound of weight loss is roughly the equivalent of 3,500 calories.) The hidden benefit is that people who exercise often feel more energetic and exert themselves more vigorously throughout the day. The result: higher than normal caloric expenditures throughout the day, leading to greater weight loss.

The third reason concerns "body composition." Body weight is not nearly as important as body composition for assessing obesity. It's how much fat you are carrying around rather than how much you weigh that determines whether or not you are obese. Most diet-only plans make you lose lean mass (including muscle and bone) more than fat. So you may still end up being classified as obese even though you have shed a year's worth of holidays. Exercise helps you retain lean body mass while losing weight. Not only does this place you in the minority (of non-overweight Americans), but it boosts sagging ego and flab at the same time.

Prevention of Coronary Heart Disease (CHD)

Coronary heart disease is the major form of cardiovascular disease in the United States, accounting for over fifty percent of cardiovascular deaths and approximately one-third of all deaths.[8] Scientists believe the underlying atherosclerotic process (fatty deposits in blood vessels) begins in childhood and that severity of CHD is related to such factors as blood cholesterol levels, blood pressure, cigarette smoking, dietary intake of saturated fat and cholesterol, *and* physical inactivity.

There are four major changes or mechanisms that have been proposed to explain how exercise might prevent the development of CHD:[9]

1. *Maintaining or increasing myocardial (heart muscle) oxygen supply* — Exercise is thought to keep the heart healthy by maintaining or increasing the oxygen supply to heart muscle.

2. *Increased myocardial function* — Regular exercise increases the amount of blood pumped by the heart with each beat. This is called *stroke volume output*. The increased output results in greater efficiency of the heart during periods of rest and exercise.

3. *Decreased myocardial work and oxygen demand* — This is due to the effect of exercise just discussed. With an increased amount of blood pumped per heart beat, the heart will beat less often in order to deliver the same amount of blood. This decrease in heart rate represents a reduction in the work of the heart. This occurs both at rest and when you are exercising or working.

4. *Increased stability of the myocardium* — Although this mechanism is not well understood, there is a strong possibility that exercise serves to regulate the nervous impulses to the heart muscle. This results in more rhythmic contractions and the reduction of irregularity of heartbeats (dysrhythmias).

Evidence on exercise and the prevention of coronary heart disease is far from conclusive. We are beginning to understand the mechanisms by which exercise helps us, but questions about the proper *dosage* of exercise remain unanswered. The general thesis, however, that exercise is a sensible if not necessary preventive measure has been endorsed by the American Heart Association's Subcommittee on Exercise/Cardiac Rehabilitation.[10] Members of this subcommittee wrote:

> Evidence suggests that regular moderate, or vigorous occupational or leisure-time physical activity may protect against CHD and may improve the likelihood of survival from a heart attack.

They indicated that exercise not only helps reduce such primary risk factors as cholesterol abnormalities, hypertension, and obesity, but also serves to influence such other risk factors as cigarette smoking and emotional stress through encouraging healthier lifestyles.

Other Health Benefits

There is good evidence suggesting that participation in regular aerobic exercise helps prevent such conditions as osteoporosis (through increasing bone density) and the onset of diabetes in adults (through improved metabolism and reduced body fat). Another significant health benefit has less to do with disease entities than with the quality of life. People who exercise regularly experience more energy and vigor in their daily lives. As noted in Chapter 3, the psychological gains from exercise are impressive and no doubt contribute to the maintenance of a healthy body. This is not to say that people who don't exercise are unhealthy or have a lower quality of life. There are many paths to health and emotional contentment. It's just that exercise happens to be a particularly good one.

Summary

If we strip away excessive claims about exercise benefits, we would at the very least have a basis for prevention and treatment of two of America's most pressing health concerns: coronary heart disease and obesity. With more than half of the American population suffering with weight problems and more than one-third of all deaths attributed to coronary heart disease, we would be foolish to ignore this opportunity for health enhancement.

The Rationale for Traditional Exercise Prescription

The methods used to evaluate fitness and prescribe exercise can be directly linked to concerns about flab and coronary heart disease. When President Dwight D. Eisenhower established the President's Fitness Council in 1956, he was responding to strong evidence of the physical unfitness of American youth. At about the same time, mortality statistics portrayed a disturbing incidence of deaths attributable to coronary heart disease.[11]

Exercise scientists addressed these growing problems of fitness and CHD by promoting standardized methods for assessing fitness and improving physiological functioning. They also began to look more closely at the body's internal reactions to exercise. In order to correlate exercise with internal body reactions, clear-cut exercise procedures had to be employed. What evolved was a rather mechanical and limited view of exercise.

Scientists concentrated on the physiological parameters of exercise, for example, how much oxygen you consumed, how fast your heart was beating, or what your blood pressure was. These measures of work or effort were best gauged under controlled laboratory conditions with subjects running on treadmills or pedaling stationary bicycles.

The laboratory results were translated into practical exercise prescriptions. Scientists, having found that maintaining a certain heart rate for a specified period of time produced beneficial physiological effects, would advise people to exercise to specific levels of intensity for a certain number of minutes in order to profit from exercise. It didn't matter how the person achieved this level of exertion—primary emphasis was on reaching specified physiological criteria.

One of the most common recommendations for getting your heart beating faster for a specified period of time is to go out for a run. Running is a simple movement that most people can do without training. It is cheap; you just need a good pair of shoes. And it is convenient—right outside your door—unless, of course, you live on a boat.

Other simple exercise programs were recommended. The stationary bicycle became almost as ubiquitous as the television. Its raison d'être derived from the logic of exercise physiology. The goals of exercise were not pleasure, fun, enjoyment, personal growth, or peak experiences (all of this came later). They were improved heart rates, oxygen consumption, blood pressure, and other physiological changes. It was as if we could disconnect our minds from our bodies for a period of time in the interest of health.

This approach was based on the *Rational Model* of psychology. Its core principle was that, an individual who knows something is good for her will do it out of rational self-interest. This sounds pretty absurd today, but the rational model was fundamental to many behavioral theories. Of course, if this model were valid, no one would smoke, alcohol would not be abused, obesity would be a rarity, and psychoanalysts would be out of work.

In the exercise scientists' zeal to get our heart rates up, the quality of the experience mattered very little — until about ten years ago when the phrase "exercise adherence" began appearing in the exercise literature.[12] What this signaled was the growing awareness of high dropout rates among exercise converts. Within a few years, the evidence was irrefutable — the rational model simply didn't work. Attaining physiological goals was not enough incentive to keep most people exercising, even if it was supposed to be good for them. Despite this awareness, the rational model prevails. Exercise prescription continues to be based on physiological considerations. Psychology and personality issues are given superficial attention at best.

Let's take a closer look at the exercise prescription process as it is commonly practiced today.

Are You "In Shape"?

The expression "in shape" has little specific meaning.[13] Exercise scientists prefer the term "physical fitness." But even here, there is ambiguity. Passing a physical fitness test is *not* the same as getting a clean bill of health. A person can be fit but not healthy; that is, he can have some disease but still be classified as fit. A tragic example of this distinction was Jim Fixx, the running guru and author of *The Complete Book of Running*,[14] who was exceptionally fit, but with severe coronary heart disease was not very healthy.

Practically, what this means is that a fitness evaluation will only measure fitness, not health. For this reason, it is generally recommended that you go for a thorough medical checkup before scheduling yourself for a fitness appraisal. This lets you know your state of health as well as advising a fitness appraiser of any special conditions that would affect your evaluation.

So what is fitness? According to Reid and Thomson in their book, *Exercise Prescription for Fitness*,[15] fitness is "a level of bodily efficiency" encompassing five important parameters:

A. Body measurements including height, weight, and percentage of fat
B. Posture

C. Flexibility

D. Muscular endurance and strength

E. Aerobic capacity

Let's consider each of these separately to understand how fitness evaluations are usually made.

Body Measurements

There are two sets of measurements that fitness evaluators concentrate on. The first consists of basic *anthropometric measurements*, which include height, weight, and girth measurements of the arm, chest, abdomen, hips, and thigh. These measures give the evaluator an idea of body proportions, so that fitness prescriptions might include exercises, for example, to develop the arms or to reduce the waist.[16]

A more critical measurement is percentage of body fat. Obesity is determined more by the percentage of your total weight that is body fat than by the number of pounds you may be over your ideal weight according to life insurance industry height-weight charts. Technically speaking, body fat consists of most of the unmetabolized energy foods (excess carbohydrates, animal fats, and protein) stored in the body in the form of triglycerides.

How much body fat should you have? The answer will vary, depending on your age and sex. For example, if you look at the percentages of body fat for men and women at different ages (Table 4.1), you can see that as you get older, you tend to have a greater proportion of body

TABLE 4.1
Percent Body Fat for Classification as Obese, Average, Ideal and Slim

	Age:	17–19	20–29	30–39	40–49	50+
Obese	M	23+	25+	27+	32+	35+
	F	29+	29+	30+	31+	33+
Average	M	12–17	15–19	19–22	22–26	23–28
	F	19–23	19–23	20–24	21–25	22–26
Ideal	M	7–11	9–14	15–18	16–21	17–22
	F	14–18	14–18	14–19	15–20	16–21
Slim	M	≤6	≤8	≤14	≤15	≤16
	F	≤13	≤13	≤13	≤14	≤15

M = male; F = female
Courtesy of Fitness and Amateur Sport Canada

weight that is fat. Men start out slimmer but increase markedly in body fat over the years, while women have a more gradual increase.[17]

The numbers shown are averages. They do not tell us what percentage of body fat you need for survival. According to one estimate, the percentage of body fat believed to be essential for life and normal physiological functioning amounts to three percent for males and twelve percent for women.[18] Essential fat is substantially lower than the usual amounts modern people have.

How do you measure body fat? If you think about trying to measure all the fat in muscles, under the skin, in bone marrow, in cell membranes, and in the internal organs, you will realize that the best you can do is estimate. There are no direct ways of measuring the amount of fat in the human body.

The preferred way of measuring percent body fat is hydrostatic, or underwater, weighing. This involves weighing a person while he is submerged in a tank of water. It is a difficult and expensive procedure.

An easier method of estimating body fat involves measuring folds of skin with special instruments known as skinfold calipers. Skinfold measurements require gently pinching and pulling the subcutaneous (beneath the skin) fat away from the body in various locations and measuring the thickness of the fat with calipers. These measurements are then combined in an equation to calculate the percent body fat.

Another method described in the book *The Marine Corps 3X Fitness Program*[19] uses a tape measure and a set of conversion tables. This is a relatively simple procedure, but is less exact and requires conversion tables to make the estimate.

While we can't offer a simple way of estimating percent body fat, a measure called the *Body Mass Index* is considered to be a good indicator of your proportional weight. It is based on your weight (in kilograms) divided by your height squared, or multiplied by itself (in centimeters). If your body mass index is greater than 27.2 for men or 26.9 for women, you are considered obese and, in this formula, your weight is considered a potential health risk.[20]

Posture

Posture analysis is an important component of fitness evaluations, particularly as related to the prescription of activity. Unfortunately, a good many evaluators ignore this component.

What is good posture? If you strip down to your underwear and arrange the mirrors in your house so you get a front, back, and side view of your body, you can analyze your posture. According to Reid and

Thomson,[21] there are ten body areas where you can evaluate posture. Each area is evaluated on a 10-point scale, where 0 is poor, 5 is fair, and 10 is good. Ratings of 2, 3, 4, 6, 7, 8, or 9 are also possible. While analyzing your posture, be sure you don't make artificial adjustments. For example, don't tuck in your stomach or force a military posture. Stand naturally with your feet a few inches apart and your arms relaxed at your sides. Now for the ten areas:

Head (view from the back): Is your head naturally erect or does it tilt to the side? If it appears squarely placed and upright, you rate a 10. If it is turned or tilted to the side, your rating is lowered by the degree of tilt.

Shoulders (view from the back): Do your shoulders look even or is one lower than the other? If they are exactly even, you are a 10. If one is lower than the other, your rating goes down.

Spine: Is your spine straight or curved? If you drew a line from your hips to your neck, tracing the path of your spine, would it be straight? If so, you are a 10. If your spine curves to either side, your score drops.

Hips (view from the back): If you placed a finger on top of your hip bone on either side of your body, would the fingers be at the same level or would one side be lower than the other? If the left side of your hip bone is at the same height as the right side, you are a ten. If one side is lower than the other, you lose points.

Feet: Are your feet pointed straight ahead or do they turn in or out? If they are straight ahead, you are a 10. If they turn in or out, deduct points. Deduct more points if your ankles sag.

Neck (view from the side): Is your neck erect, chin in a vertical line with your face, and head squarely above your shoulders—or do your head and neck jut forward? If neck, chin, and head are straight up, you are a 10. If your head and neck protrude forward, you lose points.

Upper back (view from the side): There is a natural curvature of the upper spine, causing a slight roundedness of the upper back. If the upper back has a slight, natural roundedness, you are a 10. If it rounds so that your neck and head are pushed out of line with the rest of your body, the points you lose depend on how rounded your upper back is (and how much your neck and head project forward as a result).

Trunk (view from the side): If you drew a vertical line from your shoulder down to your leg, would your trunk or torso seem straight, or would it incline toward the rear? If it is straight, you are a 10. If it inclines toward the rear, the points you lose depend on the degree of inclination.

Abdomen (view from the side): Without holding your stomach in, what does it look like in the side mirror? Is it flat or does it protrude? If it is naturally flat, you are a 10. If it protrudes, and more so if it sags, you lose points.

Lower back (view from the side): The lower back has a natural curve. If your lower back has a normal curve, you are a 10. If it seems to be overly curved and hollow, the points you lose depend on the extremity of curvature or hollowness.

If you add up your points, you get an overall score for posture. The highest score would be 100 and the lowest 0. The fitness appraiser uses this information in prescribing exercises to correct postural problems. For example, abdominal exercises help align the back, or neck strengthening exercises help realign the head. This is helpful but somewhat shortsighted. There are psychological as well as physical reasons for poor posture. Changing physical posture affects you psychologically. It is good to know what postural problems indicate and what might be changed if you do seemingly innocent calisthenics.

Flexibility

When you think about body flexibility, you may have images of graceful dancers or, to the contrary, muscle-bound body builders. Flexibility refers to the ease and range of movement in different joints of the body. You may be startled by people who are "double-jointed" (an expression used for people who are able to hyperextend certain joints in their bodies). Or you may marvel at people who have as much dexterity with their toes as you have with your fingers.

A full evaluation of flexibility would require assessing the ease and range of movement in all the major joints of the body, including ankles, knees, hips, back, shoulders, arms, wrists, and neck. Fitness appraisers generally use only two measures to reflect body flexibility:[22]

1. *Trunk flexibility.* The actual test of flexibility is known as the "sit-and-reach" test. It involves sitting on the floor with your legs together and straight out in front of you, bending forward at the waist, and reaching as far as you can toward your toes without bouncing.

The fitness evaluator uses a special measuring device and a set of conversion tables for this test. Without these aids, how can you evaluate yourself? If you are not able to touch your toes while seated on the floor, your flexibility is below average. If you can wrap your fingers around your toes, it is about average. And if you can reach beyond your toes without bouncing, you have good flexibility.

2. *Shoulder flexibility.* This test involves trying to touch your thumbs behind your back by reaching one hand up and over the shoulder and reaching the other behind and up from the hips. You get to do this twice—once with the right hand reaching behind the head, and once with the left hand reaching behind the head. If your thumbs touch

both times, you score one hundred percent. If your thumbs are some-where around ten centimeters or three inches part (averaging the two sides), you are about average. Less than that and your flexibility rating declines into the "poor" category.

How adequate are these two tests? Fitness appraisers only use them as a guide. They recognize there is a lot more to flexibility than is indicated by these tests. When we look at the "psychology of muscle" and "movement analysis" in upcoming chapters, we will see just how much more there is to the assessment of flexibility.

Muscular Endurance and Strength

Strength and endurance are different, but related. Strength is deter-mined by how much resistance or weight you can lift, push, or pull. Endurance is measured by how many times or how long you can per-form an activity. In any movement, there will always be some resis-tance — unless you are working in a gravity-free environment.[23]

There are many standardized tests of strength and endurance. Some require specialized equipment. In this section, we will look at two popular endurance tests. We will skip the strength measures because they require special equipment and, more importantly, endurance meas-ures are thought to be better indicators of fitness. The two tests are the one-minute sit-up and the push-up tests.

1. *One-minute sit-up test.* You will need someone to hold your an-kles and time you for this test. Lie on your back, knees up, with feet about ten inches apart, and fingers clasped behind your head. Touch your elbows to your knees (returning to the floor each time) as many times as possible in a minute. Do not try this test if you have any problems with your back. Your score depends on your age and sex. Table 4.2 shows the number of sit-ups necessary to score in excellent, above average, average, below average, and poor categories.[24]

2. *Push-up test.* There is no time limit on this test. With legs to-gether, body straight, and hands under the shoulder and pointing for-ward, the push-up begins with chin touching the floor and arms straight-ening each time you raise yourself. For women, push-ups use the knees as the pivot, and for men, the legs are straightened with the feet as the pivot. Table 4.3 shows the number of push-ups needed to score in excellent, above average, average, below average, and poor categories.[25]

It's interesting to see that, as people age, the norms for women begin catching up to the norms for men, suggesting that, over time, women become relatively stronger compared to men.

What have you evaluated with these tests? Primarily, you have as-

TABLE 4.2
Norms for Number of Sit-Ups in One Minute

	Age	15–19	20–29	30–39	40–49	50 +
Excellent	M	≥ 48	≥ 43	≥ 36	≥ 31	≥ 26
	F	≥ 42	≥ 36	≥ 29	≥ 25	≥ 19
Above average	M	42–47	37–42	31–35	26–30	22–25
	F	36–41	31–35	24–28	20–24	12–18
Average	M	38–41	33–36	27–30	22–25	18–21
	F	32–35	25–30	20–23	15–19	5–11
Below average	M	33–37	29–32	22–26	17–21	13–17
	F	27–31	21–24	15–19	7–14	3–4
Poor	M	≤ 32	≤ 28	≤ 21	≤ 16	≤ 12
	F	≤ 26	≤ 20	≤ 14	≤ 6	≤ 2

M = male; F = female
Courtesy of Fitness and Amateur Sport Canada.

sessed your endurance in a limited set of muscles, including the arms, chest, back, and abdomen. There are over six hundred muscles in the human body[26] and it would be impractical, if not impossible, to test them all.

Are these tests adequate? Exercise physiologists look at the degree

TABLE 4.3
Norms for Number of Push-Ups (No Time Limit)

	Age	15–19	20–29	30–39	40–49	50 +
Excellent	M	≥ 39	≥ 36	≥ 30	≥ 22	≥ 21
	F	≥ 33	≥ 30	≥ 27	≥ 24	≥ 21
Above average	M	29–38	29–35	22–29	17–21	13–20
	F	25–32	21–29	20–26	15–23	11–20
Average	M	23–28	22–28	17–21	13–16	10–12
	F	18–24	15–20	13–19	11–14	7–10
Below average	M	18–22	17–21	12–16	10–12	7–9
	F	12–17	10–14	8–12	5–10	2–6
Poor	M	≤ 17	≤ 16	≤ 11	≤ 9	≤ 6
	F	≤ 11	≤ 9	≤ 7	≤ 4	≤ 1

M = male; F = female
Courtesy of Fitness and Amateur Sport Canada.

of correlation between tests of one muscle group and all other tests of large muscle groups to find out which test provides the best prediction of overall muscle endurance or strength. Unfortunately, there is no single best indicator. What this means is that tests such as sit-ups and push-ups are limited. Their results can't be generalized to all other muscles of the body. Nonetheless, they can help a fitness appraiser make recommendations about exercise. On the other hand, if you want to understand psychological concerns through muscle analysis, you will have to look beyond these tests.

Aerobic Capacity

There is no doubt that the most critical fitness parameter is aerobic capacity. Aerobic fitness is a measure of how your body responds to intense oxygen-fueled exercise. Aerobic (oxygen-fueled) exercise challenges the cardiovascular system by demanding more oxygen for the working muscles. Oxygen is transported by the blood. The heart's ability to circulate blood ultimately sets the upper limits for aerobic fitness. An aerobic fitness evaluation is a measure of how much oxygen your heart, lungs, blood, and vascular system are able to deliver to the muscles. Since it is extremely difficult to get a direct measure of oxygen that is delivered to the muscles, the most frequently used estimate is heart rate.

To estimate the maximum amount of oxygen delivered to the muscles under intense and continuous exercise, a variety of tests have been devised. Recently, these "maximum effort" tests have been criticized as being both unnecessary and potentially dangerous, especially to people who have some risk of coronary heart disease. A new trend is to test people, using "submaximal tests" that do not stress the heart and lungs to their limits.

The 12-Minute Run. As an example of a "maximum effort" test, Dr. Kenneth Cooper, author of *The Aerobics Way*[27] and head of the Aerobics Center in Dallas, advocated a full-out 12-minute run. This test was advised only for people who had been in training for at least six weeks. Following a thorough warm-up, the runner is told to run as far and as fast as possible in twelve minutes. The runner must be exhausted at the end of the run in order for the test to be valid. The distance run in twelve minutes is then compared to a table of norms for an estimate of aerobic fitness.

Other tests. There are stationary treadmill tests, bicycle tests, bench step-up tests, and a host of others administered under laboratory conditions. They get the potential athlete huffing and puffing to exhaustion or perhaps to a less extreme criterion. Heart rates during and after the exercise session are then compared to norm tables to estimate how fit the person is.

Is there a simpler and safer way to evaluate aerobic fitness? Most candidates for fitness evaluations are advised to obtain a physician's sanction before proceeding. Such medical approval is, of course, no guarantee that testing will be entirely safe. There is always some risk with testing procedures that deliberately stress the heart to determine its functional capacity. The less severe the stress, as in "submaximal" vs. "maximal" testing, for example, the less the risk.

The Walking Test. A safe approach to submaximal testing has been advanced by The Rockport Walking Institute. It is based on walking a measured mile as fast as you can and then recording your time and heart rate immediately upon completing the one-mile distance. One of the advantages of the test is that walking serves to control the degree of overexertion, making it safer than many other tests. A formula you can use to estimate your fitness level is shown in Figure 4.1. Just plug in your numbers to get your fitness score.

Putting It All Together

We have looked at five parameters of fitness: body composition, posture, flexibility, muscular endurance and strength, and aerobic capacity. Is there an easy way to put these measures together? Each measure provides information and each has implications for exercise prescription.

The most important parameter, aerobic capacity, sets the limits of the exercise program. For all practical purposes, the exercise prescription is based on the individual's aerobic fitness level. The remaining four measures (body composition, posture, flexibility, and strength/endurance) are used to prescribe specific exercises for posture, strength/endurance, and flexibility.

What does the prescription look like? According to the American College of Sports Medicine's (ACSM) *Guidelines for Exercise Testing and Prescription*,[28] there are five components to the exercise prescription:

1. *Type of Activity.* From our point of view this is a critical issue. The activity you engage in for fitness purposes has significant psychological implications, particularly if you do it over a long period of time. Yet, in the ACSM's *Guidelines* and even in the highly informative *Exer-*

FIGURE 4.1
Estimating Your Aerobic Capacity (VO_2 Max) from a One-Mile Walking Test

(The following formula is based on walking one mile as fast as possible and measuring your time and heart rate during the last quarter mile.)

To calculate . . . VO_2 MAX

Step 1. Add the following:
a) 0.091 × Weight in pounds   a)_____
b) 5.955 × Sex, inserting 1 for male and 0 for female   b)_____
c) Add the constant 69.652   c) 69.652

                                                    Score 1 = _____

Step 2. Add the following:
a) 0.257 × Age in years   a)_____
b) 2.240 × Time in minutes   b)_____
c) 0.115 × Heart rate for 1 minute in last quarter mile   c)_____

                                                    Score 2 = _____

Step 3. Subtract Score 2 from Score 1

                                        Score 1 = + _____
                             Subtract Score 2 = – _____
                             _____

                                        VO_2 MAX =

(Measured in milliliters of oxygen consumed per minute.)

Step 4. To find your fitness level use the VO_2 MAX Norms below:

	Age	15–19	20–29	30–39	40–49	50+
Excellent	M	≥60	≥57	≥48	≥42	≥38
	F	≥43	≥40	≥37	≥35	≥30
Above average	M	58–59	52–56	46–47	40–42	36–38
	F	40–42	37–39	34–37	32–34	27–29
Average	M	54–57	43–51	42–45	37–39	34–35
	F	37–39	35–37	31–33	26–31	25–27
Below average	M	44–53	40–42	38–41	34–37	31–33
	F	35–37	32–34	29–31	24–25	22–25
Poor	M	≤43	≤40	≤37	≤33	≤30
	F	≤34	≤31	≤29	≤23	≤21

M = male; F = female
Courtesy of Fitness and Amateur Sport Canada.
Formula taken from Kline, et al.[29]

cise Prescription for Fitness by Reid and Thomson, psychological factors are ignored.[30] According to ACSM, one activity is as good as another as long as the cardiovascular work rate is matched. Principal qualifications for the activity are given as follows:

> Any activity that uses large muscle groups, that can be maintained for a prolonged period, and is rhythmical and aerobic in nature, e.g., running-jogging, walking-hiking, swimming, skating, bicycling, rowing, cross-country skiing, rope skipping, and various endurance game activities.[31]

In *Exercise Prescription for Fitness* the "personal fitness prescription" advocated by authors Reid and Thomson is built around the aerobic activity of running. In a follow-up chapter, the authors present "alternative activity prescriptions" in the form of a table that allows you to convert the number of minutes you might spend in some alternative activity (like swimming) to the standard of running time. The only comment offered regarding why an alternative activity might be chosen over running is that alternatives "are designed for persons who do not wish to follow the personalized running prescription."

This attitude of nonchalance about the choice of aerobic activity characterizes the fitness field. At best, we find progressive trainers telling potential fitness devotees to "choose an activity that you like." While in many ways this sounds like good advice, do we always choose what is best for us?

2. *Intensity of Conditioning.* The second part of the prescription specifies the intensity of the aerobic fitness activity. This is usually measured by heart rate. The standard formula is as follows: Start with 220 heart beats per minute (BPM) and deduct your age. (Example: a 40-year-old would end up with $220 - 40 = 180$ BPM.) This is an estimate of your maximum heart rate. Now, depending on your level of fitness, the advisor may recommend that you exercise at anywhere from sixty-five percent to ninety percent of this maximum capacity. (Example. Our 40-year-old with a 180 maximum heart rate: $180 \times 65\% = 117$ BPM or $180 \times 90\% = 162$ BPM.) This range of sixty-five percent to ninety percent of the maximum age-adjusted heart rate is known as the *training zone*. (For our 40-year-old, the training zone would be 117 BPM as the lower limit and 162 BPM as the upper limit.)

3. *Duration of Conditioning.* Generally, it is recommended that the aerobic activity last for about thirty minutes or, more broadly, within a range of fifteen to sixty minutes. The lower your fitness level, the most likely the prescription will be low-intensity (for example, walking at an

intensity of sixty-five percent of maximum heart rate) for thirty minutes to one hour.

4. *Frequency of Conditioning.* Aerobic fitness activities are recommended three to five times per week. Daily aerobic workouts generally are not advised. Some trainers will suggest nonaerobic workouts, such as weight lifting, on alternate days.

5. *Rate of Progression.* The program you start with will need to be revised as your fitness improves. You will have to move faster in your aerobic workout to achieve the same level of cardiovascular intensity. Many of the popular running books, for example, have weekly progression schedules for beginning runners so that conditioning takes place at a safe and injury-free pace.

Variations

Fitness appraisers attend primarily to your physiological data, for example, heart rate, lung capacity, and muscular endurance. Based on this information, an aerobic activity is prescribed. It makes little difference what the activity is as long as you engage in it for the prescribed length of time and at the proper intensity. The appraiser may also recommend certain flexibility and strengthening exercises, with the stipulation that the most important factor is getting your heart rate into the "training zone" for a designated amount of time. If you like to run, then run. If you want to swim, do that. It's basically up to you—as long as you meet the physiological requirements.

What About Psychology?

Most trainers believe they are taking psychology into account when they ask you to choose an activity. And, in fact, there is good reason for trainers to ask for your input. You are more likely to stick with something that you select than with an activity that has been imposed on you without explanation.

Within the traditional fitness framework, there are a few variations on the "do what you like" approach. In their intriguing book, *Sportselection*, Arnot and Gaines[32] tell us what the *physical* requirements are for different sports and how we can determine whether or not we will be good at a particular sport. Their approach is primarily physical—they ignore any personality considerations. They help the reader understand a sport's requirements in terms of motor abilities, perceptual skills, heart and lung requirements, and body composition. The idea is to find the sport that best matches your physical makeup so that you can excel at it.

This approach has little to do with improving or modifying how you function psychologically.

Another variation that is similar to *Sportselection*'s uses "body types" for prescriptions. It is based on the works of William Sheldon, who identified three primary body types: the ectomorph (thin, wiry), the mesomorph (square, muscular), and the endomorph (round, fat). Curtis Pesman adapted Sheldon's model to illustrate how a particular body type is better geared for some sports than for others. For example, mesomorphs would be best at sports like football and racquetball, while ectomorphs might be better at long-distance running. Although Sheldon's theory connects body types to psychological types, Pesman's use of Sheldon's theory ignores the psychological implications.[33]

What Have You Learned?

While this is *not* a book on how to evaluate your fitness level, we want to tell you what you might happen if you schedule a fitness evaluation.

With the information presented, you can obtain a general idea of what kind of shape you are in, although we strongly recommend that you undergo a formal evaluation of your fitness level at an approved clinic or training center.

The traditional approach to exercise prescription is based on the idea that aerobic exercise is good for you. Exercise is believed to help prevent coronary heart disease and to manage weight problems. This emphasis on physical health outcomes of exercise led to the advocacy of *any exercise* that met certain physiological criteria, *and* to the neglect of important psychological considerations.

The physiological principles underlying the prescription of exercise are good ones and should be applied to any exercise prescription that comes out of your reading of this book. This means that your aerobic capacity should be evaluated before you embark on a fitness program — and you need to keep the program in check by adhering to sensible guidelines of *intensity, duration, and frequency* as outlined in the American College of Sports Medicine.[34]

Before going deeper into the psychological side of exercise prescription, we wanted to acquaint you with basics: the basics of how exercise prescription is typically done, the reasons for this physical emphasis, and the guidelines for implementing a training program. Remember — whatever you do for fitness should be based on an understanding of the physical limits of your body, and this is best achieved through sound medical advice and a professional fitness evaluation.

5

What Type of Fitness Personality Are You?

Did You Know That . . .

Sports psychology is a relatively new field. It wasn't until 1986 that the American Psychological Association established a special division for members interested in the topic. Even so, psychological studies of athletes have been going on since the 1940s.[1]

One frequently asked question is about the personalities of athletes: Are athletes like normal mortals or are they a breed apart? Another popular question is, are there sport-specific personalities? For example, do football players have a certain personality?

There are no simple answers to these questions. Studies of athletes are hard to interpret because researchers use different techniques in their studies. For example, some researchers use interviews, others employ measures like the famous Rorschach inkblot test, and still others administer objective personality inventories. Some reports are based on Olympic-class athletes, while others are drawn from high school students in physical education classes. Numerous studies compare athletes at different levels of performance, as in a comparison of winners and losers. Investigations span more than four decades, making it hard to know whether studies of yesterday's heroes have any validity for under-standing today's athletes. These different approaches make it impossible to draw solid conclusions about the personalities of athletes.

In spite of these problems, let's look at what sports psychologists and other investigators tell us about athletes in general and about particular types of athletes.

Athletes In General

One of the first studies to demonstrate that athletes are different from one another was published in 1941. The investigator compared track athletes, physical education majors, student pilots, and students enrolled in weight-lifting courses. The track athletes and student pilots were found to be less "hypochondriacal" (they complained less about imaginary physical ailments) and introverted than the weight lifters, but they had more symptoms of emotional difficulties than the physical education majors.

Since the publication of this 1941 study, there have been literally hundreds of studies of school athletes, recreational athletes, Olympic athletes, and even professionals. Reports on the personalities of athletes have identified some interesting trends.[3] Some of the major differences between athletes and nonathletes are listed in Table 5.1. There seems to be abundant evidence that athletes differ from nonathletes. Where there is question is on the issue of cause and effect.

Many investigators have taken the position that athletes, by nature, are different from nonathletes—which means they were either born that way or their personalities formed early in life and were not changed by athletic participation. Others say they are not sure which came first—participation in athletics (which shaped the personality), or personality (which influenced the choice of athletics). Our position is clear: Personality and sports influence each other—it's not a one-way street!

Another question is whether athletes are "better" than nonathletes. The lists in Table 5.1 would suggest they are, but there is debate. Research findings have not been as definite as the lists imply. One of the great personality theorists of our time, Hans Eysenck, reported in a 1982 review that athletes tend to be more extroverted, less neurotic, less anxious, more assertive, more competitive, less inhibited, and seek a higher level of stimulation than do nonathletes.[4] Eysenck, however, did not believe his evidence completely supported the hypothesis that sports benefit personality. His review also noted that some athletes had negative personality changes from sports. We are entirely in agreement with this.

TABLE 5.1
A Comparison of Athletes and Nonathletes

Compared to nonathletes, those who regularly engage in athletic activity have been found to be:

MORE	LESS
extroverted	inhibited
dominant and skillful as leaders	anxious
self-confident	compulsive
emotionally stable	depressed
aggressive	neurotic
sensation seeking and adventurous	dependent
competitive	
tolerant of discomfort and pain	
impulsive	

In a recent study of aerobic dancers, body builders, and runners, the psychological profiles of these exercise enthusiasts reflected some uncomplimentary characteristics. They were generally found to be joyless, and a majority showed signs of instability and feelings of inferiority. Most of these fitness buffs had narcissistic leanings. The study concluded that fashionable fitness activities do not necessarily promote well-being, but may foster self-preoccupation.[5]

This study highlights the issue. Exercise represents both an expression of personality and a means by which personality may be modified — positively or negatively, depending on the choice!

Athletics and Exercise — A More Specific Profile

Ideally, what we would like to develop is a personality profile for different athletes. We can find plenty of studies of weight lifters, cyclists, judo experts, dancers, archers, hang gliders, basketball players, rowers, runners, or hockey players, but there is no simple way of comparing findings from one group with another.

In one study, cyclists' personalities were compared to those of hang gliders. The hang gliders were found to be more depressed than cyclists.[6] A second study found swimmers to be less depressed than basketball players.[7] Can we say that cyclists are less depressed than basketball players? No. Can we say that swimmers and cyclists are equally nondepressed? No. Different methods were used to measure depression in the two studies. In addition, swimmers in the second study were high school competitors while cyclists in the first were professional racers.

Depending on the methods used, the people studied, or the year of the report, we may get results that are quite different and in some cases contradictory. When one group of athletes is compared to another group of athletes, we don't know how they stack up to normal mortals nor do we know how they fit into the bigger picture of all sports. It is impossible to establish a pecking order when all the chickens aren't in the same coop.

Let's examine this more closely. We'll take swimmers for a start. In one study, champion swimmers were found to have a dominant personality and to be moderately extroverted.[8] The finding of high levels of dominance was supported in a second study, which also noted that swimmers were high on autonomy (or self-direction) and achievement motivation.[9] A third report on Olympic-class swimmers indicated they were the only group of Olympic athletes who showed below-average scores on anxiety.[10] When compared to basketball players, football players, and wrestlers, swimmers in a fourth study came out as the least neurotic group.[11] But then a study of British swimmers found that these athletes scored high on introversion and neuroticism[12] and yet another report labeled swimmers as self-centered and individualistic.[13] Obtaining a clear profile of the swimmer's personality from these data is not easy. There are contradictions about whether swimmers are introverted or extroverted, neurotic or well-adjusted. Although the weight of evidence argues for a healthy portrait of the swimmer, it isn't as straightforward as we would like.

Runners are even more problematic. What is a runner? There are short-distance, mid-distance, and long-distance runners. There are champions and there are recreational runners. And then there are joggers! What does the research say? Well, there are studies that label regular runners as compulsive,[14] depressive, inhibited,[15] introverted,[16] taciturn, cautious, deliberate, and suited to monotonous, repetitive situations.[17] Yes, you guessed it; on the other hand, runners seem to be more sociable, optimistic,[18] sexually active,[19] and have better life adjustment.[20]

A Common Yardstick

What we need is a common yardstick or, more accurately, a common set of yardsticks that makes sense! When we read that runners are hypochondriacs or that weight lifters suffer from feelings of masculine inadequacy, we might first of all reach for the dictionary to find out what the authors are talking about and afterward wonder how these traits relate to running and weight lifting. We may also wonder why one investigator studied masculine inadequacy in weight lifters and the other explored runners' hypochondriacal complaints. Did the researchers have an axe to grind or were the studies part of a theory?

We need measures to describe sports and exercise that are not professional jargon and that make sense in terms of what the sport or exercise program is all about. We also need to have all fitness pursuits measured with the same standards so that we can compare them.

That's what this chapter will address. By the time you finish reading it, you will know what psychological traits make sense in the sports and exercise world. Moreover, you will have completed a self-assessment on these traits.

Before tackling this sizable task, we should be clear about what we are doing. Since our goal is to measure sport-related personality, we will start by defining the term "personality" itself.

What Is Personality?

The term "personality" is a central concept in psychology, yet there is little agreement about it. From Freud to Fromm and Erikson to Rogers, we find such wide variations in the definition of personality that it seems the theorists are talking about completely different things.

Everyday language provides two principal meanings.[21] First, we talk about people who "have personality" as individuals who possess a kind of charisma, a positive style that attracts others to them. For example, we say, "Wow! Has she got personality!" meaning that she somehow excites a positive reaction in those around her. The second definition is based on the idea that each of us has a dominant characteristic that more or less rules our lives. So, we talk about a person having "an aggressive personality," "a domineering personality," or "a submissive personality."

In trying to understand how personality is influenced by sports and exercise, we first have to agree on a workable definition of personality. The common definitions of personality we just described are not very useful. The first one is more a measure of attraction than it is of personality and the second identifies us as unidimensional creatures who are either aggressive, submissive, or shy.

Sports psychologists have typically adopted what is known as the *trait approach* to personality.[22] In this school of thought, personality is made up of a number of traits that each person has more or less of. Personality is identified by numerical scores on these traits that, when taken as a whole, constitute the individual's personality profile. The number of traits varies from one theory to another. Sometimes sports psychologists will only look at part of the profile because they don't expect athletic activities to have much to do with the remaining parts. For example, a psychologist might measure aggression and self-confidence in athletes, leaving out other traits because they are not relevant to her study.

The personality model we developed avoids being either too broad or too narrow. We don't want to imply that fitness activities will affect every aspect of our personalities — that would be too broad. Of course, if you change one part of an individual's personality, you are likely to at least minimally influence all other aspects, but this doesn't mean the effect is very strong.

It would be equally misleading to consider only one or two personality traits. This is the narrow approach. As we shall see, there are many dimensions of personality that are called into play when we engage in fitness programs. To say that we are only influencing such aspects as self-confidence or aggressiveness would limit our appreciation of sport's potential for personality development.

With these preliminary ideas, let's move to a definition of personality before identifying what dimensions of your character you are "exercising" in your fitness program.

Personality Defined

Personality represents the active and dynamic interplay of "psychophysical" dimensions that determine our unique adjustment to the environment. Personality can be seen in the relatively enduring and consistent patterns of behavior that characterize how we perceive, learn, and adapt. We might say it is our style of life.

There are some important aspects to this definition. For one, personality is not passive. We have purposes or objectives that are more or less explicit in our behaviors. These may be needs we are trying to satisfy, including those for food, shelter, sex, love, or a feeling of self-worth. Whatever needs we try to satisfy or directions our behaviors take represent the active expression of personality.

Personality is dynamic, or interactive. Each personality dimension influences all others. You cannot look at one dimension in isolation from the broader profile. You cannot say a person is "an achiever" and expect that she will look like every other achiever. The way we express a drive such as that for achievement will depend on how much we have of other traits and how we mix and stir this unique concoction.

The function of personality is to help us work out individual adjustments to the conditions of our lives. Even the madman's seemingly bizarre behavior has meaning and represents a form of adaptation to the conditions of his life. A person who is aggressive is this way for a reason.

The original causes of his behavior may no longer exist, but he persists in this personality style because it has become habitual.

Personality is enduring. It is not something that changes overnight. In fact, some theorists argue that it changes very little after the first few years of life. Others take a more optimistic view and suggest that personality changes throughout life, but that it does so ever so slowly. Deliberate, consciously directed personality change takes considerable effort. This is a key point for our work.

Today's culture holds out promises for all kinds of personality transformations through experiences ranging in length from a few hours to a few weekends. It is much more complex than that. In talking about personality change through exercise, we do not wish to imply that if you jump on your exercycle three times a week for a month, you will experience the "new you." This is nonsense.

People today are embarking on lifelong commitments to exercise and fitness as part of their lifestyles. We believe these long-term involvements will have a wide range of effects on physical and psychological functions. Over the course of a few years of running five times a week, an individual will be emphasizing certain personality traits more than others, and this will produce a transformation: slow, almost imperceptible, but nonetheless substantial in its long-term consequences. The enduring nature of personality will shift.

A peculiar aspect of personality is that it is consistent. We have a self-image that is strongly ingrained. As a result, we perceive the world in biased ways. We selectively attend to or ignore certain kinds of information. Usually what we take in is consistent with how we see ourselves and what we ignore is inconsistent. This doesn't mean we only listen for the good news about ourselves. In fact, if we grow up with the self-image of a failure, we will search through our experiences to find evidence supporting this failure definition, and we will ignore signs of our success. Another way of saying this is that we will go to great lengths to ensure self-consistency — even at the cost of being effective, right, or happy!

This idea of consistency is particularly important in determining a sports/exercise activity profile. We avoid activities that threaten our self-image. For example, if we see ourselves as shy and withdrawn, we will stay away from social situations in all aspects of life — including sports and exercise. If we see ourselves as active and outgoing, we will gravitate toward gregarious, dynamic activities and avoid ones that seem solitary and passive. We build on one set of characteristics over the course of life and neglect development of other traits. This is the concept of consistency in operation, and it is one reason we need to take a closer look at personality with a view toward prescribing activities that may not feel right (because they are inconsistent), but that can help us develop more balance in life.

We have left for last that part of the definition that tells us personality is based on the interplay of mind and body. The idea of psychophysical characteristics in personality theory is more than a theme of the "enlightened eighties." In fact, one of our most prominent personality theorists, Gordon Allport, incorporated this concept in his definition of personality in 1937. It was his way of reminding us that personality is "neither exclusively mental nor exclusively physical." As he put it, the organization of personality involves "the operation of both mind and body, inextricably fused into a personal unity."[23]

The Psychosocial Activity Dimensions (PAD)

Now that we know what personality is, let's look at personality dimensions most likely to be involved in sports, exercise, and fitness programs. Based on a comprehensive review of the literature and intensive interviews with athletes and fitness experts, we have identified seven major dimensions. They are labeled *psychosocial activity dimensions* to convey two core ideas. The first is that the dimensions are both psychological and social in nature, therefore the word *psychosocial*. As human beings, we are never fully isolated from interactions with other people, whether this is in actual exchanges or just our imaginings. We function in a social world.

The word *activity* forms the second core idea. It comes from the fact that these are the dimensions most likely to be involved when we engage in activities and sports.

Some of these dimensions are quite broad, meaning that it may seem there is more than one aspect to some traits. Others are more limited or specific. All of them are subject to nuances of interpretation—that's just the way personality measures are. You may find it a little hard to give a precise answer to some questions, but your estimates will be more than sufficient.

As you read through these psychosocial activity dimensions, or PADs, be sure to answer the questions honestly and thoughtfully. Later on, we will give you an opportunity to link your PADs Profile with different exercise programs. Your personality evaluation at this point, however, will be general—more like a style or a way you go about life. So take out your pencil and get ready for a self-evaluation.

PAD 1—*Social/Nonsocial Style*

"Bill" likes the quiet hours of the morning to run. He is usually out on the streets before 5:30 A.M. — rarely does he encounter other runners, and when he does, there is minimal exchange of greetings as they streak on their separate paths. He's not a great talker; his friends describe him as "a man of few words," and those words tend to be carefully picked. As a programmer/analyst he spends much of his day working on his own, solving obscure problems that nonetheless challenge and reward him. He's not much for parties, but he has a passion for old movies and classical music.

"Sally" runs to keep in shape, and for the fun of it. Her favorite time is the lunch hour and she typically arranges to run with a friend or two. In fact, it's her way of keeping up with friends or even working on a business deal. As a real estate broker she spends a lot of time with people and really seems to enjoy it. She's a born organizer, always trying to get people together, whether for business or pleasure. She enjoys art and usually finds time to visit a gallery during her busy week.

Bill and Sally are both runners, but they have different styles of exercise. Bill likes to run alone, as he prefers to do most things, while Sally makes running a social event. What we see in both individuals is a pattern of consistency: as they exercise, so they live their lives. We are not all like this. Some of us may try to balance our needs by being alone for some things and with people for others. It's when we become lopsided that problems may crop up.

There is a commonsense understanding of the words *social* or *sociable*. What do we mean by the PAD Social/Nonsocial Style? We can look at it in two ways: the first is our *preferred behavior* and the second is our *actual behavior*.

Do you prefer to do things on your own or with other people? Would you rather go to a movie by yourself or with a friend? Do you like going to parties or would you rather spend a quiet evening at home? Would you rather work closely with other people or do you prefer working on your own? To any of these questions, you might say, "Well, sometimes yes and sometimes no — it depends." What you would indicate by this kind of response is a degree of balance. So the questions might be better phrased as "What percentage of the time do you prefer to be alone or with others?" So far, all we have talked about is what you like to do. We have no idea how you go about life, that is, your actual behavior.

How much of your time do you spend interacting with others vs. being alone? This question needs clarification. There are lots of ways of being alone even though you may be in the midst of a crowd. For example, a person working on an assembly line certainly isn't alone (that is, all by himself), but this individual is not interacting. The key is interaction. Do you spend your time talking with others, exchanging ideas, philosophies, stories? Do you interact with others nonverbally or through physical contact? Do you engage in cooperative projects where you help one another accomplish a task? Once again, you may answer, "It depends" or "Some of the time." So, you may need to look at the percentage of time that you are actually interacting with others versus the percentage of time alone (not counting the time you are sleeping, unless you sleep to excess as a way of avoiding people).

There might be a big difference between how much time you actually spend with people and the time you would *prefer* to spend with people, and you should be concerned if this discrepancy is strikingly large. You might have some good reasons why you like to be with people but just can't find the time to do so. Nonetheless, behavior is often a good barometer of inner needs, so you may have to ask whether you are being honest with yourself.

Questions about your PAD Social/Nonsocial Style (Table 5.2) measure a mix of wish and action. Your style has to do with your orientation toward people, both in terms of what you like and what you do. Bear in mind that this dimension does not evaluate the nature of your interactions, which could range from competitive, aggressive, and controlling to noncompetitive, passive, and following. You could spend a lot of your time arguing with people or you could be the world's greatest listener—it matters little for your score on this dimension.

PAD 2—Spontaneous/Controlled Style

"Michelle" researched every possible vacation option before making her plans for a winter holiday. Once she had decided, she wanted to know everything she could about scheduling, activities, and potential deviations. She left nothing to chance. Her friends thought she was the one who invented the concept of time management. Everything in her life was scheduled right down to the time it took her to shower and dress after her morning aerobics class. She was office manager for a law firm and everyone knew that if it weren't for her, the place would fold tomorrow.

"Wally" thought of himself as a product of the sixties, but that was just a convenient excuse for his lifestyle. He did everything on the spur of the moment and was known to friends as "a wild and crazy guy." He was good at what he did and had the good fortune of being in a creative profession where colleagues passed off his excesses as artistic license. His idea of exercise was a night of disco dancing in as many bars as he could get to before closing time. He was "into" jogging for a day, but the fad passed. In fact, he had been "into" almost everything—including skydiving on a dare—at least once.

Table 5.2

PAD SOCIAL/NONSOCIAL STYLE
For each question, circle the WORD that best describes you.

MOSTLY—I am this way *most of the time.*
OFTEN—I am *often or frequently* this way.
SOMETIMES—I am *sometimes or occasionally* this way.
RARELY—I am *rarely or never* this way.

1. I prefer doing things alone.	MOSTLY 1	OFTEN 2	SOMETIMES 3	RARELY 4
2. I feel a strong need to be with other people.	MOSTLY 4	OFTEN 3	SOMETIMES 2	RARELY 1
3. I like to work alone.	MOSTLY 1	OFTEN 2	SOMETIMES 3	RARELY 4
4. I feel anxious when I meet new people.	MOSTLY 1	OFTEN 2	SOMETIMES 3	RARELY 4
5. I like parties and social affairs.	MOSTLY 4	OFTEN 3	SOMETIMES 2	RARELY 1
6. I keep my thoughts and feelings private.	MOSTLY 1	OFTEN 2	SOMETIMES 3	RARELY 4
7. I make friends easily.	MOSTLY 4	OFTEN 3	SOMETIMES 2	RARELY 1
8. I talk to strangers on buses, planes or trains.	MOSTLY 4	OFTEN 3	SOMETIMES 2	RARELY 1

SCORING:
Add up the points *under* each of your answers. Then, write your total score in the space provided. Identify your **Social/Nonsocial Style** in the list below.

Category	PAD Style	Score Range
1	Highly Social	28–32
2	Moderately Social	23–27
3	Intermediate	18–22
4	Moderately Nonsocial	13–17
5	Highly Nonsocial	8–12

Your Total Score _____   **Your Rating Category** _____

When you hear words like "spontaneous" and "controlled," there is a risk that saying you are one or the other implies you are either a fun person or a deadbeat. Being labeled as controlled conjures up images of rigid, almost mechanical behavior, while the notion of being spontaneous is something that seems at least culturally desirable. After all, isn't that what the "new therapies" and self-actualizing programs promote? Well, it's not that simple. From the descriptions of Michelle and Wally, you might think you would rather spend an evening with a wild and crazy guy than with a precision instrument, but there are pros and cons we have to examine more closely.

Spontaneity can be a good thing, in the right circumstances, or it can really gum up the works. We need a certain amount of control and, indeed, doing things on a whim can get us into a lot of trouble. Michelle's planned vacations may sound like "no risk-no fun" ventures, but having controlled things that we can control might also be a way of creating a certain freedom—at least from worry.

There are two other words corresponding to spontaneous and controlled: namely, intuitive and analytical. Although they are not equivalent, we may look at them as the *inside representations* of the spontaneous or controlled behavior we see on the outside. Control often comes as the result of a lot of thought and analysis. On the other hand, when we do something spontaneously, it often occurs because it "just feels right." There is an intuitive sixth sense about the action. Sometimes we mistakenly label intuitive judgments as good judgments because our emotions are accorded a higher status than our reason (as in the adage, "trust your heart!"). We glorify people who are intuitive as if they have a power the rest of us were born without.

An example of how we might be fooled in identifying spontaneity and intuition can be found in Arthur Conan Doyle's Sherlock Holmes. Holmes would dash out of a room in pursuit of some new clue. His behavior would seem quite spontaneous and intuitive. Only later would we discover that what seemed intuitive resulted from analysis and carefully controlled observation. "Elementary, my dear Watson—a simple deduction!"

To clarify the issue, let's investigate your style. If you ask yourself why you did something in the past, you might come up with a list of logical-analytical reasons, or you might say, "I don't know—I just did it—it seemed right." Spontaneity and control have a lot to do with how we do things. A controlled person spends a fair amount of time in mental activity going over pros and cons, and can produce upon request a full array of explanations for choices and actions. This approach to situations is often accompanied by a sense of restraint and self-management, a feeling of being in control.

A spontaneous individual would not be inclined to come up with justifications or explanations. He would just pass it off as a hunch or something that was perhaps "in the stars." Getting this person to go through the rigorous process of critical analysis and flow-charting of activities might in fact induce instantaneous burnout.

So, where would you rate yourself? How much of you operates by control and analysis and how much by intuition and spontaneous behavior (Table 5.3)? You need to be careful in assessing this not only because of the value of spontaneity in our culture, but also because you may think you are pretty spontaneous when a little study of your lifestyle would lead you to discover that you do the same things at the same time each day and what passes as spontaneity is in fact a very controlled pattern.

PAD 3 — Disciplined/Undisciplined Style

"Charlie" makes himself get to the pool every morning for a six o'clock workout no matter how late he stayed up the night before, and he pushes himself through a grinding workout without the benefit of a prodding coach or even a kindred soul to swim with. "He's just a hard worker—he's got a lot of self-discipline," says his wife. At work, it's pretty much the same. He tells his coworkers, "The job's gotta get done, and it doesn't get easier looking at it," as he plows into what might be a distasteful, boring task to most people. He doesn't take excuses for too many things—at work, at home, and at play (if you can call it that).

"Christie" describes herself as the world's most practiced dropout. She just seems to get bored easily. If it doesn't excite her, it will quickly be added to her "Oh, I tried that once" list. It's as if she expects things to draw her like a magnet. In her defense, she tells friends, "At least I try!"—which is true. The problem has more to do with her expectations. She puts her body somewhere and says in effect, "Here I am! Make me enjoy it!" Needless to say, she has a rather checkered occupational history. And as for romance, once the bloom is off the rose, well . . .

It may seem from these examples that we are talking about stoicism and hedonism gone amuck—and in the extreme this may be what it's about. We can wonder whether Charlie just likes to do things that are hard because in a perverse way he enjoys them like this. And that

Table 5.3

PAD SPONTANEOUS/CONTROLLED STYLE
For each question, circle the WORD that best describes you.

MOSTLY—I am this way *most of the time.*
OFTEN—I am *often or frequently* this way.
SOMETIMES—I am *sometimes or occasionally* this way.
RARELY—I am *rarely or never* this way.

1. I do things on the spur of the moment.	MOSTLY 4	OFTEN 3	SOMETIMES 2	RARELY 1
2. I look very carefully before I leap into something.	MOSTLY 1	OFTEN 2	SOMETIMES 3	RARELY 4
3. I make decisions based on careful, rational analysis.	MOSTLY 1	OFTEN 2	SOMETIMES 3	RARELY 4
4. I let my emotions guide my actions.	MOSTLY 4	OFTEN 3	SOMETIMES 2	RARELY 1
5. I plan my day's activities in fine detail.	MOSTLY 1	OFTEN 2	SOMETIMES 3	RARELY 4
6. I act based on my intuition.	MOSTLY 4	OFTEN 3	SOMETIMES 2	RARELY 1
7. I like to surprise people with gifts and visits.	MOSTLY 4	OFTEN 3	SOMETIMES 2	RARELY 1
8. I am disturbed by last-minute changes in plans.	MOSTLY 1	OFTEN 2	SOMETIMES 3	RARELY 4

SCORING:
Add up the points *under* each of your answers. Then, write your total score in the space provided. Identify your **Spontaneous/Controlled Style** in the list below.

Category	PAD Style	Score Range
1	Highly Spontaneous	28–32
2	Moderately Spontaneous	23–27
3	Intermediate	18–22
4	Moderately Controlled	13–17
5	Highly Controlled	8–12

Your Total Score _____ **Your Rating Category** _____

Christie's behavior is solely governed by the pleasure principle: If it feels good, do it—if not, don't!.

Certainly, we can see the liabilities in both approaches. A person who is undisciplined would need a large bank account or be fortunate enough to live in a world that, motivationally, was an ideal fit. It might be harder to see the downside of the disciplined person, but there is one. This person often gets hooked on the rigor and demands of life and has difficulty doing things simply, or simply enjoying. These are extremes, of course.

For most of us the pattern is less exaggerated. We may look for tinsel and glitter to draw our attention and get us going. We may occasionally need some pats on the back or social support. Or we may just decide that something is worthwhile and with a kind of internal gyroscope keep ourselves pointed in the same direction no matter how the wind is blowing.

There is another aspect to the PAD Disciplined/Undisciplined Style you may have sensed. Just as Christie's behavior seems governed by the "pleasure principle," there is the opposite of a "pain principle." Researchers have found that people, notably athletes, have varying tolerances for pain. And dictionary definitions of discipline include concepts like punishment and enforced behavior. Discipline implies that we don't always do things we like or want to, but we do them because they are supposedly good for us or because of something we are trying to achieve.

Little boys are supposed to be raised so they are tough and not too sensitive, whereas it is quite the opposite in the traditional emotional training of little girls. What happens in our early years frequently deviates from this standard so that our tolerance for pain may have little to do with gender. Over time some of us learn to become comfortable with things that are difficult, to become more disciplined. This isn't to say that we necessarily like it this way, but merely that we have acquired a higher tolerance level.

How would you evaluate yourself (Table 5.4)? Do you have trouble sticking with things you find unpleasant or trying? Or do you persist at things you choose regardless of the obstacles, regardless of the pain? Do you need to be supported by friends, by rewards, by gimmicks that make what you are doing seem novel and exciting? Or do you just get to it—on your own, without props and aids—by the force of your will?

PAD 4—Aggressive/Nonaggressive Style

"Billy" had practically bashed the jammed door out of its frame when

Table 5.4

PAD DISCIPLINED/UNDISCIPLINED STYLE
For each question, circle the WORD that best describes you.

MOSTLY—I am this way *most of the time.*
OFTEN—I am *often or frequently* this way.
SOMETIMES—I am *sometimes or occasionally* this way.
RARELY—I am *rarely or never* this way.

	MOSTLY	OFTEN	SOMETIMES	RARELY
1. I can make myself do hard or difficult things.	4	3	2	1
2. I have a high tolerance for pain and discomfort.	4	3	2	1
3. I need lots of emotional support when I have to do something difficult.	1	2	3	4
4. When something doesn't come easily, I force myself to stick with it.	4	3	2	1
5. I operate on the belief, "If it feels good, do it—if it's too hard, stop it!"	1	2	3	4
6. I am easily discouraged when results don't come right away.	1	2	3	4
7. When I want something, there are no limits to how hard I will work.	4	3	2	1
8. I give myself lots of little rewards to help me do something I dislike.	1	2	3	4

SCORING:
Add up the points *under* each of your answers. Then, write your total score in the space provided. Identify your **Disciplined/Undisciplined Style** in the list below.

Category	PAD Style	Score Range
1	Highly Disciplined	28–32
2	Moderately Disciplined	23–27
3	Intermediate	18–22
4	Moderately Undisciplined	13–17
5	Highly Undisciplined	8–12

Your Total Score _____   **Your Rating Category** _____

he suddenly realized he had forgotten to release the lower latch. That was typical. He came on strong, regardless of the circumstances, and although friends had become accustomed to his bluster, strangers were often put off. He didn't necessarily mean any harm, it was just his style to give things a push when they only needed a tap, or to get real "hyper" when a softer approach might have gotten him what he wanted. His girlfriend attributed it to too many summers spent in football camp.

"Jeff" was your typical "nice guy," but he didn't necessarily "always finish last." He got his way without being forceful, and that surprised a lot of people. To some he seemed passive. He didn't take offense when he was criticized and if a waitress might bring him a tepid cup of coffee, he would typically drink it without complaint. He said it didn't bother him. There was one rather amusing incident during the 1987 Superbowl when the TV suddenly blanked out and one of his friends began banging the set. Jeff seemed lost in thought for a few moments, but then walked over to the VCR and jiggled a loose electrical connection—the game came roaring back into the room.

Aggression is an often misunderstood term. Depending on its context, it can sound downright nasty or it can seem quite heroic. We generally think of aggression in an interpersonal context, as when one person aggresses against another and, of course, in this context we don't think of it as a particularly friendly action.

Other views posit aggression as a necessary force for living, as a kind of energy required to take charge of our world and satisfy our needs. Modern-day psychology has given us a new word, a substitute for aggression, to avoid the negative interpretations. The new word is "assertiveness" and it implies a more socially acceptable way of manipulating our world.

What we should do is remove the excess associations attached to aggression. This can be done by going back to basics. The word aggression is generally defined as "a forceful action intended to dominate or master." It may be interpreted as hostile or destructive, but it does not necessarily imply action taken against another human being—it can be kicking a wall or breaking a dish. Aggression may involve necessary effort or undue force. It may result from frustration when attempts to get something are blocked and sometimes it may represent a way of being. Sometimes it is a constructive response, for example, in moments where survival is at stake, and sometimes it is unjustifiably destructive. An aggressive act may be effective in getting you what you want, but it might also be just one of many paths to the same goal.

How aggressive are you (Table 5.5)? How often do you try to control and master through forceful action? Or do you go about life in a less aggressive fashion? How do you respond to frustration? Do you quietly think things through? Or do you feel a surge of energy that just needs to be expressed? Do you like situations where you have to pit yourself against some obstacle to overcome resistance and to dominate? Or do you shy away from situations that call for forceful action?

Before you conclude your self-analysis, it's important to recognize that while the aggressive end of the continuum is fairly well defined by the use of force to master, the nonaggressive end is not so clear. You may perceive a nonaggressive person as being passive and meek, or easygoing and calm. It's not certain what is underneath. The person could be trembling with anxiety or feeling quite unruffled. For the present we will just have to tolerate this ambiguity and try to resolve it in the process of matching personality profiles with sports and exercise programs.

PAD 5 — Competitive/Noncompetitive Style

"Marilyn" always had to have the best, to be the best. Competition wasn't a part of life, it *was* her life. She had to ask better questions in graduate school lectures, get better grades, have the best job offers, and so on. Her car had to be faster, more efficient, more attractive, and, of course, purchased at a better price. She could be "relaxing" on vacation and there would still be a competitive edge — a better resort, a better tan. You name it, she would do you one better. She wasn't the greatest athlete, but she made sure she was better than whomever her companion was. It made her happy.

"Harvey" couldn't figure out what was wrong with him. He was bright, talented, not bad looking, but for whatever reason he was just one of the worker bees in his law office. When openings occurred for exciting projects, someone else got them. It was always that way — in school, in sports, even in romance. Friends told him, "It's a dog eat dog world," but he wouldn't play that way. He was a team man, a collaborator. He abhorred competition. He said he didn't need to have the laurels; he just wanted to do his best and it didn't matter if anyone knew.

Competition is such a popular word that it gets confused with other concepts. We hear people talk about competition in three ways: 1. competition against oneself, 2. competition against a standard of performance, and 3. competition against another. The first two interpretations do not conform so much to the idea of competition as they do to the notion of achievement motivation or self-striving. Competition, in its purest sense, has to do with *rivalry*, with the process of competing against one or more individuals who are perceived to be vying for some desired outcome.

Table 5.5

PAD AGGRESSIVE/NONAGGRESSIVE STYLE
For each question, circle the WORD that best describes you.

MOSTLY—I am this way *most of the time.*
OFTEN—I am *often or frequently* this way.
SOMETIMES—I am *sometimes or occasionally* this way.
RARELY—I am *rarely or never* this way.

	MOSTLY	OFTEN	SOMETIMES	RARELY
1. No one pushes me around without getting pushed back.	4	3	2	1
2. If I don't get what I deserve, I become aggressive.	4	3	2	1
3. I back away whenever I feel an argument coming.	1	2	3	4
4. I have a hard time standing up for my rights.	1	2	3	4
5. I complain if I get bad service in a store or restaurant.	4	3	2	1
6. When I am under a lot of pressure, I become irritable and easily lose my temper.	4	3	2	1
7. If someone does something that bothers me, I am the first to let him/her know.	4	3	2	1
8. I break things or slam doors when I get mad.	4	3	2	1

SCORING:
Add up the points *under* each of your answers. Then, write your total score in the space provided. Identify your **Aggressive/Nonaggressive Style** in the list below.

Category	PAD Style	Score Range
1	Highly Aggressive	28–32
2	Moderately Aggressive	23–27
3	Intermediate	18–22
4	Moderately Nonaggressive	13–17
5	Highly Nonaggressive	8–12

Your Total Score _____   **Your Rating Category** _____

In Marilyn's case, there was always someone she was trying to better, always a rival. It might have been friends at school, officemates, or even people she met on vacation. What made her competitive rather than simply an achiever was that she was fueled by her reaction to others. The absolute standard was less critical than the desire to have more than or be better than some other person.

Competition does not necessarily require conscious participation of the rival. You can be playing a game for social reasons while your partner is doing her best to beat you. Your goal is friendship. Her goal is winning.

Another angle on competition comes from Harvey's case. We would define Harvey as an achieving individual. He always wanted to do his best—in school and on the job. But he was noncompetitive. He would not allow rivalry to define his relationships. He became a team player as a way of avoiding competition. By denying the competitive realm, he had difficulty understanding things that happened to him. He couldn't figure out why he was always being passed over.

In your self-assessment on the PAD Competitive/Noncompetitive Style, the central theme is whether or not you compete with others. The combination of liking to compete plus active engagement in competitive situations yields the highest score. Let's take an example to clarify. Imagine you run alone every morning for five miles. Is this competitive? Not yet. Now, add the fact that you time yourself and try to improve your time each week. Is this competitive? No. So far, we have identified self-striving or achievement orientation. Add one more fact. You have a friend who also runs five miles and who times his runs, and you casually extract information from him about his running times. You feel up or down depending on whether your times are better than his. Is this competitive? What do you think?

Competition is rivalry. Sometimes we are more up front about it than other times. Sometimes our rival is fully aware of the competitive dimension, other times not. In the example, the other runner may have been hooked into the competition or he could have been oblivious that his friend was competing against him.

Do you like competitive games? Or are you bothered by situations where there are winners and losers based on some expression of skill or talent? Do you feel as if you are always trying to do better than another person, or do you try to make everyone into colleagues and collaborators? Does the adrenaline flow a little faster and do you perform better when there is a challenger? Or does the competitive dimension throw you into a frenzy of self-doubt and emotional turmoil?

These are questions you might ask in determining how competitive you are. You may hedge and say, "I'm competitive in some situations but not in others." While this is possible, we would ask you to look closer. We often carry whatever style we have wherever we go (Table 5.6).

PAD 6 — Focused/Unfocused Style

"Shirley" had a one-track mind, which meant that whenever she was working on something, it was almost impossible to get her to attend to anything else. It even made her uncomfortable to talk when she was driving, especially if there was traffic. She would get lost in a book and, as her mother would say, "The house could be burning and she wouldn't know it." In many ways it was a real advantage. She could tune out the radio or the TV and concentrate on whatever she was doing. But if she was pressured and had to try to do more than one thing at a time, she would frazzle.

"Mel" was a juggler. He liked keeping lots of balls in the air at the same time. Of course, he occasionally dropped one, but he figured he was batting better than .500. Friends found him more than a bit distractable — he couldn't keep on one topic for too long. Either he got bored or something else pulled him away. In his office he could be found on the phone with another caller on hold, his secretary pushing letters under his hand to sign, a colleague seated by his desk, and another waiting by the door. At home, the TV, radio, and whatever else were all going at the same time. He just seemed to like it that way.

We each have preferences for activity levels and tolerances for stimulation. We also have styles of attending to our agendas. Some of us work sequentially — one thing at a time. Others prefer to handle things simultaneously — everything at once. Most of us are somewhere in between with times when we buzz along like an octopus with eight arms and other times when it's more like, "Can't you see I'm busy?"

Shirley had an advantage in being single-minded. She had high powers of concentration and a way of screening out distractions. Mel, on the other hand, craved distraction. When the world didn't provide enough, he created his own. On the downside, Shirley wore out under demands to do more than one thing at a time while Mel flourished under these conditions. Each style has its benefits and liabilities; each style works well under some circumstances and not so well under others.

People who are highly focused don't necessarily have to change. It is only an issue when the world constantly demands another style and the individual can do little to alter her environment. Learning how to juggle, how to respond quickly to a variety of stimuli, or how to shift

Table 5.6

PAD COMPETITIVE/NONCOMPETITIVE STYLE
For each question, circle the WORD that best describes you.

MOSTLY—I am this way *most of the time.*
OFTEN—I am *often or frequently* this way.
SOMETIMES—I am *sometimes or occasionally* this way.
RARELY—I am *rarely or never* this way.

	MOSTLY	OFTEN	SOMETIMES	RARELY
1. I enjoy competitive games and sports.	4	3	2	1
2. I perform better when I am competing against someone equally skilled.	4	3	2	1
3. I avoid situations where there are winners and losers.	1	2	3	4
4. I get anxious or upset when friends start acting competitively.	1	2	3	4
5. I find competitive situations very stressful.	1	2	3	4
6. I like to challenge friends when we play social games.	4	3	2	1
7. Competition motivates me.	4	3	2	1
8. It bothers me to watch people fighting each other to get ahead.	1	2	3	4

SCORING:
Add up the points *under* each of your answers. Then, write your total score in the space provided. Identify your **Competitive/Noncompetitive Style** in the list below.

Category	PAD Style	Score Range
1	Highly Competitive	28–32
2	Moderately Competitive	23–27
3	Intermediate	18–22
4	Moderately Noncompetitive	13–17
5	Highly Noncompetitive	8–12

Your Total Score _____   **Your Rating Category** _____

attention from one thing to another and back again represents a skill a person has to practice in order to become more comfortable in a demanding world.

The individual who has difficulty in focusing other than for very short periods of time also runs into difficulty. Sometimes it is hard to shut the machine off. There are times when a person has to concentrate or to slow the mind to one focus. But if the mind is constantly geared to working in overdrive, it may be nearly impossible. The style needs to be counterbalanced. The person has to learn to concentrate, to narrow attention to one thing, one experience.

How do you rate on the PAD Focused/Unfocused Style (Table 5.7)? Do you find it easy to concentrate or to do only one thing at a time? Or does your mind jump around a lot, almost looking for distractions? Is your life a juggling act that you enjoy and feel stimulated by? Or do you get worn out by demands to attend to more than one thing at a time? Do you prefer to work on only one thing, finishing it before moving on to the next project? Or do you bounce from one activity to another before finishing the first? These are indications of the focused/unfocused style that may characterize your approach to life.

PAD 7 — Risky/Safe Style

"Phil" lived life on the edge. He enjoyed taking risks, although he probably thought things were a lot safer than they were. After all, not that many people die skydiving in a given year! He knew the odds and he also had formulas for beating them. He liked games where he could influence the outcome, where his skills would come into play, so you wouldn't find him at the roulette wheel in Las Vegas, but maybe at a poker table. His friends saw him as adventurous; his mother thought he was reckless. Phil just figured he was an exciting kind of guy who liked an element of risk, or occasionally danger, to get the adrenaline flowing.

"Kathy" didn't walk out of the house without checking the extended weather forecast, and she was usually the first one in town to get snow tires on her car. She just thought of herself as cautious. She didn't like the idea of being hurt or getting sick, so she took precautions. Sometimes this meant not going along with the gang and, therefore, being alone. But she reasoned, "I'd rather be a live chicken than a dead duck—or even a lame duck!" Her way was okay for her—no cavities, no broken bones, no scars, no messy romances. Maybe someone else would think she was dull, but she was comfortable with herself.

There are lots of risks in life: physical risks, emotional risks, social

Table 5.7

PAD FOCUSED/UNFOCUSED STYLE
For each question, circle the WORD that best describes you.

MOSTLY—I am this way *most of the time.*
OFTEN—I am *often or frequently* this way.
SOMETIMES—I am *sometimes or occasionally* this way.
RARELY—I am *rarely or never* this way.

	MOSTLY	OFTEN	SOMETIMES	RARELY
1. I find it easy to concentrate.	4	3	2	1
2. I prefer to work on only one thing at a time.	4	3	2	1
3. My mind jumps around a lot from one thing to another.	1	2	3	4
4. I finish projects that I start.	4	3	2	1
5. I have trouble sticking to the point in a discussion.	1	2	3	4
6. I take on more tasks than I know I can finish.	1	2	3	4
7. I have no difficulty shutting out noises and other distractions.	4	3	2	1
8. I get bored easily.	1	2	3	4

SCORING:
Add up the points *under* each of your answers. Then, write your total score in the space provided. Identify your **Focused/Unfocused Style** in the list below.

Category	PAD Style	Score Range
1	Highly Focused	28–32
2	Moderately Focused	23–27
3	Intermediate	18–22
4	Moderately Unfocused	13–17
5	Highly Unfocused	8–12

Your Total Score _____ **Your Rating Category** _____

risks, financial risks, and so forth. And there are lots of styles of risk-taking, from being utterly careless, almost suicidal, to a more calculated risk-reducing strategy. Some people like to buy tickets in lotteries where skill has little to do with the outcome, whereas others prefer games of chance where skill is involved, such as in card playing. Of course, there are many who refuse to gamble at all.

Risk-taking can be thrilling or it can be terrifying. We can be energized by a sense of adventure or frightened into a posture of extreme caution. Sometimes, when we are very skilled at something, we don't define what we are doing as risky. Consider, for example, champion slalom skiers. So, identifying a person's risk-taking comes partly from the things she does and partly from *how* she does them.

To clarify, skydiving is inherently risky, and while skill level in diving may reduce that risk, it will not bring it down to the equivalent statistical safety of sitting in your living room. Driving a car is also risky, but given the travel needs of our society, we think of driving as a necessary and acceptable risk. Skill and caution significantly affect our safety and help to lower the odds of an accident. So, in the case of skydiving, a risk-taking characteristic would be largely identified by the fact that a person chooses to skydive, whereas in the case of driving, it has more to do with how a person drives rather than the fact that she does drive. Yes, we are saying that skydivers are risk-loving creatures, recognizing, of course, that some are quite reckless and others extremely safety conscious.

How do you rate on the PAD Risky-Safe Style (Table 5.8)? Do you enjoy adventurous activities? Or are you more cautious in your recreational choices? Does an element of danger give you a positive charge? Or does it frighten you so that you avoid it? Are you a gambler? Do you like playing games of chance? And what kinds of odds attract you the most—1 in 100, 50-50, or only sure things? In what areas of life are you more likely to be cautious or risky? Or is your style pretty consistent across the board? These questions will help you explore your style and come up with a realistic appraisal.

Your PADs Profile

You have just completed your PADs analysis. We hope you got the message that there is nothing inherently wrong with either high or low scores on any of these dimensions—it's more a matter of how well-suited your personality is to your lifestyle. If you are a risk-loving creature in a security-oriented job, you may feel a bit frustrated. If you are a real social animal but your job requires you to spend long periods alone, you may get pretty dissatisfied.

Table 5.8

PAD RISKY/SAFE STYLE
For each question, circle the WORD that best describes you.

MOSTLY—I am this way *most of the time.*
OFTEN—I am *often or frequently* this way.
SOMETIMES—I am *sometimes or occasionally* this way.
RARELY—I am *rarely or never* this way.

	MOSTLY	OFTEN	SOMETIMES	RARELY
1. The element of danger in things appeals to me.	4	3	2	1
2. I have to be sure about my physical safety before I do something.	1	2	3	4
3. I avoid taking chances with my emotions.	1	2	3	4
4. The more daring an activity is, the more I am drawn to it.	4	3	2	1
5. I immediately go for a medical exam if I notice something unusual with my body.	1	2	3	4
6. I keep a close watch on the potential hazards of daily living.	1	2	3	4
7. I test the limits of my physical capabilities.	4	3	2	1
8. I enjoy doing things in new and exciting ways.	4	3	2	1

SCORING:
Add up the points *under* each of your answers. Then, write your total score in the space provided. Identify your **Risky/Safe Style** in the list below.

Category	PAD Style	Score Range
1	Highly Risky	28–32
2	Moderately Risky	23–27
3	Intermediate	18–22
4	Moderately Safe	13–17
5	Highly Safe	8–12

Your Total Score _____   **Your Rating Category** _____

Another way of looking at these scores is to consider the idea of living a balanced life. This means having time alone and time with others, being wild and crazy and also being plans-conscious, having self-discipline to get a job done yet not always being stubbornly persistent, having an aggressive push but being able to back off, enjoying a competitive game and also being a good teammate, being single-minded and also possessing the skill of a juggler, having a spirit of adventure but taking necessary precautions.

When we become too extreme about anything, chances increase that we will run into problems. By honestly evaluating your PADs Styles, you should have a better understanding of your strengths and liabilities, and your excesses and deficits.

In Chapter 8 you will learn about the PADs Styles emphasized in different fitness activities. Sports and exercise programs will be rated on the same seven dimensions you just used in your self-evaluation. This will allow you to compare your profile to each fitness and sport profile. Then you will find out how well your style matches the styles of different fitness pursuits. And, if you consider yourself too extreme on

Figure 5.1

YOUR PADS GRAPH

TRANSFER YOUR INDIVIDUAL PADS RATINGS TO THIS GRAPH
FILL IN THE APPROPRIATE CIRCLES AND CONNECT THEM WITH A LINE.

IN BETWEEN
MORE ← ● → MORE

RATING CATEGORY	1	2	3	4	5	
SOCIAL	O	O	O	O	O	NONSOCIAL
SPONTANEOUS	O	O	O	O	O	CONTROLLED
DISCIPLINED	O	O	O	O	O	UNDISCIPLINED
AGGRESSIVE	O	O	O	O	O	NONAGGRESSIVE
COMPETITIVE	O	O	O	O	O	NONCOMPETITIVE
FOCUSED	O	O	O	O	O	UNFOCUSED
RISKY	O	O	O	O	O	SAFE
RATING CATEGORY	1	2	3	4	5	

some of your PADs scores, you may come to realize that the sports you are drawn toward will not necessarily help you curb your excesses or develop your deficits. This means looking for another activity to supplement your fitness program and to help redirect your personal style.

Before going on, transfer your individual PADs scores to the PADs Graph (Figure 5.1). This will enable you to make direct comparisons with the Fitness Profiles. Keep them ready for the matching process that begins in Chapter 8.

6

Understanding Your Muscles—Psychologically!

"I'm having a bad day. I can barely drag myself from the house. It must be written all over my face. My chest feels collapsed . . . I can hardly breathe. Am I depressed or what?"

"Wow! What a day! MMMmm, do I feel good. A little pep in my stride, smile on my face. Breathe that air. Chest out, shoulders back—watch out world, here I come!"

Body Language

Body language. We know all about it. Crossed arms equal a defensive posture. Head cocked to the right, skeptical attitude. Slouched posture, defeated attitude. Is this what the psychology of muscle is all about? The simple answer is no.

Body language is one way to open the topic, to make the connection between body and mind. From books like Edward Hall's *The Silent Language*,[1] Julius Fast's *Body Language*,[2] or Desmond Morris's *Manwatching*,[3] we have learned how culture and attitudes shape our nonverbal expressions. We have become astute body readers interpreting the signals of movement and gesture. We look for meaning in the wrinkling of faces and contortions of the body. And we know that more is said without words than with them. Body-reading has become something of a game, like watching people in a restaurant and guessing what's going on. We don't take it too seriously—but then, we are also reluctant to dismiss it entirely.

Psychosomatics

The connection between body and mind may be seen in the psychosomatic theory of illness. As far back as 1956, Dr. Hans Selye expressed the belief that most diseases are influenced by psychological factors.[4] With the accumulation of evidence, it has become almost impossible these days to maintain a position that viruses or disease entities just attack us at random. At a minimum, we endorse the possibility of psychological susceptibility to illness.[5]

Whether it is allergies, arthritis, heart disease, or even cancer, we are told psychological factors are at work.[6] The concept of *stress* is often invoked as a catchall term to explain the nonphysical dimension of disease. Stress researchers regularly produce data to suggest that people who are psychologically stressed become physically ill and, conversely, that when one is physically ill, there is a major psychological dimension that must be addressed.[7] These studies make it hard for us to separate mental illness from physical disease. In a positive way, they make us attend to the psychological side of the physically sick and the physical side of the psychologically troubled.

The interaction of mind and body is not just a philosophical issue. It has real consequences and must be appreciated for all the ways mind and body mutually influence each other.

The Mind-Body Problem

The relationship between mind and body has long been a basis for philosophical debate. Arguments about whether the mind and body are truly separate, are one and the same or, indeed, that one or the other is nonexistent have occupied philosophers for centuries. René Descartes (1596–1650) is perhaps best known for his theory of dualism, whereby the mind and body represent separate entities that interact via the pineal gland (a small structure in the center of the brain). While our sophistication about the human body has progressed vastly since Descartes's time, we have perhaps come no closer to identifying exactly how or where mind and body interact.

Some have tried to skirt the issue. The early behaviorists suggested that mental activity is irrelevant and that human beings are mindless. At the opposite end, the subjective idealists completely denied the existence of matter. They proposed that reality is only a perception; what is claimed to be the physical world is just an exceptionally vivid and coherent hallucination.[8]

A recent resolution of this debate is found in a position known as Identity Theory. It suggests that mental and physical processes are identical and that the concept of separate mind and body has arisen only because human beings are consistently looked at from two differing points of view. Identity Theory has been largely adopted in the field of psychiatry, where it forms an indispensable part of the holistic approach. As represented in the World Health Organization's Expert Committee on Mental Health, the following position was taken:[9]

> When we speak of psychological processes and physiological processes, we are speaking of different ways of approaching one phenomenon.

Chickens and Eggs

There are theories of how to diagnose your personality from the bumps on your head (known as phrenology), or others that link ear-lobe length to criminal tendencies. Theories like these can make you just a little bit skeptical. (Is your head cocked to the right at this moment?) So, it helps to establish at the outset that body-mind interest is not simply a twentieth century fancy and, more importantly, that evidence is mounting for the position that body activities affect the mind, and vice versa.

If we look at causality, or what causes what, the most reasonable position for understanding body-mind relations comes from Systems Theory, which tells us that if you change any one dimension of a system, you influence all others. As human systems, any change in one aspect of our existence will produce changes, large or small, in all other aspects.

Let's consider the effect of change in economic status. You may remember a rather ancient TV drama called "The Millionaire," where unsuspecting people were anonymously given one million dollars. Viewers watched the sudden and sometimes startling personality transformations that resulted. So too, you can understand why feeling depressed over a long period of time might have a variety of effects on social, economic, and even physical planes. This is the message of Systems Theory.

In this chapter we will try to understand how muscles form and what effects these muscle developments have on personality. We will emphasize psychological theories of body development to highlight the mind-body interplay. This doesn't mean that psychology is the major influence on body shape. Genetics, environment, nutrition, and physical activity have powerful effects on growth and development. We stress the psychological side because it is so poorly understood. Most people simply don't think about psychology as a factor in physical development.

The Body-Type Game: Constitutional Psychology and Clinical Insights

Endomorphs, Mesomorphs, and Ectomorphs

Of all the body-mind theories, William Sheldon's (1899–1972) constitutional psychology represents the most systematic exploration of how personality and physical characteristics mesh.[10] Most of us have some familiarity with the three somatotypes (or body types) Sheldon established: endomorphs, mesomorphs, and ectomorphs. *Endomorphs* are fat and round. Muscles are weak and underdeveloped and the digestive viscera are dominant in the body. *Mesomorphs* have hard, muscular bodies with a rectangular shape. Blood vessels are large and skin is thick. *Ectomorphs* have long, fragile bodies with delicate bones and slender, poorly muscled arms and legs. The ectomorph's nervous system and sensory tissue have poor protection and seem overly exposed to the world. Although the methods Sheldon developed to identify somatotypes were complex, simplified formulas involving the ratio of height and weight can be used as estimates.

A pure type is rare. Most of us have characteristics of each of the three types. Sheldon established a seven-point rating scale for each type, so that an individual's profile would include scores on all three types. For example, a 7-1-1 would be an extreme endomorph, a 1-7-1 an extreme mesomorph, and a 1-1-7 an extreme ectomorph. A person could have ratings like 3-5-2, where the dominant feature is mesomorphy (5), but there is some degree of endomorphy (3) and even ectomorphy (2).

Independent of the ratings of physical structure are evaluations of personality. Sheldon developed three scales that measured characteristics of *viscerotonia, somatotonia,* and *cerebrotonia.* An individual who scores high on viscerotonia loves comfort and is a glutton for food, people, and affection. He is relaxed in posture, slow to react, even-tempered, tolerant of others, and highly sociable. A high scorer on somatotonia loves risky adventures and has a strong need for vigorous physical activity. He is aggressive, callous toward others' feelings, over-mature in appearance, noisy, courageous, and given to claustrophobia. Action, power, and domination are of primary importance to such an individual. A high scorer on cerebrotonia is restrained and inhibited. A cerebrotonic person is secretive, self-conscious, youthful in appearance, afraid of others, and happiest in small enclosed areas. He reacts over-quickly, sleeps poorly, and prefers solitude, particularly when troubled. He diligently avoids attracting attention to himself.[11]

Once again, seven-point scales were established for each personal-ity component so a person could be characterized according to how much of the traits of viscerotonia, somatotonia, and cerebrotonia he possessed. When the personality traits were correlated with the three body types, Sheldon found a strong correspondence between endomor-phy and viscerotonia, mesomorphy and somatotonia, and ectomorphy and cerebrotonia.

These scientific findings support common beliefs that fat people (endomorphs) love comfort, are sociable, and seem to have insatiable needs for people, food, and affection (viscerotonia); or that muscular people (mesomorphs) are daring, adventurous, aggressive, and perhaps callous toward others (somatotonia); or that skinny people (ectomorphs) are nervous, shy, and inhibited (cerebrotonia). Yet, we have to be careful in applying these traits to fat, muscular, or skinny people because the measurement of body type according to Sheldon's scheme is compli-cated, and because pure types are rare. Most of us possess a mixture not only of body types but also of personality characteristics.

Extremes and Therapeutic Suggestions. When we consider the ex-tremes, the 7-1-1 endomorph, the 1-7-1 mesomorph, or the 1-1-7 ecto-morph, we can't resist imagining a personality profile that is likewise extreme and perhaps dysfunctional.[12]

If an endomorph's viscerotonia is extreme, we have a person craving an incredible amount of contact and comfort. This need originates from feelings of helplessness and isolation and results in compulsive move-ment toward people for nurturance and support. The endomorph doesn't know when enough is enough. If the endomorph were to natu-rally select activities or exercise, we predict he would choose activities with few boundaries or ones that allow indulgent expression. This would feed the endomorph's dysfunctional pattern and thereby foster behavior that ultimately is detrimental to well-being. We might imagine the endo-morph luxuriating in a swimming pool or perhaps swaying rhythmically to light rock music. More structured activities, including lap swimming or even low impact aerobics, would not attract the endomorph, even though they hold more potential for positive personality restructuring.

If a mesomorph's somatotonia is extreme, we have a person with an excessive need to aggress against and dominate others. We also have a person who is extremely impulsive. The mesomorph doesn't allow enough time for awareness to develop and guide actions. As a result, actions may appear callous or even ruthless. We can readily imagine the mesomorph happily engaged in a game of football or even some racquet sport, but once again we have to question the wisdom of this choice. It seems natural enough, but given the overdeveloped inclination toward impulsive, forceful actions, wouldn't something softer and less competitive be better? Wouldn't the mesomorph profit more from activities that reinforce sensitivity and interpersonal awareness? And wouldn't we guess how difficult it would be for the mesomorph to stick with such activities?

Finally, if the ectomorph's cerebrotonia is extreme, we have a person who hides from others. The ectomorph's tendency to be introverted and secretive means he will have difficulty expressing his needs. Unlike the mesomorph, the ectomorph is adequately aware of his needs and, given his penchant for withdrawal, he won't have the endomorph's problem of not knowing when to stop. But it will be painfully difficult for him to let his wants be known or to be involved with others in fulfilling his needs. In sports and exercise, we can imagine the ectomorph as a lonely runner or in some other solitary activity, but we would not be as likely to find him playing racquetball or taking aerobics. Would he profit from these experiences? Eventually. It would take effort and, fortunately, the emotional difficulty would be countered by the anxiety-reducing effect of exercise.

Genetics and Psychology.   For all that Sheldon's somatotypes have contributed to body-mind theory, they tell only part of the story. His studies demonstrated the correlation of objective body assessments and personality traits, but they did not show that one causes the other. In fact, Sheldon's work came from the school of constitutional psychology, which says our genes play the determining role in who we are. From his perspective, the connection between personality and body structure is mostly determined by genetics, not by the way we are raised. In this regard, it doesn't tell us how psychology can actually influence physical development. Let's look at another theory to see how this might work.

Muscles and Bone and Body Armor

When you consider the somatotype theory, something is missing.

Bodies are not only different sizes, but they also appear in a wide assortment of shapes. In Sheldon's system, measurements are taken of different parts of the body and combined for an overall index. This index doesn't allow us to see that one person may have hunched shoulders while another's shoulders are rounded, or that an individual may have a very rigid and muscular back while his front is soft and flabby. These anomalies are important. They tell us something about personality and the individual's psychological development.

One of the most influential psychological theories of body development grew out of the works of Wilhelm Reich, a student of Freud who went on to establish a unique way of viewing personality through body analysis. Reich originated the term *character armor*, which was defined as the total pattern of chronic (meaning long-term, not just temporary) muscular tensions in the body.[13] He called these tensions "armor" because they protect the individual from painful or threatening emotional experiences. They shield him from dangerous impulses within his own personality as well as from attacks by others.

One of Reich's followers, Alexander Lowen, expanded this body theory into a school of psychotherapy known as Bioenergetics. Lowen wrote a number of books on the topic of the body and its signs of psychological conflict, including *The Language of the Body*,[14] *Betrayal of the Body*,[15] and *Bioenergetics*.[16] Lowen defined *character*, a term analogous to personality, as a fixed pattern of behavior determined by the quantity and quality of controls imposed upon muscular activity. Muscles that are subject to these *unconscious* controls are chronically tense and contracted, yet somehow we are unaware of this tension. We don't realize we are tensing these muscles and holding them in contraction over long, long periods of time. To understand this, you might recall a time when you had a terribly stiff neck or tight back that only forced itself into your awareness at the end of the day, or perhaps when you woke up the next morning.

To appreciate what these chronically tense muscles do to your body shape, you first have to strip away all the muscles and organs of the body and look at your skeleton. Assume for the moment that your bones are not deformed (which happens to be true for a vast majority of the population). If you were to suspend your skeleton from the ceiling by a string attached to the top of your skull, you would find that everything hangs in proper alignment. Although your skeleton may be longer or shorter, wider or narrower than someone else's, you would be amazed at how wonderfully aligned you are with arms hanging easily by your sides, legs and feet in proper placement, back showing the natural curvatures of the spine, and so forth.

When you begin reconstructing yourself by strapping everything together with ligaments, tendons, and the chronically tensed muscles that are shorter than they were meant to be, you no longer look so well aligned. You may have your shoulder bones up around your ears, someone else's may be down toward her waist. Your back may be bowed with a slight hump, and another person may have her shoulder blades squeezed together and her chest pushed forward.

The shape of the skeleton is influenced by the pull of muscles that insert into bones. The structure of the body changes as a reflection of its muscular tensions. This, according to Lowen, not only justifies the use of the body's structure in the analysis of personality, but it also provides a basis for attempts to modify personality through the release of chronic muscular tension.[17]

Two other investigators, Kurz and Prestera, give us the same message in their book, *The Body Reveals*, when they point out that our psychological identity and our fixed muscular patterns "reflect, enhance and sustain one another. It is as if the body sees what the mind believes and the heart feels, and adjusts itself accordingly . . . The muscular pattern in turn sustains the attitude, as for example slouching forward, which makes every action more difficult and so makes life itself seem burdensome."[18]

Lowen does not look upon this kind of body reading of chronic muscular tension as a guessing game. He says, "the correlation between muscle tensions and inhibition is so exact that one can tell what impulses or feelings are inhibited in a person from a study of his muscular tensions."[19] For example, the desire to do something, which would involve the use of particular muscles, may be counteracted by feelings of guilt or fear, thereby calling into play opposing muscles. The result is a tense body or body part, which, over time, shapes itself according to the conflicting muscle tensions.

These ideas represent a popular school of clinical psychology founded on the belief in body-mind connections, or Identity Theory, as it was more formally labeled earlier in this chapter. Lowen's works, in particular, provide a basis for the upcoming section on "muscle psychology," or how muscle groups have specific psychological functions.

Psychopaths, Masochists, and Other Bodies We Have Known

It may clarify the body-mind connection if we look at some of the basic character types that Lowen identified in his clinical work. Unlike William Sheldon, who studied a normal population in the development of his somatotypes, Alexander Lowen is a practicing psychotherapist and his data come from patients in treatment for psychological difficulties.[20]

Lowen's model is developmental, in that early life traumas or conflicts are thought to give rise to psychological disturbances and corresponding body formations. In their developmental sequence, the five character types he identified, from the earliest to the latest, are: *schizoid, oral, psychopath, masochist,* and *rigid.* He believed that the type of character a person ends up with depends on the stage of development at which he is traumatized. If the trauma occurs early, then chances are the person will have trouble developing through the successive stages as well. So, the earlier the trauma, the more complex the problem. This means the schizoid type is the most complex and the rigid type the least complex.

1. *The Schizoid Character.* How would you like to feel rejected from day one of life? That's the schizoid's trauma and it has been largely related to the infant-mother relationship. The infant feels punished for existing, and as a result holds in all feelings. Emotions get tied up in knots. In body-reading the schizoid type, a great deal of body armoring is seen around the eyes, which seem unexpressive and vacant, as if they are looking through you. Generally, the whole body seems tense, with stiffness at the joints and with body parts, like the head, going off at odd angles. The body seems poorly coordinated. Energy is low in the face, hands, feet, and genitals. And the top and bottom halves of the body don't look like they belong together.

2. *The Oral Character.* What would happen if, as an infant, you cried out for food and comfort and only rarely were answered? Eventually, you might give up. That's the oral character's trauma. He is deprived and as a result is afraid to have needs. As an infant, the oral type may have been left hungry for food and comfort. He finally stops crying and starts believing that needs are dangerous because they don't get met and that no one is there for him. The oral character gets hung up on nurturance and support. Oral types have a strong need to cling, to hold on, to be propped up, but no matter how much they get, it is never enough because they can't take it in fully. Depression, disappointment, and feeling unloved are common reactions. Oral characters have difficulty asking for things. On a body level, the oral type looks immature. Muscles are poorly developed and feelings of weakness are common. The skin is often thin and pale. The oral type tends to lock his knees a lot, and frequently has narrow, flat feet. The head is tilted forward, the chest collapsed, and the abdomen is soft and protruding. The overall portrait is of an energyless, sunken body that looks propped up.

3. *The Psychopathic Character.* Do you remember your feeling as a child of being small and powerless? That's the kind of trauma the psychopath continually experienced. And what do you think the effect would be? The child feels weak and overwhelmed and develops an obsession for power. The psychopathic type grows up needing to dominate and control, but does so by denying his own feelings. There are actually two types of psychopaths: the *bully*, who takes advantage of others by overpowering them, and the *seducer*, who undermines others by being gentle and overly polite. The bully has an overdeveloped upper body, which makes his chest and abdomen look as inflated as a balloon. His eyes are often penetrating and distrustful. By contrast, the seducer has a back that is almost too flexible, and free-swinging hips that seem disconnected from his upper body. Naturally, his eyes and voice are soft and seductive.

4. *The Masochistic Character.* What would happen if, as a child, love only came to you when you obeyed, that is, you were loved conditionally? Your right to be independent would be violated. This is the masochist's trauma and it typically occurs with an overbearing mother who restricts the child's freedom and makes him feel guilty if he disobeys. In these cases, the father is usually passive. The masochist is outwardly submissive but inwardly spiteful and full of rage. He is long-suffering, whining, and complaining, but at all times submissive. He seems to be self-effacing, but underneath it all feels superior. The masochist has difficulty being aggressive or assertive. He appears hardworking, but there is a sense of awkwardness about his behavior. This character type comes across as negative, resisting almost everything. And he feeds on the anger he generates in others. It is through being beat upon that the masochist experiences release from the energy bound up in his body. Physically, the masochist has an almost gorilla-like appearance, with thick, powerful muscles, a short, compressed body, flat rear, and rounded back. Calves and the front of the thighs are overdeveloped, and the hamstring muscles are generally tight. Facially, the masochist looks innocent and naive, with soft, sad eyes showing a life of suffering. The voice, of course, has an annoying whining quality.

5. *The Rigid Character.* The traumas so far have involved mother-child interactions. What happens when the child at about age five begins to take on a sexual identity and now Daddy acts in a rejecting manner? The rigid character develops after sexual identity is set, thereby allowing for female and male variations. While the mother's influence predominates in the earlier character formations, it is the father's rejection of the child's love that triggers the rigid character's

trauma. The father pushes the child away, and for the male child makes love contingent upon performance. Yet whatever the child does is not enough. The little boy believes that performance is all that life is about and gives up on love. The rigid male seems self-confident, ambitious, competitive, and prone to action. He is also inflexible, determined, and perfectionistic. On the body side, there are two manifestations of the rigid male. There is the *phallic-narcissistic* male, who identifies with the father and is obsessive. He comes across as emotionally charged. He is sexually preoccupied, but has difficulty achieving orgasm. His body tends to be small and narrow. Although it will be proportionate in shape, it is often stiff and inflexible. The second manifestation is the *compulsive* male, who identifies with the mother because his father is so threatening. He is compulsive and has a cold, inflexible ego. His feelings are blocked. His body is relatively large and heavily muscled. He has a strong jaw that is set forward in an aggressive manner. His body looks strong and hard with broad shoulders, narrow waist, and tightly contracted hips.

What happens to the little girl whose love is rejected by her father? Because of the gender difference between father and daughter, the rejection becomes sexualized. The father may fear his sexual feelings toward his daughter and becomes rejecting. The little girl develops into a character type known as the *hysteric*. She is suggestible and has irrational emotional outbursts. Her lifestyle is chaotic. She is easily influenced and prone to high expectations and fads. Her awareness is impressionistic, and her world overly romantic and dramatized. She gets bored and often feels like she is in a rut. The hysteric is usually surprised at the outcomes of her actions. She has a quality of wide-eyed innocence that makes her appealing to men. Her relationships with men are highly sexual. Physically, the hysteric is armored in the vaginal and thigh muscles. She has a tight lower back and her hips are pulled back in a provocative posture. The hysteric often has a stiff neck and jaw, showing her pride and determination. Because her chest and abdomen are rigid, breathing and feeling are restricted. In a general view, her body appears seductive with an upper half that is childlike and a lower half that is more womanly.

Lowen's five types demonstrate how personality dynamics are translated into body shapes. Since these types come from the psychotherapist's office, you may only recognize small bits and pieces of yourself or your friends in the five character types. In reality, people are often a mixture of types with some degree of trauma at each stage of growth giving shape to personality and physique.

Diagnosing the Body

Muscle Types and Muscle Actions

As we move from general information about body-mind relations and typologies to specific diagnoses of muscles and body parts, we need to define some terms in "muscle language." We have to distinguish among the different types of muscles and the actions they perform. The value of this will become clearer as we proceed.

There are three types of muscles when we classify them according to location: *skeletal muscles,* which attach to our bones; *visceral muscles,* which are associated with our internal body structures such as the stomach and intestines; and *cardiac muscles,* which form the walls of the heart. In exercise and sports we work directly with skeletal muscles and only indirectly with cardiac and visceral musculature. For this reason, the remainder of our discussion will focus on skeletal musculature.

An important thing to know about skeletal muscles is how they make our bodies work, and this comes from understanding what they do with our bones. To simplify the picture, imagine a bundle of telephone wires wrapped in a protective covering. This is basically what one form of skeletal muscle looks like. It is attached to bone at either end, but what is most important is that, with few exceptions, skeletal muscle stretches across one or more of our bony joints, such as the elbow, wrist, hip, or knee.

If you think of a muscle beginning in the upper part of the arm, around where your bicep muscle bulges, and ending somewhere on the forearm, you have an example of a muscle crossing a joint, in this case, the elbow. When this muscle contracts or shortens, what do you think happens? You would be right if you pictured the forearm flexing. Now, applying this principle to all of the joints in the body, you not only know how the body moves but also have a clue about how bones are temporarily held in position, as when the wrist is held in a tennis serve, or more chronically, when the body shape becomes distorted through muscle tension over a long period of time.

To better understand this muscle-shortening principle, let us refer back to our model of telephone wires all bundled together and covered by a protective sheath. This sheath in muscle anatomy is known as the *fascia* and, although at birth it is pretty elastic stuff, by the time we are adults it has lost some of its elasticity. In fact, when muscles are chronically tense, the fascial sheath tends to harden around the muscle fibers, keeping them in place and preventing the muscle from relaxing into its full length. You see this in people whose tense muscles cause their movements to be short and rigid.

Let's take this analysis one step further by examining different muscle actions. So far we have seen that it is the contractions or tensing of skeletal muscles that cause the body to move. Some muscles *flex* the joint they cross (as in bending the elbow). Others are positioned so they *extend* the joint (as in straightening the elbow). Some muscles move a part of the body to the side and away from the midline of the body (*abduct* it). Others move the part back toward the midline of the body (*adduct* it). And some muscles *rotate* certain joints. To bring about these movements, muscles often work in conjunction rather than individually.

Muscles responsible for a particular movement are called *prime movers*. But for every movement there are always muscles, generally situated on the opposite side of the joint, that oppose the movement. Muscles that resist the movement are called *antagonists*. When prime movers contract and produce a movement, the antagonists are stretched. For example, when muscles like the biceps bend the arm at the elbow, other muscles like the triceps, at the back of the arm, are stretched. It is important to realize that muscles can serve either as prime movers or antagonists, depending on the action. So, in our example, the biceps would be a prime mover and the triceps an antagonist when the forearm is flexed, but this would be reversed when the forearm is being straightened from a flexed position.

In addition to prime movers and antagonists, most joint movements involve muscles that act as *synergists*. Synergists are muscles that indirectly assist a movement by steadying a joint, thereby allowing the prime movers to function efficiently. When a synergist immobilizes a joint or a bone, it is called a *fixator*. The muscles that immobilize the wrist, for example in a tennis serve, function as fixators.

This completes our brief anatomy lesson.

What does all of this have to do with psychology? Chronically shortened muscles pull your skeletal structure out of alignment and restrict both the range and the quality of your movements. You develop a particular posture that may be described as deflated, repressed, tense, or suspicious. And your interactions with the world become limited by how the different muscles in your body work.

Knowing about muscle actions helps you understand how different muscles accomplish different things. Some arm muscles, for example, allow you to pull the world toward you, others let you push it away. Some leg muscles ground and connect you to the earth, while others push you away, giving you a sense of freedom. Depending on muscle strength, you can assess where you are weak and where you are strong. Are you more capable of pushing away the world than taking it under your control? Are you more accustomed to flight and freedom than to holding your ground? Do your shoulders support the weight you must bear or do they collapse under the strain of your life?

Appreciating the distinction between prime movers and antagonists enables you to understand conflict as it is enacted by the body: one force moving forward, the other pulling back; one wanting to take, the other wanting to push away; arms that yield and arms that control; legs that rise to the occasion and those that sink; chests that expand in pride and those that collapse in defeat. When you are in conflict, this gets represented in the opposing tensions of prime movers and antagonists locking in a battle of wills.

Body Analysis Dimensions (BADs)

We now move into the formal evaluation of your body. What should you be looking for? Much of what we will ask you to describe about your body will come from a history of use. How does your body work? Where is it strong? Where is it weak? Where is it flexible? Where is it tight? Another part of the description comes from looking at it. What does it look like? Is one arm different from the other? Does it appear shapeless or well-defined? Does it look healthy or lifeless? Depending on what you see, there may be other words to describe your body.

We will ask you to make three evaluations of each area of your body:

1. *Strength:* How strong is this area? Is it adequately strong for all the things you need to do with it as well as for things you would like to do? You may find this area is overdeveloped or underdeveloped, meaning it has either too much or too little strength. For some areas, like the stomach or back, you may have little direct way of measuring strength, but you will know indirectly by certain symptoms; lower back pain, for example, may be related to weak muscles in both the abdomen and back. Another thing to keep in mind when measuring strength is the *comparison* of this area with other areas. Are your arms relatively weaker than your legs, for example?

You can rate each area of your body on a five-point strength scale:

5 = Massive/Overdeveloped
4 = Overdeveloped
3 = Adequately developed
2 = Underdeveloped
1 = Weak

This is a subjective rating. You have to judge strength in terms of what you need for your life and reasonable standards of fitness. A body builder will usually fall into Categories 4 or 5 (Overdeveloped or Massive/Overdeveloped) because muscular strength goes beyond what is needed for life and is in the ninety-ninth percentile of standards for adult fitness. At the other extreme, a person who has difficulty jogging a mile would rate his legs muscles in Categories 1 or 2 (Weak or Underdeveloped).

2. *Flexibility:* How rigid, tight, or restricted is this area? Flexibility involves movements around joints of the body, but as we saw earlier, muscles are the main culprits in restricting range of movement by being too tight or chronically contracted. Sometimes massive muscles restrict movements, but thin, tight muscles can have the same effect. So, flexibility is not the same as strength or degree of development. A person who is flabby and weak can still have stiff or contracted muscles (a muscle that is short and weak). People who overdo their stretching exercises and neglect muscle strengthening may have the opposite problem, that of being too flexible and weak, like a rubber band that stretches but can't hold itself up.

We will use a five-point flexibility scale:

5 = Overly Flexible
4 = Flexible
3 = Adequately Flexible
2 = Inflexible
1 = Rigid/Tight

If your body feels like a piece of wet spaghetti or if you move like a weed in a windstorm, you may rate in Category 5 (Overly Flexible). You may have little control over your movements and be a bit too pliable for this world. Category 3 (Adequately Flexible) means you have enough range of movement for most things you do, but could improve some. Category 1 (Rigid/Tight) is an extreme rating where an area of your body is bound with rigidly tight muscles that prevent free movement.

3. *Shape:* The final evaluation is the most subjective; it is qualitative rather than quantitative. It involves looking at your body and describing, in your own words, what you see based on some idea of what this body part should look like. There is a risk of being overly idealistic in evaluating shape. You may have a well-shaped stomach, but because you don't have that washboard muscled look, you see yourself as less than ideal. We will provide guidelines for assessing shape with each area of the body we review. We hope this will curb excessive criticisms.

There is a body chart provided (Figure 6.1) so you can record observations about your body as you read through this material. We will take

YOUR BADS PROFILE

STRENGTH RATING:
5 = MASSIVE/OVERDEVELOPED
4 = OVERDEVELOPED
3 = ADEQUATELY DEVELOPED
2 = UNDERDEVELOPED
1 = WEAK

FLEXIBILITY RATING:
5 = OVERLY FLEXIBLE
4 = FLEXIBLE
3 = ADEQUATELY FLEXIBLE
2 = INFLEXIBLE
1 = RIGID/TIGHT

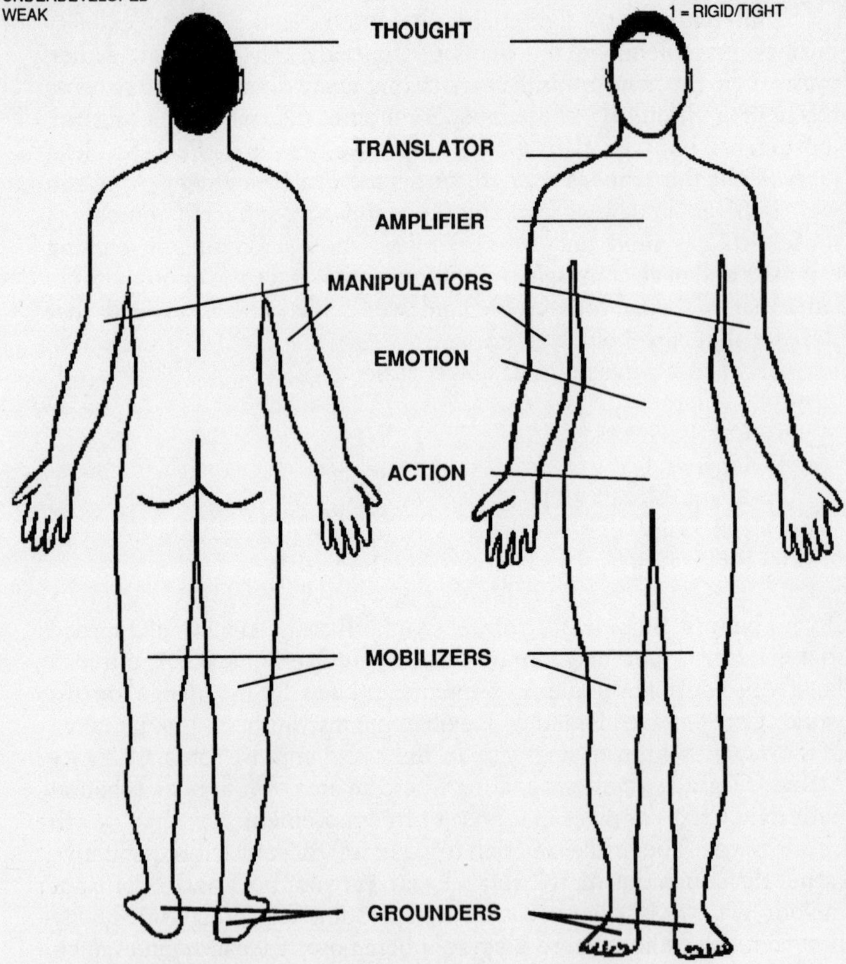

THOUGHT

TRANSLATOR

AMPLIFIER

MANIPULATORS

EMOTION

ACTION

MOBILIZERS

GROUNDERS

RATE YOUR STRENGTH AND FLEXIBILITY FOR DIFFERENT AREAS OF YOUR BODY.

USE THE RATING SCALES IN EVALUATING YOURSELF.

MAKE NOTES ABOUT SPECIAL FEATURES OR SHAPES OF YOUR BODY PARTS.

Figure 6.1

this step by step, going from more general features to more specific ones. As a suggestion, you might first read through the rest of the chapter and then go back over it while looking at your body in the mirror (and, of course, without your clothes).

Diagnosis: Body Splits

The first technique for analyzing your body is based on "body splits." This approach was described by Dr. Ken Dychtwald in his popular book, *Bodymind*.[21] Dychtwald split or dissected the body in particular ways to provide insights into body psychology. Three body splits of special relevance to exercise and sports are (Figure 6.2):

(1) Top and bottom halves of the body
(2) Front and back of the body
(3) Right and left sides of the body.

1. The Top/Bottom Split. When you contrast the upper and lower halves of the body with a dividing line drawn an inch or so below the navel, you are comparing significantly different psychological functions as well as different body regions.[22] What functions does the upper body serve? And the lower body?

The upper body houses all those functions of social contact, including speaking, touching, tasting, smelling, and hearing. You engage the world with your upper body; you interact, manipulate, and control; you think and analyze; and you reach out or hold back.

The lower body serves different functions. If the upper body is your social half, the lower body represents your animal half. It includes your sexual organs. Through hips and legs, it connects you to the ground, enabling you to feel support and a sense of roots. You also move about or stand your ground with your lower body.

How can you compare the upper body to the lower? One way to make the contrast is to ask whether the two halves go together. Much like the childhood game of constructing figures from a variety of plastic parts, if you were to take a bunch of nude photos of different people, cut each in half at the waist, and then mix and match, would the upper bodies always correspond to the lower bodies? Or would you find instances where the upper body was a poor fit for the lower body? When you go to the beach, you see people (more typically men) with barrel chests and spindly legs or, conversely, people (more typically women) with small, underdeveloped upper bodies and massive hips and legs.

If you find disproportion or other indications of difference, will you also observe an imbalance of psychological functions? The person with a massive upper body and underdeveloped lower body might over-

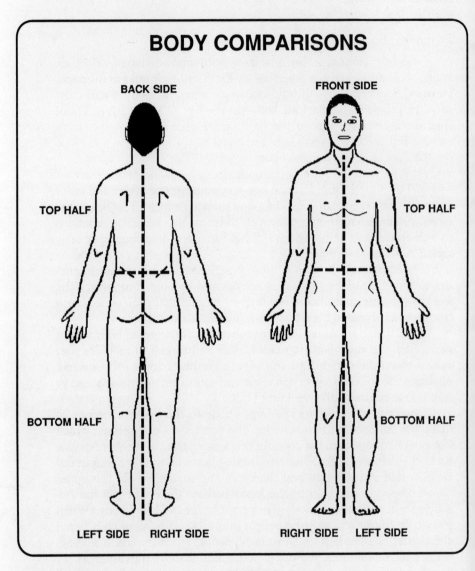

Figure 6.2

emphasize the social, expressive side of life, including excessive needs for recognition, achievement, and action. This person might lack a sense of support through the underdevelopment of the lower body and likewise have difficulty in feeling grounded. He might tend to be emotionally dependent and impulsive.

The person with an overdeveloped lower body and underdeveloped upper body might show greater comfort with the grounded, stable, or private sides of life, but could have more difficulty in social, assertive, or aggressive action. This kind of person might tend toward passivity and inertia.

In thinking about the top/bottom split, bear in mind we are dealing with a set of building blocks, each of which is necessary for appreciating the whole person. To only talk about a top/bottom split would result in a very partial analysis. And there is so much more to consider. Hold onto this piece of data about your body and let's move to the next split.

2. *The Front/Back Split.* The front side of your body is what you present to others. It is both literally and figuratively your "front." It is the area of your body you are most aware of. The front reflects your social and conscious self. Usually, the softer emotions—happiness, sadness, loving, longing—are represented in the muscular development of your front. The back side has more to do with the private and unconscious. Unwanted or socially disapproved feelings may be housed in the back of the body. Anger, cruelty, hardness, and hatred are more likely to be reflected in the development of the back than the front.[23]

We see people whose fronts look like jello, but their backs are surprisingly hard with bunched muscles distorting the shape. In this contrast between a soft, vulnerable front and a rigid, tense back, we find evidence of a personality split. The weakness and vulnerability of the front masks all the privately held, unconscious drive and anger that the individual has stored. (Remember Lowen's description of the masochistic character for an example of this kind of split.) While such a person may seem to be easygoing or a pushover, it is only through seeing the backside—the withheld, negative emotions—that we can fully appreciate how this person might act.

3. *The Left/Right Split.* Imagine a line dividing the body into right and left sides. Theorists from Carl Jung to Alexander Lowen have discussed the psychological differences of the two sides of the body. These differences are thought to exist regardless of whether you are right-handed or left-handed. Some of the major observations about this split derive from notions about cerebral control. For example, the left side of the body is controlled by the right hemisphere of the brain, which is primarily responsible for orientation in space, for creating holistic, inte-

grative impressions, for pattern recognition, for sensory perception and spatial relations, and for visual memory. The left side of the body is also seen as the emotional side. It is thought of as being more receptive and passive.

By contrast, the right side of the body is controlled by the left hemisphere of the brain, which predominantly controls logical, analytical thinking, verbal and mathematical thought, language comprehension and memory. It represents the expressive and aggressive side of our personality operating primarily on reason and logic.[24]

If you compare your two sides, you may find more development on one side than the other, more tension, more flexibility, and so forth. These contrasts can tell you where your emphasis seems to be stronger, and where you may be underdeveloped psychologically.

Sometimes we see people who have tremendous tension and even pain on one side of the body but not the other. Although this may result from overuse of that side (for example, tennis elbow is typically found only in the playing arm), it may also represent psychological conflicts, or too much emphasis on one aspect of the personality over another. A balance of assertiveness and receptivity, of rationality and emotionality, is reflected in a body that looks equally developed on the right and left sides. An imbalance along these dimensions will display itself in lateral differences of body shape and musculature.

Diagnosis: The Psychoanatomy of Muscle

We are now going to connect each major area of the body with psychological functions they serve. For this diagnosis, you will want to keep in mind the three ratings of strength, flexibility, and shape. Also, note any differences you find from one side of the body to the other. For example, what differences do you see between your right arm and your left arm? Is there a difference in the shape of one side vs. the other? You will be developing your own psychoanatomical map in this section. It will tell you how you use your body, how you store tensions, what you emphasize in your daily interactions, what you undervalue or underuse.

We will proceed from bottom to top, beginning with the feet and ending with the head. An overview of the areas and their psychological functions can be found in Figure 6.3.

Feet (or Grounders)

In one foot there are nineteen bones, not counting the seven ankle bones, and there are nineteen muscles intrinsic to the foot and an

PSYCHOANATOMICAL MAP OF THE BODY

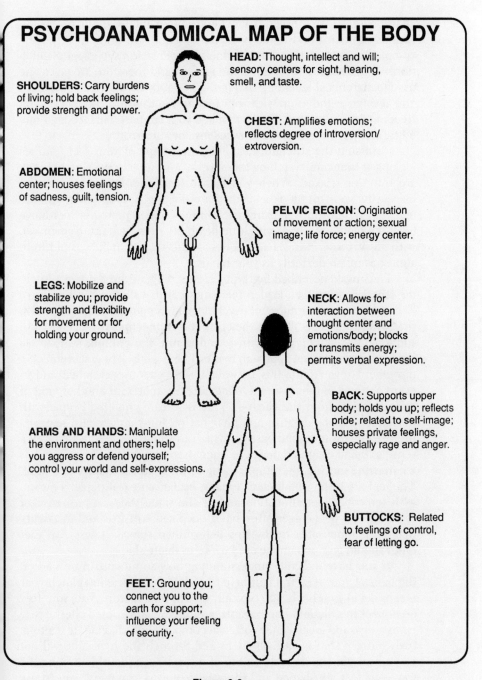

SHOULDERS: Carry burdens of living; hold back feelings; provide strength and power.

HEAD: Thought, intellect and will; sensory centers for sight, hearing, smell, and taste.

CHEST: Amplifies emotions; reflects degree of introversion/extroversion.

ABDOMEN: Emotional center; houses feelings of sadness, guilt, tension.

PELVIC REGION: Origination of movement or action; sexual image; life force; energy center.

LEGS: Mobilize and stabilize you; provide strength and flexibility for movement or for holding your ground.

NECK: Allows for interaction between thought center and emotions/body; blocks or transmits energy; permits verbal expression.

BACK: Supports upper body; holds you up; reflects pride; related to self-image; houses private feelings, especially rage and anger.

ARMS AND HANDS: Manipulate the environment and others; help you aggress or defend yourself; control your world and self-expressions.

BUTTOCKS: Related to feelings of control, fear of letting go.

FEET: Ground you; connect you to the earth for support; influence your feeling of security.

Figure 6.3

additional thirteen muscles that act on the foot and toes. Add to this the various ligaments and tendons in the foot and you have an extremely complex body part that serves some indispensible psychological functions. Your feet connect you to the ground and therefore are given the psychoanatomical label of *grounders.* They provide a sense of security. You also move and jump with your feet and in this regard they give you freedom of movement. They symbolize your support, balance, and mobility, and for these reasons allow a sense of autonomy.[25]

Assessing the strength, flexibility, and shape of your feet requires looking at them and watching them work. You can observe whether they are tense or relaxed. When you habitually clutch the ground out of insecurity, your toes look as if they are digging in even when you are relaxing. When you walk barefoot, you may notice that your feet move like solid blocks of wood, with little flexibility in movement. Remember, with all of those muscles and bones in the feet, your feet could have almost as much dexterity as your hands.

Dychtwald described five types of feet.[26] There are flat feet, clutching feet, tiptoeing feet, leaden feet, and feet that dig in with the heels. Each type represents different psychological themes. *Flat feet* fail to grip the earth, they slide all over, they lack the connection you need to feel supported. *Clutching feet*, with toes dug into the ground, represent a rigid, overly controlled approach to life. There is a lack of gracefulness in movement (if you doubt this, try walking with your toes clutched) and an overly rational emphasis in life. *Tiptoeing feet* represent another kind of disconnection from the earth—a kind of dreamy quality. People with these feet may be creative and imaginative, but they are also removed from reality, from a solid base on which to stand. *Leaden feet* convey a sense of being weighted down, of stagnation and decay. The person has a hard time moving, overemphasizing stability and reliability to a fault. The feet are heavy and lifeless. Finally, *heel-digging feet* depict a person with too much determination and at the same time a false sense of security. The heel-digger often has a deep sense of fear and instability that he compensates for by this determined stance. These five foot types should give you an idea of how to evaluate shape.

If you have difficulty understanding how so much can be said on the basis of your feet, it might help to realize that when you clutch your feet or dig in your heels, you typically do this for a reason. Also, your feet do not act in isolation. For example, a tight jaw, constricted chest, tense hamstrings, and locked knees often accompany heel-digging. It is a total body pattern that is partially identified through the feet. You will not find a lively, energetic body on top of dead, leaden feet. Identifying the way your feet are shaped and the way they work can cause you to use them differently. And as the movements of your feet change, so do the movements of your body, *and* so will your psychology shift.

Legs (or Mobilizers)

Legs are less complex than feet with only three major bones and the patella (or knee cap). There are thirty-eight muscles that either originate or end in the leg. Sixteen of these muscles operate the thigh, nine make the lower leg move, and thirteen originate in the lower leg and connect somewhere in the foot.

In our psychoanatomical dictionary, legs are called *mobilizers* because they help you move around. They also stabilize you and keep you in touch with reality. The thighs provide strength for movement and are related to feelings of independence. The lower legs have more to do with connecting you to your feet and thereby influence the quality of your movements. Lower legs elevate you by flexing the feet, and in this sense represent your strivings.[27] Overall, leg muscles allow you to move forward or backward and from side to side. They permit you to go up and down, to leap and creep. They represent psychological issues of determination and independence, support and fear, striving and letting go.

Leg strength has a lot to do with feelings of determination and independence. If your legs are weak, you feel dependent and tentative in your movements. You may compensate by overusing other areas of the body, such as upper body functions of control, aggression, and intellectual manipulation. If your legs are overly developed, you show determination to a fault. You may be compulsive and have difficulty giving in. If your legs are tight and rigid, movements are intense but awkward. You may be erratic and unfocused in your behavior. Legs that are highly flexible but weak are like rubber bands with no supporting strength. The legs simply can't carry the body. Feelings of anxiety or being stuck may prevail.[28]

There are other variations of leg types, depending on which muscles are developed and the nature of this development (for example, short strong muscles vs. long strong ones). To complete the analysis of legs, however, we have to consider something else: the joints. Ankles and knees are critical elements in body analysis, so let's look at them for a moment.

Dychtwald called the joints *psychosomatic crossroads* to convey the idea that joints permit emotions and psychological processes to move more or less readily from one area of the body to another.[29] Joints are controlled by muscles and tendonous connections so that, as muscles become locked in tension, so too does your ability to be flexible.

The ankle joint provides flexibility to the foot and enables you to change directions, to elevate yourself, to move delicately or aggressively. When ankles are weak, energy flow from feet to legs or legs to feet is impeded. It is thought that injuries to the ankle represent psychological conflicts of pride, of progress or resistance to progress.[30]

Knees give you flexibility in getting around and they transmit feelings of stability from your feet and lower legs to the upper parts of the body. Under emotional strain knees become susceptible to injury. They give in, they fail to support you. They can also become locked and inflexible, thereby cutting off feelings, particularly those of support and groundedness. Anxiety and feelings of separation are often the result.

The Pelvic Region (or Action Center)

The pelvic region serves many functions, not the least of which is to bring about the connection between lower and upper body, between animal and social functions. The pelvic region has to do with your sexual image as well as your way of relating to others. It also has bearing on how you contain or express your life energy. When experts talk about moving "from your center," they are saying that proper body movement should originate from your pelvic region. Depending on philosophical or psychological leanings, the pelvic region can be seen as the center of power, energy, or sexuality. Anatomically, its location often coincides with your center of gravity. Although there is no easy way to capture its importance, our psychoanatomical label, the *action center*, signifies some of its functions.

Muscles in this region confirm its centrality to integrated human behavior. Some pelvic muscles connect to the upper body and others to the lower body. And then there are muscles that relate primarily to sexual, reproductive, and eliminative functions.

Theorists from Freud to Lowen had much to say about the pelvic region and how early life experience creates chronic tensions in this area. Anxieties around toilet training or genital expression are instilled early in life. The psychological character that forms from these experiences often has a psychoanatomical label such as "anal personality" or "phallic personality."

Tension and blockage of energy can be seen in the flexibility a person has in the pelvic region and in the musculature of the buttocks. When you watch someone move, how free are the hips? Are they rigidly held in place? Do they move naturally and rhythmically? Or do they move so freely that they almost seem disconnected from the rest of the body?

One way of diagnosing chronic tensions in the pelvic area is to examine how your pelvis is held. Is it cocked to the back so that the genital region is held back and muscles of the lower back are shortened? (Imagine the classic Playboy bunny pose.) Dychtwald indicates that this posture represents a kind of sexual overcharge, where feelings are held in check and there is a fear of letting go. Concomitant with this posture is a life attitude of unassertiveness and an inability to fully express needs.[31]

What about when the pelvis is curled under, causing the buttocks to flatten and the genitals to press forward? According to Dychtwald, this posture represents a constricted life attitude where emphasis is on achievement, where the feeling of energy from the legs is cut off and life is directed more from the head than from the emotions.[32] With energy from the legs being cut off, the legs are often either rigid or undeveloped. This position, with the buttocks tucked under, resembles a dog with his tail between his legs. There is a fear of aggression from behind and an attitude of appeasement rather than confrontation.

The pelvic region does not function in isolation. For example, when the pelvis is curled backward, back muscles are shortened, the abdomen is expanded, and the legs become overly developed. When the pelvis is curled forward, the buttocks muscles may be squeezed together, suggesting a tight and controlling approach to life. Feelings are controlled and the person may have difficulty giving in and taking in.

Abdominal Region (or The Emotion Center)

The abdomen is one of the most unprotected and vulnerable areas of the body. Vital organs, including the liver, stomach, and intestines, have only muscle and skin as protective coverings. The rib cage protects heart and lungs but not these other organs. This region is given the psychoanatomical label of the *emotion center* because it has so much to do with emotional experience. We often talk about not being able to "stomach" something or getting hit in the "gut." And when we are emotionally upset, we may report this as stomach upset. We stuff food into our bodies to keep emotions down. We clutch our stomachs when we hear a story that evokes strong emotion. And we curl up in a ball, protecting the abdominal region, when we are sad or hurt.

How can you diagnose this region? No doubt you have seen abdomens that look soft and all too vulnerable—young children are good examples. They often have protruding stomachs, suggesting they relate to reality with their feeling centers in the lead. (For contrast, you might picture an adult with his head in the lead as he goes through life.) You have also seen overly large abdominal regions that suggest the person may be stuffing too much emotion (and food, too) into this area. If you recall the earlier discussion of endomorphs, you might remember how the obese endomorph is gluttonous as a way of fending off feelings of isolation and helplessness. When the abdominal region is fat and weak, you experience a kind of helplessness in dealing with your emotions. You have little emotional control and you feel vulnerable. At the opposite end, you have seen abdomens that are rigidly protected with washboard musculature guarding the emotions from unwanted intrusion. The mesomorph would illustrate this pattern with his insensitivity to feelings and emotional concerns.

In response to the question, "How do I lose weight around my belly?" a yoga teacher told her student that when she was psychologically ready to let go of her emotions, she would lose weight around her waist. The basis for this assertion derives from the fact that your emotional stance toward the world is reflected by your abdominal structure. If you consider how you sit, how you stand, how you hold your body, you will find your stomach muscles called into play more or less. You may understand how you "stomach" your reality.

The lower back is related to the abdominal region. If the abdominal muscles are weak, the back has to do more than its share of work. If the muscles that keep the spine erect are contracted, the pelvis curls back, causing a pull on the stomach that lengthens and expands the abdominal region. Oftentimes, when a person suffers from lower back pain, doctors prescribe exercises to release tension in the lower back *and* strengthen abdominal muscles.

Lowen proposed a rationale for lower back pain that goes like this: The back acts as a mediator between psychological issues of the upper body and those of the lower body. From the upper body come demands of authority, duty, guilt, and the burdens of life. From below come feelings of support, sexuality, self-control, and stability. The lower back is caught in a maelstrom of conflict, passion, and psychosomatic struggle.[33] In such a view, is it so surprising that many people carry tension and stress in the lower back?

Lower back tension has also been used as a barometer of how compulsive or impulsive you are. People who are extremely compulsive have tight lower back muscles, whereas impulsive people have flexible lower backs. One diagnostic test is to try to touch your toes without strain and without bending your knees. The more readily your lower back yields and allows the torso to bend forward, the less compulsive you are. If the body just flops forward with no resistance from the muscles along the back, this would suggest more of an impulsive personality.[34] (Anatomically, we should note that this diagnostic test also calls into play muscles along the back of the legs. In this sense, the diagnosis really involves the whole body and not just one muscle group.)

We need to look at one more muscle to complete the discussion of the abdominal region. The *diaphragm* is a large dome-shaped muscle that rests below the lungs and above the stomach. It cannot be observed from the surface of the body. However, its psychological function is paramount. The diaphragm is essential to breathing and, therefore, a rigid or tense diaphragm will impede respiration. Looked at from another angle, if you think of energy flowing up and down the body, the diaphragm serves as a gateway allowing feelings to come and go. As you breathe in, the diaphragm contracts—as you breathe out, it relaxes. As you allow emotions to be expressed, you do so through your breath. The diaphragm affects breathing, and in so doing it regulates feelings.[35]

Breathing is critical to emotional management and the diaphragm is without question the principle muscle involved in breathing. When the diaphragm is free from chronic tension, energy flows freely. When it is tight and constricted, there is a limitation of feelings and energy. The diaphragm becomes rigid partly in defense against feelings we don't want, against emotions we may be afraid to experience.

You may ask, "How do I work on this muscle that I can't see?" Or, "How do I even know whether I need to work on it?" If you have breathing problems that are not disease related, if you have a habit of taking shallow breaths, if your abdomen barely moves when you inspire, if you feel an emotional blockage in your chest, you probably have an indication of tension in the diaphragm. As a cue to cure, you have to relearn how to use the diaphragm. It's a muscle that, like any other muscle, can be developed. The way it develops is through use. And this means full diaphragmatic breathing. And it matters little whether you develop this muscle through something like yoga breathing or the full breathing that often accompanies solid aerobic workouts.

The Chest (or Amplifier)

What function does the chest serve? It is the part of the body that focuses feelings, that amplifies and shapes them. Therefore, we call it the *amplifier*. The chest muscles and rib cage form a protective covering for heart and lungs. Expansion of the lungs within the rib cage is more or less facilitated by the density and flexibility of this covering. Chronic muscular tension in the chest decreases the capacity of the lungs and also serves to promote anxious feelings. Anxiety, which underlies so many psychological difficulties, is affected by breathing irregularities.

Armoring the chest through overdevelopment may serve the function of protecting the heart and our "heartfelt" emotions. Muscular armoring that might result from body building guards us against emotional pain, but it also blocks the experience of emotional warmth and nourishment.

According to Dychtwald, a wide range of emotions are focused and amplified in a freely functioning chest, but when the chest is blocked, certain emotions in particular tend to get stuck in this region. These are the tender feelings of sadness, sorrow, longing, grief, and depression. Because the heart is on the left side, it is typical that more armoring or tension is found on the left than on the right side of the chest.[36]

When the chest is chronically tense, the pectoral muscles are usually underdeveloped and a minimum amount of energy and feeling flows through this region. If you were to exhale fully and hold the chest in contraction after you exhaled, you would have an idea of what this posture is like. Then try breathing while contracting your chest muscles. It is difficult to sustain strong emotion with this posture, to experience passion or to feel aggression. In fact, a person with a contracted chest is more prone to depression than to anything else. Action will be based on fear and feelings of inferiority.

At the opposite extreme are people with chests that look inflated. It would be like taking a deep breath, fully expanding your chest, and holding it. Emotions tend to be overblown. Aggressive, assertive feelings rule to the detriment of softer, more tender emotions. Toughness and power are conveyed by this posture, but in fact a person with an overly expanded chest is cut off from feelings and is likely to experience chronic anxiety or even hypertension.

Overdeveloped, expanded, or contracted chests are less than ideal for healthy psychological functioning. A balance where the chest muscles permit a free flow of energy through the chest cavity is far more advantageous. By appreciating the extremes you can become more aware of the function of the chest and how armoring it can affect you.

Shoulders, Arms, Hands (or The Manipulators)

The shoulders, arms and hands represent the expressive, active dimensions of personality. Shoulders carry the burdens of living, whether they are real or imagined, and arms and hands reach for the world—they hold, embrace, carry, and sometimes refuse it. As a group these parts have to do with control and expression and, therefore, are labeled the *manipulators.*

Shoulders are relatively easy to diagnose; their varied shapes are evident upon inspection. When they are round or bowed, they tell us the person may be feeling the "weight of the world." People with these shoulders may take on more responsibility than they can handle. If you see someone with raised shoulders, you might suspect she has lived a life filled with fear, and perhaps paranoia. Shoulders that hunch forward represent a life position of self-protection, as if the shoulders are rounding forward to protect the heart, to ward off emotional pain. When the shoulders are pulled back, it is as if the person is holding back feelings such as anger and hatred. You may also see people with square shoulders who approach life with self-assurance and who shoulder their responsibilities.

Arms and hands provide the means by which we express emotion, by which we transmit action to the environment. We hold, we take, we give, we reach, we caress, we push, we shove, we stroke, we feel, we accept, we reject. According to Dychtwald, rigid or tight arms display an attitude of clutching and grasping, an inconsistency in the ability to hold on, to control. The arms tire and let go, and then they reach out again, almost in desperation. Fat, underdeveloped arms are sluggish and lacking in energy. They are heavy with their own weight so that when the person does reach out, the action is too much for the arms to handle. Arms that are overdeveloped have a surplus of strength, resulting in transactions that lack grace and sensitivity; the world is controlled by force rather than cooperation.[37]

To understand your arms, you need to be aware of what they look like, how strong they feel, how adequately muscled they are for carrying out the transactions in your life. How gracefully do they move and how easily does energy flow from the rest of your body into your arms? You need to contrast the right with the left. You might study where energy gets blocked. It might be that as one set of muscles extend the arm in reaching out, the antagonistic group resists the movement so that your arm becomes frozen in midstream. Think of a time, for example, when you hesitantly extended your hand in a handshake, only to find it frozen in a conflicted greeting. You might compare the upper arm with the forearm and hand to detect whether the strength in the upper arm has adequate means in the forearm and hand for its expression.

In talking about shoulders and arms, we have to include some discussion of the upper back. The upper back is partially represented by the shoulder girdle, including the shoulder blades, but also incorporates the thoracic region of the spine. Emotions that are housed or represented in the back are usually ones that we have conflicts about express-ing, emotions that may not be as socially acceptable as others. For this reason, feelings of anger, rage, or even hatred get deposited in the upper back, and if this area is chronically constricted, a great deal of the individual's energy gets diverted to keep these strong emotions in check.

The Neck (or Translator)

As feelings seek release in verbal expression, the neck becomes involved. Emotions passing from the abdominal region through the chest are translated into words and sounds as they move through the neck. When the brain sends communications to the rest of the body, these messages move through the neck. The neck must mediate be-tween the thought center and the feeling center of the body and is given the label of *translator*.

When you are unwilling to let your feelings out, to make public your emotions, you swallow, you eat, you keep them down. When you want to keep out some thought or idea, you refuse to swallow, to allow it to affect your feelings. Conflicts around emotional expression often find themselves caught in your throat. You get a "pain in the neck" when you are exposed to situations you can't confront directly. Chronic neck ten-sion can be your way of blocking emotions from coming out, as in the case of a person with a stout, bull neck who rigorously denies himself access to his emotional world. Overly weak necks not only have difficulty supporting the weight of the head, but also do little to prevent the unfiltered, unchecked impulsive expression of virtually any and all emo-tions.[38]

The Head (or Thought Center)

Much has been written about the functions of the head, the sen-sory organs located there, and the intellectual character of this region. It has often been said that eyes are "windows to the soul" and more eso-teric opinions include views about the nose as a symbol of sexuality and power, about the mouth as the locus of oral eroticism, and about the jaw as the residence of pride, power, and control. For our purposes, atten-tion to this region will be limited.

In sports and exercise, vision and hearing become more or less involved. You may need to be constantly alert and watchful during rac-quet games, whereas you need to be far less vigilant when you are out running through the park. Although you may grit your teeth in various sports, you don't work directly on the jaw muscles as you do when you bite and chew. And an acute sense of smell is rarely an asset on the sports field.

You may hold a great deal of facial tension throughout your day and find opportunities for its release through recreational exercise and sports pursuits. Depending on the nature of the activity, however, you may continue to employ cognitive, rational decision-making powers of the *thought center*, or you may switch to an emotional lead. As one runner said, "I don't like any activity where I have to think too much . . . I do enough of that all day long!"

Perhaps the most critical diagnosis to make of the head region derives from how much you are locked in your head or how much your face portrays an image of tension. If you find it difficult to escape the inner world of thought and analysis, you are likely to see contractions in facial muscles—around the eyes and particularly in the forehead. Eventually, these become ingrained in lines and wrinkles of the face. And if this is the case, you should have some idea about what is needed; in essence, to move away from leisure pursuits that occupy you in the same mental patterns and to move toward activities that allow you to take the lead from your emotional center or from a more focused, almost meditative mental attitude.

Completing Your Diagnosis

This is a lot of information to digest. You might want to go back over the chapter, piece by piece. As you do so, use the body diagrams provided for your analysis (Figure 6.3). There is a diagram for the front of your body and one for the back. What you need to do is to fill in descriptions of each area according to what you have observed in your body. We have included the psychoanatomical labels as a reminder of the psychological issues represented in each region. Your task will be to evaluate according to the three ratings of *strength, flexibility,* and *shape.* And then you will need to look at the splits: the differences between top and bottom, right and left, and front and back. You might want to note any other observations about your body that distinguish it, locating these observations by region. For example, you might note that when you examine your body sideways, your head always appears to be in the lead.

The analysis of muscle strengths and functioning will help you know where you need to work. Since different sports and exercise programs emphasize development of different areas of the body, you will be able to find an appropriate match, once again working on the principle of "opposites" or developing areas of weakness rather than further developing your strengths. It may be that your whole body needs toning or that you are too muscle-bound and may need to work on flexibility. We will help you translate your body diagnosis into action strategies later on. For now, be as thorough as possible in your assessments. When in doubt, you might want to ask a friend whom you consider a reliable observer.

7

How Your Movements Reveal Your Personality

> If we accept that the way people sit, walk and make gestures
> has any relevance to how they are thinking and feeling, then it
> is only a short step towards the idea that a more subtle and
> deep analysis of the composition of the movement can lead
> towards a greater understanding of the personality.
>
> *Marion North*[1]

Bodies in Motion

We have just seen how body structure reveals personality traits. Now let us look at what movement can tell us. Imagine an invisible man had a camera focused on you from the moment you got out of bed in the morning until you went to sleep at night—for an entire month. You never saw the man or the camera, in fact, until this moment you were completely unaware you were being filmed.

Aside from wanting a sizable percentage of royalties from whatever this invisible Peeping Tom produces, what do you think you would discover about yourself from watching these films? Would you expect to find particular patterns in your actions, or do you think your motions would differ from day to day?

Well, if you answered that a lot of your movement patterns would look the same from day to day, you would be right. Not only would the way you brush your teeth look the same, but your *movement style* in so many activities would have the same qualities.

Most of us are aware of our unique movement patterns. Friends may have commented on the way we gesture when we talk, or we may have learned something about the way we walk from a shoe salesman who remarked about how we wear out shoes. We may also be attuned to our repetitive rituals of daily life: the way we roll out of bed, our bathroom ceremonies, and other things we do before leaving the house each day.

What we may be less aware of are the more microscopic patterns in our action sequences: the way we move our bodies, the speed of our movements, the delicacy of our actions, our use of the space around us, and so forth. These patterns betray our inner emotions much more so than whether we brush our teeth before or after our morning shower — or is it bath?

Movement Is Communication

Intuitively, we know that what a person says may be far less truthful than what he does. "Actions speak louder than words," as the expression goes. The problem comes when we try to interpret these actions. Spoken language has syntax and grammar; we have, for example, a subject, verb, and object in a sentence. But what about the syntax of our unspoken language?

Scientists who study body language have created systems for understanding gestures and movement. These movement experts refer to their specialty as *kinesics*. Dr. Ray Birdwhistell is credited with naming this field of study in his pioneering book *Introduction to Kinesics*, published in 1952.[2] He believed that all human gestures and movements had meaning and that a skilled observer could decode these imbedded meanings with the aid of a complex syntax of movement.

As the study of kinesics broadened during the 1960s and 1970s, popular accounts of movement and body language began appearing in local bookstores. From the sociological end we had books like Erving Goffman's *Interaction Ritual*[3] and *Behavior in Public Places*.[4] The popularized anthropology angle could be found in Desmond Morris' *The Naked Ape*,[5] *Manwatching*,[6] and more recently *Bodywatching*.[7] Pop psych had its representatives in authors like Julius Fast *(Body Language)*,[8] and

Bruce Vaughan *(Body Talk).*[9] These books were entertaining and informative, but they fell short of giving us a coherent system for interpreting
movement.

Instead, they created new pastimes like "body reading at happy
hour" and they poked fun at our curious habits, such as staring at the
floor indicator as soon as we step into an elevator. But the individual got
lost in the analysis. Somehow we were all alike. We all crossed our arms,
tilted our heads, or read the elevator's floor indicators for the same
reasons.

Movement Myopia

A fascinating footnote to the scientific study of movement is revealed in the bibliographies of body language, or movement analysis,
texts. It comes under the category of "the right hand not knowing what
the left hand is doing." Rarely do we find mention in the works of
psychologists, sociologists, or anthropologists of the contributions of
Rudolph Laban and his followers in dance/movement therapy.

You are probably asking, "Who is Rudolph Laban and what is
dance/movement therapy?" Briefly, Laban was a dance choreographer
who invented a system of analyzing and recording movement. And
dance/movement therapists are people who use movement as a tool to
promote health and psychological well-being.

Going back to the question of why Laban's work was ignored, the
most likely answer is sheer ignorance. What respected academician
would think to look to the writings of dancers to find a scientifically
respectable system for understanding movement? After all, dancers
dance—they don't write. Wrong!

While most social scientists studied movement out of interest in
communication, dancers started more purely: they were interested in
movement itself. Of course, they believed that dance was a form of
communication, but their primary concern was movement, not movement as an appendix to something else, like verbal communication.

What did Rudolph Laban do? As a dance choreographer during the
first quarter of this century, Laban recognized the need to describe
movement in a convenient shorthand. In those days, film was expensive
and videotape was not yet available and a struggling young choreographer needed a way of saying, "That's my dance—not yours!" As a first
step, Laban had to develop a vocabulary of movement. Then, he had to
design a practical method of recording his observations. This was a more
direct approach than the social scientist's search for symbolic meaning

in movements and gestures. And, as it turned out, it was a far more useful one.[10]

After Laban developed his vocabulary and recording system (known as Labanotation), a critical connection was made. With his language of movement, Laban began to notice that people had particular movement habits; that is, they preferred certain actions over others. In fact, people could be characterized by their repeated use of certain qualities in their movements and by the absence of others.

Laban and his followers used this information about movement habits in a variety of settings, including the selection of employees and executives in large corporations. More clinical applications also became popular, where dance/movement therapists would diagnose which styles of movement a psychiatric patient preferred and which ones he avoided. Based on this, a therapy session would be designed to help the patient learn new movements to facilitate the healing process.[11]

Let's take an example. A movement therapist notices that a patient usually moves in a slow, heavy manner with arms limply hanging and the body shrinking toward the floor. What kind of diagnosis do you think would fit this patient? If you said, "Depression," you would probably be right.

Now, the usual approach to working with depressed patients is to give them some kind of drug treatment or psychotherapy. In the extreme, they may receive electroconvulsive shock treatment. The movement therapist, however, works with movement, recognizing that the patient has a kind of deficit in his movement repertoire. The treatment would consist of teaching this patient new movement patterns, including ones that are quick, light, and expanded. This would take place in individual or group sessions. As the patient learns to move in a lighter, faster manner, some of the emotional "heaviness" of depression would also lift.

Making the Connection

What does this have to do with exercise? It may seem strange to take this detour to make a point about exercise, but Laban's work and the movement therapist's approach are directly related to our purposes. Let's sum up the rationale for connecting movement analysis to involvement in sports and exercise programs:

First, you have unique movement habits that can be analyzed.

Second, your movement habits are related to your personality.

Third, sports and exercise emphasize particular movement patterns.

Fourth, by emphasizing particular movement patterns, sports and
    exercise reinforce certain personality traits.
Finally, by knowing what your movement habits are, you can select
    fitness programs that will help you reduce or develop spe-
    cific personality characteristics.
That, in brief, is the argument for studying movement patterns and for
trying to identify your preferred styles and movement deficits.

Movement Fundamentals

The body speaks clearly. We just don't know how to interpret what
it is saying. The more educated we are, the more we devalue the language of the body, the more we rely on the spoken word. We then have
to take special courses to help us understand what children and many
street smart people know intuitively: we have to relearn how to separate
words from actions, how to close our ears so we truly sense what a
person is saying.

We have to become more astute observers. This means far more
than "tuning into another person's vibes." It means developing a language and a system for decoding the body's messages. Sure, some people do it naturally, which means they spend years correlating what they
see with what people do. And the result is they seem to instinctively
read people. But it's not instinctive. It comes from trained observation.
If we haven't spent years developing our own observational system, we
can at least rely on guidelines offered by movement experts.

Basic Ideas

Where do we start? What should we look at first? Is everything we
see equally important? Just as in the example of the imaginary camera-
man following you for a month, we know that each person has movement habits that occur over and over. So, if we miss it the first time, we
will be sure to see it again. We also know that there is far too much for us
to take in at any moment in time. There are large movements and small
movements. There is the flutter of an eye and the swing of an arm. It is
impossible to see it all and to know which is most important. We have to
rely on approximations, which are nonetheless quite useful in understanding personality dynamics.

Based on what we know from movement experts, we can draw the
following conclusions about movement patterns:[12]

1. The body is clear in its communications.

2. There is a language that can describe the body's communications.
3. Each person has unique movements that, nonetheless, can be described according to a common movement language.
4. Just as in speech, some people have a broader movement vocabulary than do others. This means some people have more variety in movement.
5. Movement patterns are, by definition, repetitive. If the movement is part of the individual's makeup, we will see it repeatedly.
6. Movement patterns are meaningful: they tell us something about the person's inner life.
7. By observing these repeated or habitual movement patterns, we can identify elements of the individual's personality.

Building Blocks of Analysis

Marion North, a student of Rudolph Laban and head of the Movement and Dance Department at Goldsmith's College, University of London, has given us one of the most complete descriptions of movement analysis in her book, *Personality Assessment Through Movement.*[13] She divided an individual's movement makeup into three broad aspects:

1. How a person uses his body.
2. Where the person moves in the surrounding space.
3. The general style and qualities of the person's movements.

Let's look at each of these components separately.

1. *How do you use your body?* If you were to watch those imaginary silent films of your daily movements, what would you learn about how you use your body? You could readily identify what parts of your body you use the most. It might be that you use the right side of your body more than the left. When you talk, you might gesture entirely with your right hand, while your left hand burrows into your pocket. In your sedentary world, you could be surprised at how little you use certain parts of your body, such as your legs compared to your arms. So, on a global level, you would notice *how much* of your body is involved in particular actions and *which parts* you seem to use the most.

Another aspect of body use is *range of movement.* If you watched yourself on this imaginary film, would you be surprised at how restricted your movements are, or would you observe a relatively full range of movements in bending, stretching, or twisting? You could rate yourself on the range of movement you show for different parts of your body, observing perhaps that you have a lot of flexibility and range with your arms, but that your legs move stiffly.

2. *Where do movements originate in your body?* If you are sitting down and need to stand up, which part of you moves first? And what happens next? As you move toward another person, is your head the first part to move or is it your hips? This is another aspect of how you use your body that provides clues about internal emotional states. Of course, there will be variations from time to time and from one situation to another. You have to look for the consistencies in the way you use your body. Knowing this can help you discover what your underlying personality dynamics might be.

3. *How do you use space?* Imagine you have a small light attached to your head, hands, and feet, and that you photograph your movements in a series of still shots. Would your movements be circular or would they be angular? Would they be small or would they be generous? Would they be contorted or would they be smooth?

Not only could you identify shapes but also directions. Where do you go and where do you avoid? Little children jump up and down, move backwards and forwards, and even roll around on the floor. As an adult you may find you generally move straight ahead, rarely to the side, and never do you roll around. While you may think it inappropriate to move like a child, recognize that many adult games and sports give you opportunities you may unconsciously crave for acting in just such inappropriate ways. In fact, a number of large corporations have developed "adult play pens" for executives to bounce up and down, do somersaults, and otherwise — through movement — stimulate their creative juices.

What's your movement style?

If you put together how you use your body and where you move in space, you will begin to form an idea of your movement style. You will see shapes in your movements and you will identify patterns. You might notice that many of your movements are strong and quick, or they may be light and slow. You may find that you show a lot of flexibility, so much so that you avoid being direct.

What do these qualities have to do with personality? Imagine a person who shows a consistent pattern of fast, direct, forceful movements and who never moves with slow, light, flexible qualities. What would you guess about this individual's personality? Do you think she would be passive and easygoing, or aggressive and demanding? If you can't answer right away, keep reading. It will become evident by the time you have finished this chapter.

Think of another person who has a consistent pattern of fast, light, indirect movements. Do you get an image of an anxious, evasive person?

If not, the problem may be one of language, of understanding the vocabulary of movement. We will solve this problem in the next section, where you will learn a basic vocabulary for interpreting movement.

Up to this point, the intention has been to get you thinking about movement in very simple ways, to have you describe what you see, leaving the interpretation for later. According to the model developed by Marion North, we know we can observe the parts of the body you use, where your body moves in space, and such qualities of movement as speed, direction, strength, and shape. In the upcoming section we will take these observations and help you understand what they imply about your approach to life and your personality.

Your Movement Personality

The first step to analyzing personality in your movements is to learn a movement vocabulary. As we do so, we will connect movement patterns and personality style. The special advantage of this vocabulary is that it can be used not only to describe you but also to analyze typical movements of sports and fitness activities. This means you will be able to match your movements to those required by different sports and exercise programs to determine whether you are *reinforcing* (doing more of the same), *balancing* (doing the opposite), or *avoiding* (neglecting certain dimensions) with your exercise program.

Five Movement Analysis Dimensions (MADs)

What is the vocabulary of movement? The system we will use to analyze your movements and those required by sports and exercise programs is based on five dimensions: *force, control, linearity, speed,* and *extension.* As you review each dimension, evaluate yourself by considering your typical style. If you are not sure, ask friends to help you with the assessment. Your style will change from time to time and from situation to situation, but you will notice that you tend to move with certain typical qualities more so than with others. This is what we will designate as your style.

MAD 1: *Force*

Strong ——————————————— Light

Strong	Light
Striding into the room	Tiptoeing through a room
Giving someone a bear hug	A delicate kiss on the cheek

Punching the air	Waving a wand
Waxing a car	Dusting knickknacks
Hitting a baseball	Putting a golf ball two inches
Pounding the desk	Tentatively sitting down

As you read these examples, you should get some appreciation for the movement dimension of force. It has a lot to do with strength and pressure. In extremes it is overpowering or light as a feather. We often identify people based on the force they use to accomplish things. One person may be seen as overbearing while another is hypersensitive. Some people have difficulty doing anything that requires delicate movements, but give them a hammer and the world becomes a nail. Others have problems being forceful. They tiptoe around, hardly disturbing the air as they move.

What if your movements are appropriately forceful, that is, you use just the right amount of pressure or strength to suit the situation? In this case, your movements have a wide range: they cover the spectrum from light to strong, from soft to hard. If this is the way you use force, then you have the capability of being strong and forceful when necessary or light and delicate as the situation demands.

What if you only use light movements? It may be that at most you muster up moderate levels of strength, but you never go stomping around or use extreme force. Then your rating would be more toward the light side. If you ever were to use more force in your actions, it might give you a lot of emotional release. (It might also frighten you.)

What if you use only strong movements? This would be the case if you have difficulty being delicate or resisting the opportunity of giving a stubborn machine a good kick. You might be the type whom downstairs neighbors complain about because you shake the house when you move. You might also be the type that friends intercept when you volunteer to fix something because they know it will end up in pieces.

Caution! Force is not the same as weight. Fat people can be as delicate or indelicate as skinny people. Force involves the flexion and extension of muscles. If you punch something or lightly touch it, you have to contract your muscles, whereas when you slump around, there is a relative absence of strength or lightness—the muscles are not working. It's what we call dead weight. Force is largely missing when someone moves heavily through a room. We often see this when a person is depressed. Movements are heavy, not strong and not light.

Force and Personality. The obvious linkage of force and personality is to the PAD Aggressive/Nonaggressive Style. How a person uses force is a large part of an aggressive or nonaggressive style. We don't want to say that force and aggression are the same, but there is a high correlation. It is hard to imagine a person who tiptoes, moving like a feather and delicately touching life, being a very aggressive person. Conversely, a person who stomps around, smashing things due to the overuse of force, would not be considered a very passive individual.

Your Self-Assessment. Based on the description of force, evaluate yourself. Take into account your predominate use of force. If you feel you use force appropriately, with an ability to be light or moderate or strong, as the situation requires, then you would shade in the entire scale. If you tend to be light only, then shade in that end of the scale. If you tend to be strong only, just shade in that portion. Similarly, if you tend to use moderate to light pressure or strength, then you would shade in both of these portions. Shade in all areas of the scale that characterize your *typical* action style. Use heavier shading for the one area that is most descriptive of your use of force (Figure 7.1).

YOUR FORCE RATING

SHADE ALL PATTERNS TYPICALLY USED. DARKEST SHADING FOR MOST CHARACTERISTIC PATTERN.

STRONG	VERY	STRONG	MODERATE	LIGHT	VERY	**LIGHT**

Figure 7.1

MAD 2: *Control*

Precise ——————————————— Imprecise

Precise	**Imprecise**
A diamond cutter at work	A child tumbling down a hill
Hitting a golf ball	Rock and roll dancing
Threading a needle	Tossing confetti
A military walk	A drunkard's swagger
Painting by the number	A child with finger paints
Taking a photograph	Mixing a salad

Reading these examples will tell you something about *control*. It has a lot to do with being precise and exacting as opposed to being imprecise and perhaps sloppy. Control requires precise muscular movements and a careful attitude. Movements are managed through painstaking effort rather than being allowed to wander or stray. When you think about a child running with abandon or a skiier tumbling down a slope, you have movement samples that are deliberately unmanaged (the child) or unintentionally out of control (the skiier). Both are imprecise. By contrast, a surgeon's movements are exact and precise, requiring great mental effort and muscular control.

The examples may seem to imply that, by nature, certain acts can only be done with precision while others can only be performed haphazardly. This is not the case. Precision is a quality of your movements—it is not inherent in the tasks you perform. Some people fold laundry with great precision, while others create a stack of laundry that looks as if it were just pulled from the dryer. A child throwing a baseball differs considerably in precision from a major league pitcher.

Precision is not just an attitude. A drunk who wishes to walk a straight line cannot do so, no matter how hard he tries. Precision requires mental effort and muscular control. You have to pay attention in order to control your actions. Sure, you can thread a needle by chance, but it might take weeks before you succeed.

Life's tasks demand varying degrees of precision, but even when we are instructed to be precise, there is variation from person to person. An example can be found in the way people complete computerized answer sheets. The instructions tell you to mark your answers between the two dotted lines. If you look at answer sheets from a class of students who read the same instructions, you will be amazed. Some people are habitually sloppy. When they scramble eggs, some of the mix always pours over the edge of the bowl. When they pour coffee, they miss the cup. It appears as if their body parts are moving in different directions all at the same time.

Others are habitually precise, almost compulsively exact, even when it isn't necessary. People like this fold their napkins neatly *after* dinner, move carefully, and touch things with exacting attention. We trust them instinctively with our most delicate possessions and we might even recruit them to remove a cinder from a child's eye.

A person can be working at a job that requires precision but perform it poorly. Of course, such on-the-job movement experience might improve the individual's level of control, but it would be at great expense to the company. On the other hand, a person could be a ditch digger and yet perform the task with great precision.

In evaluating yourself, recognize we have been talking in extremes. You may be a moderate slob or a moderate compulsive. You may only spill the coffee half the time or you may be only moderately exacting and controlled. Another possibility is that your movements are controlled when they need to be and uncontrolled and unmanaged at other times.

Control and Personality. Unlike the movement dimension of force, where there was a neat link with the PAD Aggressive/Nonaggressive Style, control has no easy match-up. Control has some relation to PAD Disciplined/Undisciplined Style in that controlled movements require mental discipline, an attitude of attentive care. Control can also be seen in the PAD Spontaneous/Controlled Style in that spontaneity in movement may appear quite uncontrolled and abandoned while emotional control may come across in movement as precise and exact. We can see another aspect of control in the PAD Risky/Safe Style. A psychological emphasis on safety and caution would no doubt be accompanied by movements that are more controlled and precise. Finally, we see a link between control and PAD Focused/Unfocused Style. When an action is precise, it typically involves a high degree of focus, or single-mindedness. When it is imprecise, attention can wander.

What we are saying is that the movement dimension of control is multifaceted, from a psychological perspective. Improving the precision of your movements will have wide-ranging effects on your personality.

Your Self-Assessment. Your self-assessment on movement control may not be an either/or proposition. You may be more or less controlled and precise in your movements. On the scale, shade in those areas that represent typical or habitual movement preferences. Keep in mind that different life tasks demand different levels of precision. Do you typically do things with too much or too little precision? Are you moderately precise in your style, meaning you don't go overboard and you permit yourself a margin of error (or sloppiness) in your efforts? You may feel that sometimes you are precise and other times just moderately precise — rarely do you see yourself as being imprecise. In this case, you would shade in the *precise* and *moderate* categories. Since *imprecise* is not a typical style, you would not shade it in. Taking all your activities into account, if you have shaded more than one category, give a heavier shading to your predominant movement style (Figure 7.2).

MAD 3: *Linearity*

Linear ——————————— **Non-linear**

Linear	Non-linear
Running to first base	A drunkard's swagger
Hammering a nail	Playing with your hair

YOUR CONTROL RATING

SHADE ALL PATTERNS TYPICALLY USED. DARKEST SHADING FOR MOST CHARACTERISTIC PATTERN.

PRECISE | VERY | PRECISE | MODERATE | IMPRECISE | VERY | **IMPRECISE**

Figure 7.2

Throwing a javelin	Playing ice hockey
A direct handshake	A wave of the hand
Charging into an office	Jumping on a trampoline
Chopping wood	Snuggling on the couch

The adjective *linear* is defined as "relating to, or resembling a line: straight." Implied in a linear movement is progression toward some point or goal. In evaluating movement we want to know whether an action is straight or direct, that is, moving from Point A to Point B without deviation, or whether the action is *non-linear,* that is, flexible and indirect. Non-linear movements take many shapes, including wavy, circular, or even zigzag.

Imagine a sprinter running the 100-meter dash and you see linear motion. If you think of an angry man marching toward a confrontation, you again see straight movement.

Non-linear movements are more evident when you think of people playing soccer or a football player running an interference pattern or a man staggering home after an office party. Hand movements as we trace our way through a maze are also non-linear. Non-linear movements go off in a variety of directions: they are curved and wavy and frequently change direction. These movements may or may not be oriented toward some end point. When someone is non-linear or indirect in speech, we say they are "beating around the bush," meaning they are not getting directly to the point.

If you attached lights to a person's head, arms, and legs and asked that individual to move linearly, you would see straight lines of light and a forward progression of the body. If you now asked that person to move non-linearly, you might see wavy, flexible lines of light, movements to the side, up and down, backward, and perhaps even circular patterns.

Linear movements appear to be going somewhere directly, whereas it is unclear whether the meandering flexible course of non-linear movements are going anywhere in particular, or perhaps whether they are aimless, undirected actions. To clarify, imagine a person stumbling home over a winding rocky road and a tourist gawking and gazing as he wanders aimlessly through a foreign city. Both represent non-linear movements, but in the first case there is a clear goal, while in the second there is an absence of a specific objective.

The distinction between goal-oriented and goal-less non-linear movements may not be something you see right away, but after the fact the relation of action to its goal becomes apparent. Consider a person's hand movements when she is doodling. They may be circular and wavy, resembling those we might use in figure drawing. But there is no clear purpose in doodling, whereas in figure drawing there is a clear purpose. The hand movements in figure drawing may look like doodling movements, but they have a goal or end point.

Why is this distinction relevant? You might think of your early years as a child when you played freely. There was no objective, no end point. You may have run wildly in a field, tumbled down hills, or splashed about in the water. As an adult you might find yourself engaged in goal-less non-linear movements when you play with your hair or sift sand through your fingers while lying on a beach.

As an adult you may feel trapped by the goals you set for yourself — so much so that it is hard to get away from purposeful activity. As John Lennon put it, "Life is what happens while you are busy making plans." The idea of doing nothing, of wandering aimlessly, of simply experiencing without expectations is quite foreign to many people's lives. Depending on what you do for exercise, you may be perpetuating that trapped, purposeful pattern or truly recreating through goal-less physical expressions.

Linearity and Personality. The link between this movement dimension and personality is multifaceted. Linear actions imply an assertive or aggressive stance, such as walking straight toward an adversary without wavering. So, we expect *some* relation between MAD Linearity and PAD Aggressive/Nonaggressive Style. Why we say there would only be some relation is that linear movements are not necessarily aggressive. Think of worshippers filing down the aisle in a church or prisoners being marched down a road. We will find a higher correlation with specific personality traits when we combine all five MAD dimensions. (As a quick example, imagine a movement that is linear and strong. There is a greater chance that this kind of action will correspond to an inner attitude of aggression than one that is linear and light.)

A second personality link is between linearity and PAD Focused/Unfocused Style, in that a linear action is likely to be a focused one, whereas a non-linear one (like wandering through a foreign city) would more likely be unfocused. The relation is imperfect for many reasons. Consider a person walking in his sleep. The movements may be direct, but we could not say the mind is focused. Or imagine a person working on an assembly line whose body has memorized the required linear movement pattern so his mind can wander freely.

A third link is between linearity and the PAD Spontaneous/Controlled Style. Linear movements imply an intentionality of moving from A to B, and thereby resisting the temptation to veer off or to wander. Spontaneous movements may have a creative flavor, a flexibility in motion that moves first in one direction and then in another (non-linear). However, a movement can be direct and still be spontaneous, as when a child rushes toward his mother.

Finally, we can link linearity to the PAD Disciplined/Undisciplined Style. To keep moving directly without wandering requires a certain amount of discipline. One always has the choice of opting out. It may be a costly option, but even prisoners can refuse to walk the line. Therefore, linear actions imply a control of emotions, a harnessing of will. As noted with each of these links, the relation is far from perfect. One of the many contradictory examples can be found in the undisciplined, impulsive act of punching someone in the nose.

Your Self-Assessment. In making your self-assessment on movement linearity, consider one additional twist. Linear movements are straight and to the point—like hitting a nail on the head or walking directly from A to B. Anything other than straight movements are non-linear.

The additional distinction is whether your typical non-linear movements are *simple* or *complex*. What's the difference? It's a matter of degree. In simple non-linear movements, you may have a wave or slight curvature, as in a wave of the hand. Complex non-linear movements are much more intricate. If you have ever seen the extreme shapes and body contortions that are choreographed in many modern dance works, you would have an idea of complex non-linear movements.

What we are getting at is whether your non-linear movements are very simple waverings or very complex and extreme. An example might help. Imagine someone asks you for a favor. A simple non-linear response might be a folding of the arms across the chest and a rounding of the head and shoulders as you consider. A complex non-linear response might be a strong shrugging of the shoulders, rounding of the back, twisting of the head from side to side, and a wringing of the hands.

This distinction between simple and complex non-linear movements gets at how expressive you are with your body and how flexible your body is. If you are not expressive and your body has a limited range of movements, complex non-linear movements are less likely to characterize your style.

On the scale in Figure 7.3, there are three categories: linear, non-linear (simple) and non-linear (complex). Shade in the part or parts of this scale that strongly characterize your movement patterns. Use darker shading for the one category that most strongly represents your movement style.

YOUR DIRECTION RATING

SHADE ALL PATTERNS TYPICALLY USED. DARKEST SHADING FOR MOST CHARACTERISTIC PATTERN.

LINEAR	LINEAR	NONLINEAR SIMPLE	NONLINEAR COMPLEX	NONLINEAR

Figure 7.3

MAD 4: *Speed*

Fast ———————————— Slow

Fast	Slow
Racing	Strolling
Cracking a whip	Stirring soup
Pitching a ball	A yoga stretch
A darting glance	A sleepy yawn
An aggressive push	A gentle caress
Casting a fishing line	Picking up a sleeping baby

Speed is often a relative matter. For example, if you are jogging along the road and someone passes you, you might say that person is fast, but, in turn, as that person is passed by a faster runner, she may label herself as slow and the other as fast. Speed can also be measured quantitatively on something like a stopwatch. This allows both absolute and relative definitions of speed.

Because of the relative definition of speed, we have to guard against labeling certain actions as inherently fast or slow. Pitching a ball may be defined as inherently fast, yet we know there are fast pitches and slow pitches, as well as fast pitchers and slow pitchers!

Two people doing housework may move at very different paces. One may buzz from room to room like the "white tornado," while the other seems to be moving through jello. We don't want to say that fast is better because many times it is just the opposite.

However, we often have a concept of the appropriate speed for an action, such as picking up a sleeping baby. When someone exceeds this expected speed, we say the movement is fast, or if they move less quickly than expected, we say it is slow.

We want you to consider your movement pacing. Of course, you have some variation in speed throughout the day, but when you compare yourself to others, you may notice that you move relatively faster or slower, or you may move faster or slower than some internalized set of norms you developed in life. At some point, you may have gotten feedback about being "real speedy," or you may have been described as a "slow poke."

Speed and Personality. The dimension of speed is best thought of in conjunction with other MAD factors. For example, fast + linear- + strong movements are likely to be assertive or aggressive in nature, while slow + non-linear + light would imply more uncertainty and tentativeness in a person's inner emotional world.

By itself speed can be linked to the PAD Focused/Unfocused Style in that fast movements should involve more concentration. Even impulsive actions (which are likely to be fast) rivet our attention in the moment. Although many slow movements require our attention, as in taking a cinder out of someone's eye, the slower the movement, the greater the possibility that the mind will stray. This is why meditation training is so difficult. It takes a long time and lots of practice to quiet the mind, to make it concentrate. We do this more naturally with fast movements because the information processing requirements of the situation demand it.

Speed can also be related to the PAD Spontaneous/Controlled Style. There is a greater chance that quick actions are spontaneous or even impulsive. Slow movements often require control, as in a surgeon's slow, deliberate moves. Fast movements can also involve extreme control, as in a professional golfer's swing. But if we look a little closer, we can see how slight distractions, emotional influences of one sort or another, bring an undesired spontaneous dimension into these fast movements. To be fast and precise takes extreme mental concentration and control. On the other side, a slow movement may not be very controlled emotionally, as when a fatigued person shuffles from one place to another.

There is an element of speed in many aggressive actions (PAD Aggressive/Nonaggressive Style). We often associate quick action with a kind of assertiveness or even aggressiveness, as when one person hits another. Slowness in motion may imply a lack of certainty or perhaps an emotional passivity. When there is a giveaway sale at a local department store, we see a lot of speed in the movements of people pushing through the doors at opening time.

There is also a risky component to speed (PAD Risky/Safe Style). The faster the action, the less control we have and the more likely we are to make mistakes. Bear in mind that certain actions can only be performed quickly; a slower pace means failure, for example, in a broad jump or when hitting a baseball. A downhill skier who always goes after faster times increases the chances of error and injury. A quick change of lanes while driving may result in collision. To the contrary, the ability to move quickly can be life saving. If a car is hurtling out of control and you do not have the speed to get out of its way, you might not survive. In terms of personality inclinations, the issue is whether you choose to move quickly because you enjoy the thrill, even when such levels of speed are unnecessary.

By pointing out the linkages of speed to personality, you can see the intricate structure of movement and personality. It may at times seem confusing, particularly if you try to make a one-to-one comparison between a MAD movement factor and a PAD personality factor. It's just not that simple. If it were, you would have read about it long before this.

Your Self-Assessment. How fast or slow are your typical movements? To answer, there are two comparisons you can make. The first is to compare yourself to other people doing the same kinds of things. If you think about times you were doing a job like washing dishes, how did your speed compare to others'? (Don't worry about the precision of your work — think only about the speed.)

The second comparison comes out of norms or standard times for tasks. We grow up with a pretty good idea about how quickly or slowly certain things should be done. Are you always faster or slower than the norm?

The scale in Figure 7.4 presents five possibilities. Consider your typical speed in moving through life. If you have great variability, you may need to shade in the whole scale. If you only have one typical speed, then shade in that area. If you shade in more than one area because you think you typically move at different paces, sometimes very slowly, sometimes very fast, depending on what you are doing, give a darker shading to your predominant style.

YOUR SPEED RATING

SHADE ALL PATTERNS TYPICALLY USED. DARKEST SHADING FOR MOST CHARACTERISTIC PATTERN.

FAST	VERY	FAST	MODERATE	SLOW	VERY	SLOW

Figure 7.4

MAD 5: *Extension*

Extended ———————————— Contracted

Extended	Contracted
Stretching in the morning	Sitting curled up in a chair
Reaching for the ceiling	Huddling against the cold
Jumping to catch a fly ball	Defending your body in boxing
Walking with uplifted spirit	Walking with the weight of the world
Pushing something away	Pulling something toward you
Leaping for joy	Bound up with anger

This final movement factor is represented in the actions of stretching, as in a wide yawn or yoga movement, and contracting, as in the posture of a cringing child or a person tense with anger. With an extended movement the muscles stretch into the surrounding space. The body takes up as much room as it can. Oftentimes when you feel good about yourself, your body expands — you seem to swell up. You feel taller and your arms reach out with graceful extension.

A contracted movement comes with muscular tightness, as when you wrap your arms around yourself to fend off the cold or some unpleasant emotion. When you feel crushed by life, your body contracts — it sinks and becomes smaller. You feel weighted down and your shoulders sag. Contracted movements also occur when you pull something toward you, for example, clutching a blanket or bringing food to your mouth.

The curious aspect of extension and contraction is that some people are more comfortable reaching out or extending into the world. Others are more comfortable with contracted movements. You see this in such simple acts as handshakes, where some people reach way out toward the other, fully extending the arm in a gesture of greeting, and others barely move the arm from the body, keeping it contracted in what seems a halfhearted gesture.

This preference for movement can also be found in such daily actions as taking a jar from a high shelf. Some people get a stepping stool and crawl up on it to obtain the jar, and others reach up on their toes and extend to the tips of their fingers to grasp the jar.

There are people whose range of movement is closely confined to their bodies. Arms rarely reach out. They walk as if their bodies were compressed by the force of gravity. Others stretch and reach. They stride into a room and use expansive gestures of arms and hands.

Extension and Personality. Create an image of a woman who typically moves with extended gestures, who strides when she walks, who reaches out for a handshake, and who seems taller than she really is. Now, create the opposing image of a woman whose body seems compressed, whose movements stay close to her body and whose steps are short. What personality traits might correspond to these two types?

The woman with extended movements expresses more self-confidence, more assurance, and is probably more open and sociable. In contrast, we might assume that the woman with contracted gestures and movements is more controlled, less self-assured, and perhaps more introverted. These would be reasonable assumptions based on what we know about the correspondence of movement patterns and personality.

There is a connection between MAD Expansion and PAD Aggressive/Nonaggressive Style because assertive behavior requires extending into the environment, "reaching for the brass ring," and making your presence known instead of shriveling up in a corner.

There is also a relation with PAD Social/Nonsocial Style. People who reach out for others, who move with expanded gestures, are likely to be perceived as more open and approachable. When we move with compressed gestures, keeping ourselves closely compacted, we convey a fearful attitude, or at least a closed posture toward others.

There is a tie with the PAD Risky/Safe Style, again for the reason that with open, expanded movements, we appear more willing to risk ourselves rather than remain hidden or protected. This becomes even clearer when we think of extended movements in sports. For example, imagine a skier extending himself to the limit or a runner in full stride racing down a hill. The chance of mishap is greater—the risks of being overextended are real.

Finally, expansion is related to PAD Spontaneous/Controlled Style. The more controlled the person is, the more chance there is that the effort will be contracted. Spontaneous experiences often involve a release of tension, a leaping into life, as when long-lost lovers rush into each other's arms.

Your Self-Assessment. There are five categories listed on the scale. *Very Extended* means that your typical movements and gestures are full, reaching far into the space around your body. It means walking very tall, gesturing very widely, reaching to the limit. *Extended* is less extreme, but it does involve movements that lift and rise, extend and reach. *Moderate* describes movements that are neutral—they are neither extended nor contracted. Your body is not lifting up, nor is it compressed down. Your gestures are open but they tend not to extend beyond the length of your limbs. In a sense, your movements are contained within the anatomical dimensions of your body, whereas extended movements go beyond these dimensions and contracted movements are more restricted. *Contracted,* as we just noted, means that movements are restricted, the arm moves less than its anatomical length, the stride is shortened, the body compresses toward the ground. Finally, *Very Contracted* is an extreme of being pulled in toward yourself, of gesturing with limited movement, of keeping your limbs close to the body in various movements.

When you snuggle up with someone, your body is contracted, but unless you typically move through life with this same level of contraction, you would not shade in this area of the scale. Only shade in those areas that represent typical or habitual movement styles. If you shade in more than one category, use darker shading for the one category that represents your predominant movement style (Figure 7.5).

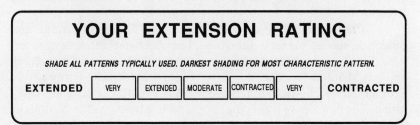

Figure 7.5

Your MAD Graph

What you need to do now is transfer the evaluations of your individual movement dimensions to the graph in Figure 7.6. Be sure to transfer all the shadings and especially make sure to note your predominant style on each MAD factor with a darker shading.

YOUR MADS GRAPH

TRANSFER YOUR INDIVIDUAL MADS RATINGS TO THIS GRAPH.

STRONG	VERY	STRONG	MODERATE	LIGHT	VERY	**LIGHT**
PRECISE	VERY	PRECISE	MODERATE	IMPRECISE	VERY	**IMPRECISE**
LINEAR	LINEAR		NONLINEAR SIMPLE	NONLINEAR COMPLEX		**NONLINEAR**
FAST	VERY	FAST	MODERATE	SLOW	VERY	**SLOW**
EXTENDED	VERY	EXTENDED	MODERATE	CONTRACTED	VERY	**CONTRACTED**

Figure 7.6

How to Interpret Your Graph

When interpreting your graph, there are two considerations to pay attention to:

1. *The Range of Evaluations on Each MAD Factor:* The more categories you shaded on each dimension, the wider your movement repertoire. Ideally, you would describe your movements with each category on each MAD factor; that is, you would have shaded the entire graph. This would mean that your movements are unrestricted and highly varied. The chances of this being the case are extremely slim. Most of us have some restrictions in our movement patterns. We prefer to move one way more than another.

By looking at the areas you left blank, you will have an idea of deficits in your movement repertoire. Some of these so-called deficits may not be very important for how you live. So what if you don't typically move very fast or in a very contracted fashion? It may not be relevant to your lifestyle. However, you should at least consider whether you could move very fast if the need arose.

Wherever there is a blank or unshaded area on the graph, give some consideration to what this means and whether, in some situation or another, it might represent a potential problem.

2. *Your Predominant Styles:* Looking at the five darkest shadings (one for each MAD factor), you have a characterization of your movement profile. Take the five descriptions that you have darkened and write them in the spaces provided.

FORCE   **+ CONTROL**   **+ LINEARITY**   **+ SPEED**   **+ EXTENSION**

_____ + _____ + _____ + _____ + _____

Given the personality correlates of each of these movement factors (summarized in Table 7.1), how would you describe yourself? If you remember, we hedged on many of the personality links when we described the MAD factors individually. But now that you have the whole profile, we have stronger evidence of the link. For example, we said that an aggressive or assertive personality trait went along with the movement styles of being extended, fast, strong, and linear. If you have all four of these words listed above, the chances of your being aggressive or assertive in your personality approach is much higher than if you only have one or two of them listed. As you might imagine, a strong movement style constitutes a critical element in the evaluation of aggressiveness.

Let's take another example. Imagine the following combination:

light + precise + non-linear + fast + extended

Does anything come to mind? You might be painting a picture of a person who moves with soft, fluid motions that extend into the world, that are exact and swift. A dancer? An actress? A hair stylist? A thief? Perhaps any of these. We might experience this person's mental concentration *(precise)* and yet be aware of a certain kind of freedom she possesses *(non-linear, extended)*. The lightness of movements may tend to erase our fears, and perhaps keep us off guard. Speed coupled with precision keeps us watching, especially as the movements show range and flexibility *(extended, non-linear)*.

Movement analysis creates images that help us form personality assessments. If we change one word in the above depiction, the whole image changes, and so too the personality implications. Let's try by changing *non-linear* to *linear*:

light + precise + linear + fast + extended

Quick, straight, precise action—with a delicate touch. A surgeon? A gourmet chef? A grocery checker? An office manager? A champion dart thrower? Any of these might fit. We see a person who extends into the surrounding space, who is fast and light in movements, and who is precisely controlled. There is a kind of assertiveness about this person, but the absence of strong movements makes it difficult for us to say she is aggressive.

Table 7.1
Summary of Personality (PADs) and Movement (MADs) Relationships

FORCE	CONTROL	LINEARITY	SPEED	EXTENSION
Strong	**Precise**	**Linear**	**Fast**	**Extended**
aggressive	controlled	focused	risky	social
assertive	disciplined	controlled	spontaneous	risky
	safe	disciplined	aggressive	spontaneous
	focused	aggressive	assertive	aggressive
		assertive	focused	assertive
Light	**Imprecise**	**Non-Linear**	**Slow**	**Contracted**
nonaggressive	spontaneous	unfocused	safe	nonsocial
passive	undisciplined	spontaneous	controlled	safe
	risky	undisciplined	nonaggressive	controlled
	unfocused	nonaggressive	passive	nonaggressive
		passive	unfocused	passive

PADs and MADs

The implications of movement assessments go beyond the seven PADs factors. PADs and MADs measures are not just overlapping and redundant. Each set contains unique information about who you are and how you function. As you review your movement assessments, consider what else might be implied by the way you typically move.

In the next chapter, we will evaluate different sports and exercise programs according to personality requirements, body structure demands, and movement patterns. Then, you can relate your own patterns to an activity's and begin to appreciate why certain fitness regimes will be far better for your development than will others.

8

A New Classification of Sports and Fitness Programs

Overview

At last! This is what you have been waiting for: the fitness activity profiles.

When we put together all the ideas about personality dynamics, body analysis, and movement, we have a fairly complete system for classifying any fitness activity or sport. Because we are mostly interested in the more popular fitness activities, we will examine in detail twelve fitness options and make brief commentaries about some other activities that are worth considering.

The fitness options we will review are:

RUNNING	DANCE
WALKING	AEROBICS
SWIMMING	RACQUET GAMES
BODY BUILDING	YOGA
CYCLING	GOLF
MARTIAL ARTS	SKIING

In each of these options are subcategories that need to be analyzed to a greater or lesser degree, depending on how much they differ from the primary fitness form. For example, skiing includes alpine and cross-country; dance ranges from classical ballet to modern and jazz; aerobics classes are available in low-impact and high-impact varieties; racquet games include tennis, racquetball, squash, and—pushing this category a bit—handball; swimming can be subdivided into freestyle, backstroke, breaststroke, and butterfly; even running might be found in forms of sprinting, middle distance, or marathon. And what about walking?

With all these subcategories we don't want to lose sight of the overall profile. Our analysis of each fitness option will concentrate on the leading form as it is practiced today by people who undertake exercise for health, enjoyment, or aesthetic purposes.

High performance programs or competitive athletics is a completely different subject. There just is not enough space to do justice to these programs or to the training of highly specialized athletes. This is why a number of other fitness options have been omitted, including such games as basketball, baseball, football, hockey, and gymnastics. They are not typical fitness outlets. It's unlikely that you could play football three times a week even if you wanted to. Aside from difficulties in locating a convenient football field, rounding up a team for regular play would be none too easy. Essentially, we are looking at activities you might find at a local health club or community recreation center—activities you can do twelve months a year, three times or more a week, with little difficulty.

How do we plan to describe these fitness options? Just as you have been evaluating yourself throughout this book in the areas of personality (PADs), body structure (BADs), and movement characteristics (MADs), we will take these same classes of information and apply them to each of the options. This will give us an evaluation of:

1. *personality dynamics* required or reinforced by the activity;
2. *musculature* developed and how these muscles relate to personality;
3. *movements* emphasized with corresponding linkages to personality.

As you read along, make notes on your charts to get a feel for how well your profile matches each activity's, and begin to appreciate what each activity might do for you—for better or for worse!

Keep in mind that these descriptions are based on the *typical* way the activities are performed. There will always be variations in style and performance based on what you bring to your exercise program, but for the present we will address ourselves to the way it is generally done.

Running

Runners have been labeled as loners, compulsives, and fitness fanatics. Yet, if it is so negative, why do so many people do it? Why is it our most popular form of exercise, next to walking? Clearly, there's more to it than these terms imply. The predominant view held by the non-running public is one of an individualistic, disciplined activity that doesn't feel like a lot of fun. We even hear runners say "I feel so good *after* my run"—but they don't say nearly as often that they feel good *during* the run. Let's look inside running to understand why it can be so good for some people, and why others should avoid it. Our analysis will take us through personality dimensions, body development, and movement analysis, concluding with a review of major points.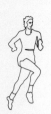

PAD/Psychosocial Dimensions of Running

Looking at the seven dimensions for evaluating exercise options and participants' personalities, here is what we find about running (Figure 8.1):

Social-Nonsocial: Rating—*Moderately Nonsocial*

Most runners exercise by themselves, setting their own schedules and paces. They relish the privacy. It's time to get away—from people, from work or family demands. The runner's gaze is mostly inward. The mind may be active with thoughts of the day or with feelings about the

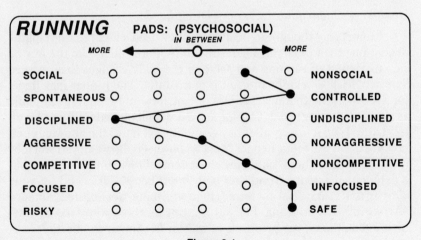

Figure 8.1

run. Scenery passes by unnoticed. Admittedly, there are people who make it a point to run with a group or with a friend. In these cases it is more likely they bring this sociability to running than that the activity makes them sociable.

Over the years that running has been in vogue, a kind of camaraderie has developed among runners. They are not nearly as detached as they once appeared. Today's runners may even go out of their way to give one another a wide wave or word of encouragement. Nonetheless, the activity does not require interaction, so we will stick to our rating.

Spontaneous-Controlled: Rating — **Controlled**

Runners are seen as being highly regimented, and the activity has few variations other than distance, speed, or pacing. Sure, you can always run sideways, backwards, or in circles, but, realistically, how often do you see runners doing pirouettes? Running requires little spontaneity or flexibility in behavior. One simply gets on the road and runs; it is a very programmed activity. It might be harder to understand how it is analytical other than by realizing that runners set goals in time and distance, sometimes increasing their pace at particular points or taking a break midway through the run. Running is very structured and corresponding mental activity during the run tends to proceed along similar analytical or logical lines. Rarely does the runner have to be spontaneous or intuitively guided, with the exception perhaps of dodging cars and outrunning aggressive dogs.

Disciplined-Undisciplined: Rating — **Disciplined**

Runners are thought to be driven. They need a lot of self-discipline to continue their program. There are few supports other than the intrinsic satisfaction of running and some of the body changes that accrue. The activity itself can be difficult if not painful. The runner may hope for a second wind that never comes or look forward to the midway mark as a mental turning point. Getting started is difficult and it takes a lot of self-talk to keep it up day after day. Sometimes it is just the knowledge of how good you will feel when it's over or, conversely, how bad you will feel if you don't run! There is little joy or excitement on a runner's face — it is a determined activity. Mind over body; do it because it's good for you! This is not a universal pattern. There are some free-spirited runners who joyfully bound along their course. But for those who take up running in adulthood, the prospects of quickly becoming an effortless and euphoric runner are slim.

*Aggressive-Nonaggressive: Rating — **Intermediate***

Aggression is based on the use of forceful action in attempts to master or dominate. Running is essentially a nonaggressive activity, but it involves forceful action aimed at mastery. As the runner progresses from one- and two-mile runs to the marathon, there is evidence of strong effort, of a push to mastery. Interestingly, some runners describe the activity as masochistic, reflecting perhaps the energy required to overcome inertia, gravity, or other forces that keep the body at rest. While we might say this about any exercise program, the discipline and tolerance of discomfort running requires add to the sense of forceful action. As a final comment, runners talk about the release of aggressive feelings through running or note that while running they may feel aggressive toward any individual or object that causes them to deviate from their path.

*Competitive-Noncompetitive: Rating — **Moderately Noncompetitive***

Runners may not have actual rivals as they go through their paces, but ask them what their times are for an average mile and they will know. Time and distance are used as gauges of progress and comparisons are covertly made with others who run. The games runners play are perhaps most evident in annual "fun runs," where egos inflate and deflate with each passed or passing participant. Why is it that your time is just a little better when you are running with a comparably skilled friend, or even when you are running on a populated jogging path instead of an empty one? Perhaps competition is one of the ways runners motivate themselves or find reward for their efforts. Running as a sport is highly competitive, but for the recreational runner it tends more toward the noncompetitive end of the continuum. The runner's goal is less to compete or to win than it is to complete, to finish a set course in a reasonable period of time.

*Focused-Unfocused: Rating — **Unfocused***

Running doesn't require concentration. The mind is free to wander, although it may be distracted by messages from the body like, "More oxygen, please!" or "Slow down, I'm tired!" Runners often use workout time to think about problems or plan activities. The release of pent-up energy while running allows your thoughts to flow. Runners feel doubly productive at the end of a workout because of what they have achieved mentally as well as physically. The mind is free to work or play. Some runners discipline their minds to focus on body mechanics or meditational thoughts, but this tends to be more the exception. In sum, the mind is not constrained by the body's actions; it doesn't have to pay attention to anything in particular.

Risky-Safe: Rating—Safe

Running is not inherently threatening. Nor is it bold or adventurous. It is a common enough activity that virtually anyone can feel inconspicuous doing. The myriad of shapes and sizes running the streets says it's an okay activity for anyone who is interested. No special skills are required. If there is risk, it is in the form of injuries resulting from running conditions, equipment (notably shoes), or the training process itself. With all the warnings coming out of sports medicine clinics these days, we might consider running as slightly more adventurous than it was seen a decade ago. However, in general, we find little threat or, conversely, adventure, inherent in running as an exercise form.

BAD/Body Psychology for Running

What you mostly develop through running are certain leg muscles. Although the arms may pump away as you run, it is essentially the legs that carry the load and propel you. Primary muscle involvements during running include muscles that extend and flex the hip and those that extend and flex the leg. Muscles that move the leg to the side and back (abductors and adductors) are used mostly as synergists (Figure 8.2).

Today's runner is keenly aware of the need for proper stretching before and after the run, but these "extraneous" efforts are often neglected. The result is that leg muscles, particularly the hamstring group (back of the thigh), get tight and shortened. A short stride adds to the problem of tight hamstrings. Unless the runner consciously works on obtaining longer stride, the leg muscles never get fully extended.

A runner's overall flexibility may also decrease because only certain leg muscles are exercised. Side steps or rotating movements that call forth the thighs' abductors and adductors, or hip rotators, are rarely used. This results in an overdevelopment of muscles that propel the body forward compared to other directions the body might take. In addition, the constant pounding that the body absorbs (approximately three times the body's weight with each step) stresses joints throughout the body, especially those in the ankle, knee, and hip. Injuries in these areas may become chronic.

What does this mean psychologically? The legs represent our so-

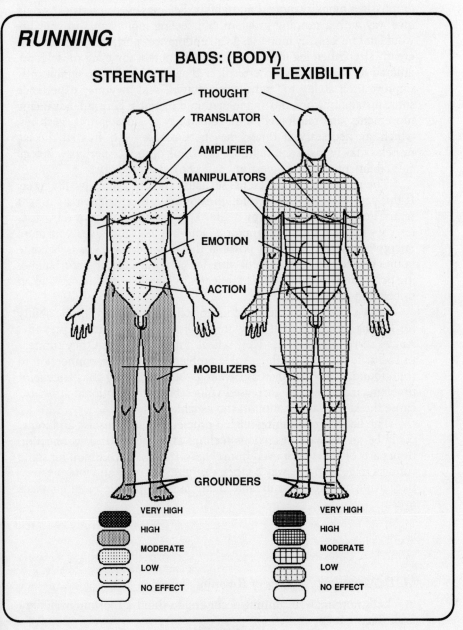

Figure 8.2

matic support and mobility system. They carry us places and they stabilize us, keeping us upright and in touch with the ground. Running emphasizes mobility more than stability. Feelings of "being stuck" would give way with a running program, but feeling more stable in your life would not necessarily increase. As an endurance sport, running does not greatly strengthen leg muscles. Plus, as we noted, some leg muscles are ignored by this activity. The result is that runners do not significantly improve their ability to "stand their ground," and they may experience some instability when moving in certain directions. Forward, advancing movements are reinforced, but retreating or sidestepping gestures, which are necessary at times, may be unstable. Also, in that the leg muscles may be rigid and tight, we can think of the runner's psychological stability or advancing gestures as having some rigidity.

The pelvic region represents sexuality and our aggressive life force. If this area is strengthened through running, we experience a stronger sexual image and more energy in life. This has been supported by studies showing that running improves your sex life and gives you more energy.[1] However, it is also possible that, should these areas become bound due to the development of rigid, tight musculature, corresponding personality dynamics would reflect a rigidity in sexual image and an unbending forcefulness.

Let's switch from musculature to joints. Knees provide flexibility for getting around, but if they are weak they give in under pressure. Ankles serve to elevate us. They reflect our strivings. And they connect us to our feet for grounding. Ankle problems reduce our connection to the ground. This can increase feelings of anxiety. So too, knee-joint problems may promote increased vulnerability to emotional stress because the knees cannot support the weight of life.

The liability of running-related problems in leg muscles and joints could be an increase in anxious feelings and a sense of disconnection from parts of yourself or even from others. It is not uncommon for some runners to get carried away by their exercise programs and lose perspective, giving up career, family, and friends as a compulsive addiction takes over.

MAD/Movement Analysis of Running

Let's now analyze running according to the five movement dimensions (Figure 8.3):

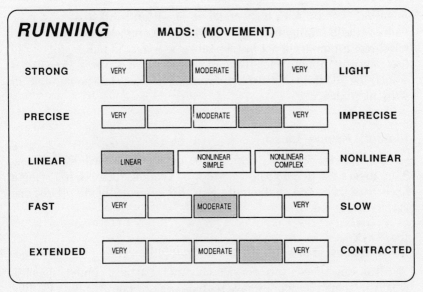

Figure 8.3

Force: Rating—Strong

Running movements range from the powerful efforts of a sprinter to the lighter ones of a marathoner. Based on the finding that three times the body's weight goes through the foot with each step, we can describe running as moderately strong as opposed to being delicate and light. The implication is that personality becomes strong-willed, resolute, and moderately aggressive. In the extreme, a quality of stubbornness develops.

Control: Rating—Imprecise

The idea that anyone can run and that it takes no special training is only part of the reason we rate the typical runner as imprecise in movements. The foot does not have to be precisely placed. The arms do not have to move in a particular fashion. The body does not have to be aligned exactly. There are runners who are more precise than others in the way they move, but in most endurance sports movements lack precision. This leads to some interesting insights. Since we rated running on PADs as disciplined and controlled, we can say that running promotes a compulsive lifestyle. Because of the rating on precision, we might add that this controlled, disciplined way of being may lack good form or precision. The runner's body could be significantly off balance, but he will continue, compensating by misaligning himself. Without good coaching, running will not instill a sense of quality in movement—or in life. Graceful runners bring this dimension to their running. Precision is something you have to strive for in running. It doesn't come naturally or without guidance.

Linearity: Rating—**Linear**

Motions are linear or direct, restricting the use of the body in space. This suggests a psychological pattern of keeping focused, following a fixed pattern or line of thought, or, in the extreme, being obsessional and narrow-minded.

Speed: Rating—**Moderate** (with range from fast to slow)

Running speeds vary considerably. For a typical runner, speed is what we would consider average with a range of slow (for the plodding jogger) to fast (for the five-minute milers). As such, the moderate-paced runner will tend to be somewhat unfocused and controlled. However, the faster you run, the more you reinforce a decisive, aggressive, and focused personality.

Extension: Rating—**Contracted**

Running is more contracted than extended. Arms and legs do not reach to their limits. Some runners have a freer, more extended flow to their movements than do others who are more bound or contracted. For instance, slow joggers are more contracted than are fast runners. The implication of these contracted motions is that the runner tends toward caution and restraint, toward an emphasis on control and emotional guardedness.

Running in Review

Running helps develop or intensify specific psychosocial dimensions. Depending on your needs, these changes may be more or less appropriate. It enables you to be more directed, more controlled, more disciplined, and more structured. It makes you move out into your world. It helps you advance in a chosen direction. It is relatively safe and nonthreatening to your ego and your physical well-being. However, it does not develop you socially or make you feel more secure and grounded in reality. In extreme cases of running addiction, you can become quite detached from your reality-based needs, and from significant others.

Because it is an unfocused activity, it does not necessarily relieve mental anxiety. Body anxiety, yes, but worry and obsessional thinking, no! However, if you learn to meditate while running, you can improve this. There is some risk of becoming overcontrolled or rigid through intense running programs, and given that the activity is highly repetitive and lends itself to an analytical lifestyle, it may not be as good as other activities for stimulating creativity.

Walking — A Variation on Running

Did you know that walkers outnumber runners by more than two to one? There are an estimated 53 million exercise walkers vs. 23 million joggers.[2] Walkers probably would not put themselves in the same category as runners, and with good reason. Many people who walk for exercise don't push themselves nearly as hard as runners do. Walking is a lot easier than running and exercise walkers are less compulsively driven. They also like company, making the social element a preferred component of their exercise. Unlike runners, they are less time conscious, so you won't find too many of them with stopwatches. And, so far, we don't have too many walking competitons spurring walkers on to a faster pace. It is no doubt safer than running both in ego and physical terms. Walking injuries are far fewer than running ones (Figure 8.4).

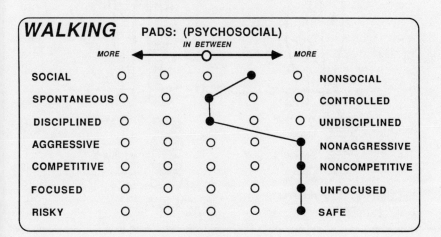

Figure 8.4

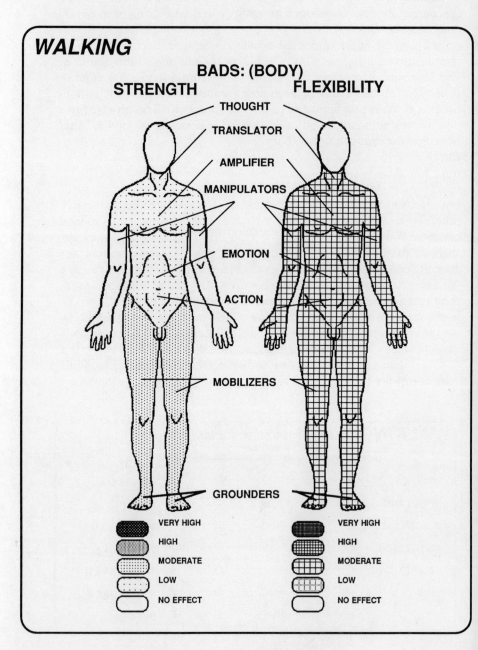

Figure 8.5

Body development in walking and running involves the same muscle groups, but of course you won't get the same cardiorespiratory benefits from walking as you do from running, unless you are a speed walker. On the other hand, you don't get the sore, tight muscle syndrome that running gives you and certainly walking creates less stress on your joints. For these reasons it doesn't lend itself to some of the body-psychology problems of running. There is less risk of becoming rigidly bound or obsessional (Figure 8.5).

Movement characteristics are also less severe. It involves less force because you don't have to leap through the air as you do in running. And the impact when your foot strikes the ground is greatly reduced. It is imprecise like running and improves along this dimension only with coaching. (Many people wouldn't even consider coaching for walking, but it can be terribly important.) It, too, is linear because walkers are not prone to doing pirouettes in the park. And for a sport or exercise program, the speed rating is slow or at best average. On extension, it can be slightly more extended than running since walkers have to develop a good stride in order to get their hearts pumping faster (Figure 8.6).

Walkers like to create interesting routes for themselves and may use their exercise as a way of getting to know their towns or different neighborhoods. This is a more creative use of walking, but since few walkers

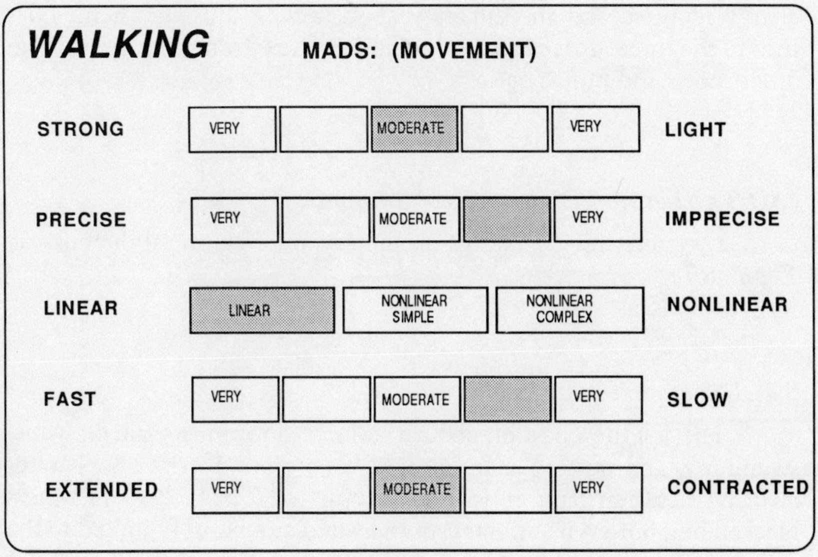

WALKING   MADS: (MOVEMENT)

STRONG	VERY		MODERATE		VERY	LIGHT
PRECISE	VERY		MODERATE		VERY	IMPRECISE
LINEAR	LINEAR		NONLINEAR SIMPLE	NONLINEAR COMPLEX		NONLINEAR
FAST	VERY		MODERATE		VERY	SLOW
EXTENDED	VERY		MODERATE		VERY	CONTRACTED

Figure 8.6

restrict themselves to the cardiorespiratory benefits of their exercise, we are likely to find this component in most walkers' programs.

You might think of walking as easy and therefore not as exercise. But it *is* exercise and its easefulness is one of its main draws. It can be a good way of getting some of the benefits of running without enduring all the hardships. And for people who want to become more active, walking is a good way to start.

Swimming

Swimmers are regarded as quiet and introspective, yet strong-willed and tenacious. They are also described as graceful, dependable, and relaxed. These common associations reveal only part of swimming's image, which on the surface seems similar to other solitary activities, such as running. Maybe it's because we can't see the swimmer's face as she does laps or perhaps it's the synchrony of movements in a good swimmer. For whatever reasons, impressions of swimmers are not like those of runners.

In our analysis, we will consider swimming as a relatively homogeneous activity represented by the freestyle stroke, or overhand crawl. The analysis would be relatively similar for backstroke and breaststroke. Butterfly probably deviates most on some factors due to the greater energy required and the difficulty of sustaining the movement. Let's turn to the three areas of analysis to find out how swimming differs from other sports and fitness options.

PAD/Psychosocial Dimensions of Swimming

We will first review ratings on the seven psychosocial dimensions (Figure 8.7):

Social-Nonsocial: Rating—Nonsocial

There is little question about the limitations on socializing while swimming, and not too many people hang around in the cool water chatting between laps. It is a solitary activity. Not only are others blocked out, but even awareness of the world around us is limited to the sensations of water. It is not a sport to develop social skills, at least not directly.

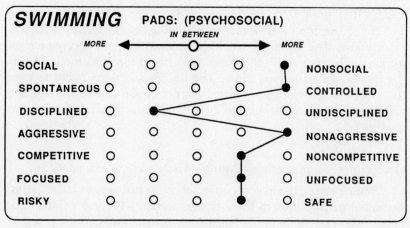

Figure 8.7

Spontaneous-Controlled: Rating—*Controlled*

Once a person has learned to swim, the movements are fairly mechanical. Good swimmers have grace and rhythm, but it comes from long hours of practicing proper arm placement, breathing, and kicking. Swimming can be more playful and spontaneous, but as represented in lap swimming it tends more toward the controlled end of the continuum.

Disciplined-Undisciplined: Rating—*Moderately Disciplined*

Swimmers are not seen as being driven or self-punishing, but they are viewed as dedicated, conscientious, and strong-minded. Why the difference from runners? Because in water the body is supported. Joints do not experience constant pounding and muscles are allowed to extend and flex more gradually. In brief, it is less painful than running. For this reason, it requires somewhat less drive and internal push. And there is something pleasurable in easy, relaxed swimming—something that is hard to achieve even when you slow to a shuffling jog. But then all of this depends on how well you swim. If you are constantly fighting the water, it takes extreme discipline to keep going. If you can glide and float, it is almost effortless. Nonetheless, a regular routine of swimming requires devotion, an ability to motivate yourself, to talk yourself through the hard spots, to make the swim a good workout.

Aggressive-Nonaggressive: Rating — **Nonaggressive**

If you use too much force in swimming, it becomes a battle you quickly lose. The swimmer has to have an attitude of acceptance, of working in harmony with the water and using it for support. The fewer the ripples, the easier you move. The deeper and more fluid the kick, the more efficient your propulsion. No doubt you can splash and flail about, but fatigue wins out and either you learn to harmonize or you give up.

Competitive-Noncompetitive: Rating — **Moderately Noncompetitive**

Adult swimmers today are more likely to belong to Masters swim clubs, but participation in these groups accounts for only a fraction of people who exercise in pools. For the most part, swimmers are prone to setting their own pace and distance. They work for self-improvement rather than competition. A major criterion swimmers use is distance counted in numbers of laps. Time is more crudely estimated with not nearly the obsession found in runners with their stopwatches. The trend, however, is toward greater involvement in competitive events as reflected in club swimming as well as the growing popularity of open-water swims. For the vast majority of recreational swimmers, however, swimming is a noncompetitive activity.

Focused-Unfocused: Rating — **Moderately Unfocused**

Although the motions of swimming become repetitive and mechanical with increasing practice, the swimmer must maintain a minimal focus while in the water, attending to the upcoming pool wall on each lap, the presence of other swimmers, and unexpected possibilities. Since swimming is an acquired skill, we must also attend at times to our stroke, kick, or breathing pattern. Aside from these small distractions, we can think about life's concerns or other preoccupations as we swim back and forth in the pool. In this regard, swimming does not fully take us away from prevailing thoughts. It simply provides a different medium, water, in which the mind re-engages. This difference created by water may nonetheless alter the way we think.

Risky-Safe: Rating — **Moderately Safe**

Swimming is not as natural as walking or running and there is always the possibility of drowning. This means there is risk in swimming. Once a person learns to swim competently, the risk is minimized. Also, the settings where most people swim, namely public pools, are usually well guarded and carefully maintained. Ego risks are also reduced when the swimmer progresses beyond about ten nonstop laps, thereby surpassing the ability of most people. Injuries in pools (with the exception of diving-related ones) are infrequent and, more on the benefits side, swimming is thought of as one of the best exercises, not only for its positive effects on cardiorespiratory and muscular development, but also because of the relative absence of strain on joints and the easing of pressure in the spinal column.

BAD/Body Psychology for Swimming

Although swimming exercises most of the body's muscles, it relies more on upper-body muscles to pull the swimmer through the water. Shoulders, arms, chest, and upper-back muscles are used extensively. The freestyle kick involves hip flexors and extensors more so than muscles of the lower leg. The result of swim training can be seen in the inverted triangular shape that characterizes many competitive swimmers. Shoulders are broad and well developed, with long, smooth muscles in the arms. Chest and abdominal muscles are strong but not overly large. Waist and hips are small, and legs are long, lean, and evenly muscled (Figure 8.8).

There is more to the swimmer in the upper half (waist up) of her body than in the lower half (waist down). Since the upper half of the body has to do with social and physical interactions, swimmers would seem to be well developed for these exchanges. Muscular development supports the capability to take charge, to control, to give, to take, to carry responsibility. However, with relatively less strength and, therefore, less stability in the lower body, the swimmer's top-heavy development may imply transactions that are not well grounded. The result would be a feeling of instability or insecurity in relating to others.

The long, fluid musculature of the swimmer suggests an ability for energy to flow without blockage throughout the body. Joints and musculature remain open as a result of swimming. They do not become rigid and tight, nor are they likely to become traumatized through exercise. Since the swimmer does not learn to work with the ground and, on a body level, does not understand the use of support, the open musculature and energy flow allow the swimmer to be quite sensitive and, in the extreme, vulnerable. Adding to this is the tendency for swimmers to have well-developed and flexible chests, permitting emotions to be am-

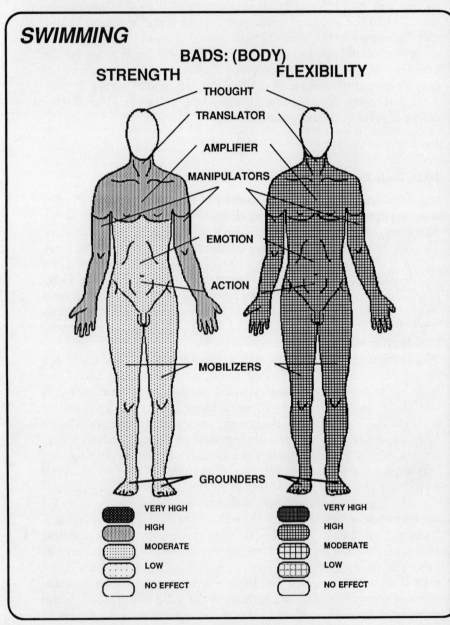

Figure 8.8

plified. The swimmer might be acutely aware of all her feelings but not have the necessary support to comfortably manage these emotions.

For the most part, muscular development in swimming has more positives than negatives. These comments highlight potential pitfalls worth considering if you are prone to any of the conditions or feelings noted.

MAD/Movement Analysis of Swimming

Swimming must be understood in context. Water provides a unique medium in which to experience ourselves. It is a different reality, one that determines how we move and how we feel. Water is a therapeutic medium found in a variety of forms from whirlpool baths and flotation tanks to soft, supporting seas (Figure 8.9).

Force: Rating—Range: Strong to Light

Swimming requires steady forceful pressure at different points of the stroke and then lighter efforts as the arm glides forward. These alternations of strong and light movements promote a balance of assertion and passivity, an ability to sense the need for strength and for delicacy. Swimming develops sensitivity to the appropriate use of force in situations along with an ability to be forceful or delicate, as required.

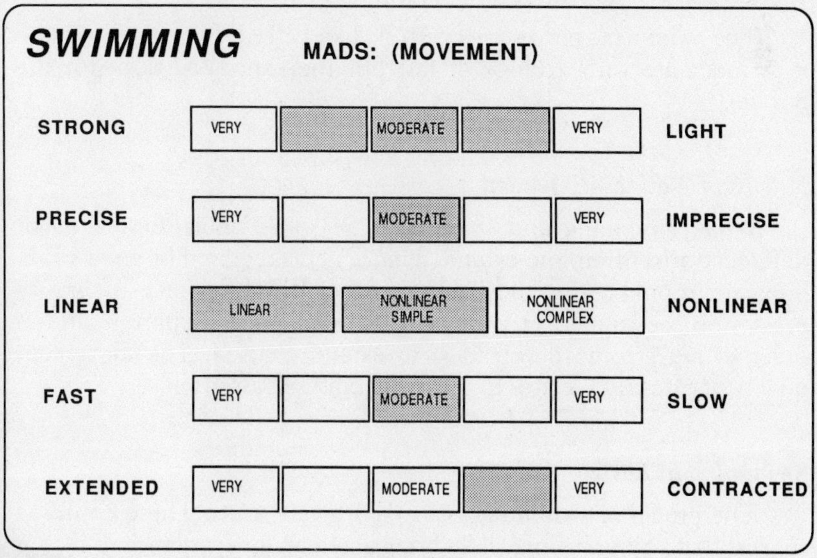

SWIMMING	MADS: (MOVEMENT)				
STRONG	VERY		MODERATE		VERY	LIGHT
PRECISE	VERY		MODERATE		VERY	IMPRECISE
LINEAR	LINEAR		NONLINEAR SIMPLE	NONLINEAR COMPLEX		NONLINEAR
FAST	VERY		MODERATE		VERY	SLOW
EXTENDED	VERY		MODERATE		VERY	CONTRACTED

Figure 8.9

*Control: Rating — **Moderate***

Much as in running, precision of movement is not required. There are plenty of sloppy swimmers. However, in order to swim well, arm placement, kick patterns, and breathing movements must be performed with some precision. Anyone who swims regularly would tend more toward greater precision over time. Otherwise the feeling of always fighting the water would become too discouraging. As an endurance sport in a medium, water, that demands respect, our rating for swimming is moderate in precision, recognizing there are some swimmers who have far better form than others.

*Linearity: Rating — **Range: Linear-Non-linear (Simple)***

Swimming motions are curved and wavy, even though the body's direction is linear and forward. Propelling movements of the arms sculpt an S as the body snakes through the water. The head twists from side to side as the swimmer breathes and the legs kick in a wavy pattern. Yet, the body moves ahead. Swimming must be seen as emphasizing both linear and non-linear (simple) movements and in this regard would foster a balance between control and spontaneity, focus and nonfocus, discipline and ease.

*Speed: Rating — **Moderate** (with range from fast to slow)*

The swimmer's pace varies with skill and effort. In general, we rate it as moderate with a range of fast (for the expert) to slow (for the novice).

*Extension: Rating — **Extended***

While swimming and running share some similarities, a major difference arises from the extended movements required by good swimming. In running, the body gets compacted as the force of gravity presses on the runner. In swimming your weight is supported, and in order to move forward you have to extend yourself. The movement quality of extension relates to sociability and self-assertion.

Swimming in Review

The profile of swimming is marked by contrasts. These contrasts suggest that swimming may help bring about an inner balance of reason and emotion. The activity requires control and a moderate degree of discipline, yet it is a relatively easygoing exercise that stresses the safe, noncompetitive, and nonaggressive ends of the scales. However, it is a nonsocial activity and as such would not be of direct value in developing interpersonal skills. The fact that the body it produces is related to the more social-interactive or controlling-manipulating parts of our being counterbalances the nonsocial nature of the sport. One problem we noted was that the development of controlling/manipulating musculature may cause some problem when we take into account how little swimming does to make you feel grounded.

These comments illustrate the potential and limitations of swimming. If you need social development or feel insecure and ungrounded, there are better activities than swimming to help you in these areas. With persistence, the sport will facilitate a moderately high level of sensitivity both to your own feelings and to others, an ability to be flexible, to sustain your direction in life, to take control, and to be organized. The element of water must always be kept in mind when considering swimming in that for many people it is relaxing, while for others it stimulates profound anxiety. This may come as much from a loss of support in the water as from a fear of drowning.

Body Building

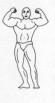

What exactly do we mean by body building? Are we talking about trainees for Olympic events where you lift the heaviest weight for your particular size category? Or are we talking about the Mr. America contest? Depending on the body builder the goals may be different: one may want a beautiful body while another may be more interested in becoming the Incredible Hulk. For the most part, body builders are image-conscious, striving for a well-proportioned *and* strong body. Aesthetic appeal is important. Our consideration of this exercise form includes people who lift heavy weights to develop big, strong, and attractive musculature. We are talking about people who want both strength and beauty. This discussion will not apply as well to "body shaping," which involves the use of light weights for muscle toning and fitness.

Psychological research on body builders offers a different profile than the one that is commonly held. Popular belief has it that body builders are egocentric and narcissistic. The idea of spending all that time building muscles and flexing in front of mirrors is a bit much for the average person to comprehend without implying a personality quirk of one sort or another. Curiously, research studies have found a high level of insecurity in body builders—not something that is generally known about these weight-room aficionados.[3]

Let's move beyond everyday impressions of body builders to a more systematic examination, starting with an analysis of the seven psychosocial dimensions and proceeding to the muscle and movement descriptions.

PAD/Psychosocial Dimensions of Body Building

We will consider body building as it occurs in a weight-training center rather than in the basements or exercise rooms of private homes. Admittedly, a large number of people dabble in body building with home-fitness equipment, but as the individual comes to define himself as a body builder, he will eventually grow out of the home gym and begin working out at a club that caters to body builders (Figure 8.10).

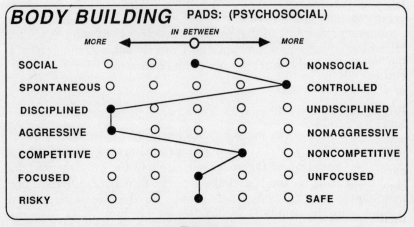

Figure 8.10

Social-Nonsocial: Rating—Intermediate

A body builder working out in a club setting has numerous verbal and nonverbal exchanges with peers. It is a semisocial environment with rules about interpersonal conduct. When using heavy weights, builders "spot" for each other to prevent accidents. In between sets, they strut around the studio commenting to friends or stopping to spot. It is virtually impossible to go to a club day after day and remain anonymous. You have to interact in order to do parts of the workout. And body builders are full of advice and information about all sorts of things: technique, diet, and steroids, as well as the daily social news of the club.

*Spontaneous-Controlled: Rating—**Controlled***

When builders get to the level of competing in contests, there may be a new element of artistry added to the exercise session, but for most body builders it tends to be a highly rational, controlled process based on records, charts, and a logical analysis of what exercises build which muscles. In the extreme, body building represents an obsessive-compulsive pattern of critically analyzing your body and, with an extreme degree of planning and regimentation, reshaping muscle groups to achieve an ideal profile. There is very little about body building itself that can be described as spontaneous or creative. The performance dimension of contests requires a choreographed routine of movements and poses, but this level of achievement is not often attained by the recreational body builder.

*Disciplined-Undisciplined: Rating—**Disciplined***

It is hard to see the inherent appeal of hefting weights in repetitive series, day after day, changing only the number of plates or the frequency of the exercises. Yet many people are hooked on body building. Perhaps it is the gratification that comes when you notice a new muscle or when you have to buy new clothes, not because your waist has expanded, but because you popped your collar button. There may also be some payoff in the social atmosphere of the club or the looks you get when you walk down the street. In spite of these potential gains, the fact is that muscles develop slowly and changes don't occur overnight. Every day or so you have to face those piles of iron plates and dumbbells and convince yourself to move them with feeling, lots of feeling. "No pain, no gain!" You have to make the muscles burn. It's no pleasure trip and there's not much to distract you from the joyless sensations of lifting. The drive, the determination, the discipline come from inside.

*Aggressive-Nonaggressive: Rating—**Aggressive***

If aggression is defined as applying force to master or dominate, there is little question that body building fits the definition. The force is used on inanimate objects but it can be nonetheless extreme. The grimace on a body builder's face tells it all. He is indeed trying to master, to dominate an oppressing weight that just won't budge while someone is screaming in his face to push harder. You can develop a lot of aggressive feelings in moments like these. Although the force is impersonal, what is critical is the nature of the effort. The body builder struggles to overcome resistance, to be in control, to fight against pressures that could crush him. It is not a passive activity.

*Competitive-Noncompetitive: Rating—**Moderately Noncompetitive***

Bodybuilders frequently play the game, "My bicep is bigger than yours" or other variations on the theme. It is mostly a friendly game with no big winners or losers. Everyone is just trying to do his best, working with whatever potential or size limitations he has. There tends to be a cooperative attitude in weight-training centers—people are genuinely helpful. Mostly, the feeling of competition comes from within: striving against yourself, trying to improve, to lift more, to develop bigger muscles. Implicit comparisons come about through observations of others. Explicit comparisons are reserved for body-building competitions.

Focused-Unfocused: Rating—Intermediate

It should come as no surprise that a body builder has to pay careful attention to what she is doing while lifting. At other times, the mind is free. The experience of lifting heavy weights requires concentration—it is not a passive mental act. By contrast, some light-weight exercises with dumbbells can be monotonous so that your attention is not demanded. In this latter case, as well as in between sets of exercises, the body builder is open to whatever internal thoughts or distractions happen along.

Risky-safe: Rating—Intermediate

Although body builders tend to be careful and analytical, lifting such excessive weights increases the likelihood of physical injury. And weight-lifting injuries can have long-term consequences. On the psychological side, ego risks can also be considerable, particularly if you are not well proportioned to begin with. Walking into a body-builders' den can be intimidating, if not frightening, because your body is dwarfed by the massive anatomies that surround you. It takes a while to feel comfortable, and the initiation period can be trying. Flab takes shape slowly. Although the rating of this activity is intermediate, it leans more toward the safe side in that the prevalent attitude in most clubs is toward safety and progressing at your own pace. Of course, there are fanatics who would try to convince you that taking steroids and megavitamin supplements is the only choice for serious body builders.

BAD/Body Psychology for Body Building

The conscientious body builder is careful to develop musculature proportionately. Although many people play around with weights to build big arms and chests, the resulting asymmetry is most unappealing. For devotees of body building, the regimen is addressed to all the major surface-muscle groups, so that legs are given as much attention as arms or abdominal muscles. There are even special exercises to get at the deeper layers of muscles, the ones that don't show but that the educated body builder knows are important for proper development (Figure 8.11).

So, what can we say about the bodies of sensible body builders? There is an emphasis on proportion and balance where the upper body is sculpted to look like it belongs to the lower body and the left side is as strong as the right. Certain imbalances will always occur, but body builders try to be aware of lateral differences and adjust their workouts accordingly.

If a body builder overemphasizes upper-body development, psychological functions of control, manipulation, and social interaction would likewise be overstressed. When body building is done on a more proportionate scale, however, what we need to consider are factors of strength and flexibility. In a sense, the body builder armors his body with excessive musculature, creating heavy protective layers that are, for the most part, unnecessary in today's world. These muscles can make him less sensitive to feeling. The body builder has trained his body to endure pain and discomfort through rigorous workouts and as a result is less aware on a body level. It simply takes more to get through all that protective covering.

Another feature of the muscles is that they tend to be less flexible than required for graceful or delicate movements. The term "muscle-bound" is not just an idle figure of speech. Muscles can become short and bulky, restricting the body builder's range of movement. There is a lack of flexibility created by excessive and contracted muscles that simply cannot extend into their full range. Along with the restricted range of movement, the muscles also bind the body so that emotions are contained or controlled. For example, the chest, which serves to expand emotional feelings, becomes restricted due to the development of heavy layers of muscle and, as a result, tender feelings can get blocked.

Psychologically, this kind of muscle structure implies a tendency to overpower one's world, of approaching with more force than necessary, and of lacking the ability to intervene more delicately. Body armoring, which makes one less vulnerable and less sensitive both physically and interpersonally, can be better appreciated in light of research findings that report an underlying insecurity in many body builders. The choice

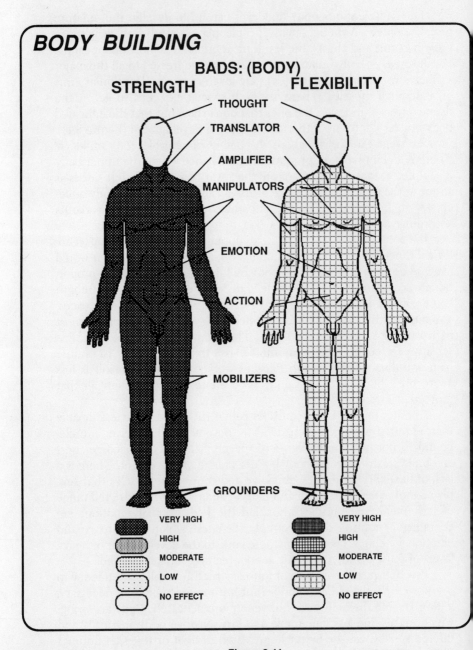

Figure 8.11

of this exercise form makes sense for someone who feels overly vulnerable.

MAD/Movement Analysis of Body Building

Movements are analyzed according to what the body builder does in the process of lifting and releasing weights (Figure 8.12).

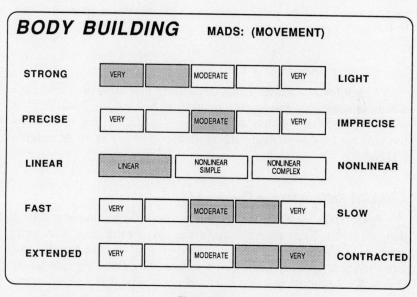

Figure 8.12

Force: Rating—Range: Strong to Very Strong

Body building requires strong, forceful action. On our scale it rates in the range Very Strong to Strong. Body building fosters overly assertive or even aggressive tendencies, as well as an attitude of willful determination.

Control: Rating—Moderate

There are many styles of lifting weights. Most require a moderate degree of precision. If you are sloppy, you get injured. If you do the exercise incorrectly, you develop the wrong muscles. Yet, you do not have to move the weights to an exact point in space nor do you have to move them with mathematical accuracy. This quality of body-building movements fosters a moderate degree of control, discipline, safety, and mental concentration.

Linearity: Rating—**Linear**

Movements in body building are direct and linear, with few exceptions. Motions are to the point. Muscles flex and then extend. Weights are lifted directly overhead and then brought down. The personality pattern reinforced by such moves are similarly direct, assertive, controlled, and focused—in the extreme, rigid and stubborn.

Speed: Rating—**Range: Slow to Moderate**

Weight lifting involves controlled efforts that range in speed from slow to average. Fast movements are likely to be harmful. Imagining the pace of hulky body builders does not bring to mind quick, darting motions but rather slow to moderate efforts that convey a sense of restraint and control.

Extension: Rating—**Range: Contracted to Very Contracted**

Body builders emphasize the contraction of large muscle groups in their workouts. Even after a workout they like to flex their muscles in mirrored studios. There is little emphasis on reaching out or extending into the space around them. The corresponding character that is emphasized is one oriented toward emotional safety. Risky engagements are not encouraged by the body builder's workout. And a certain controlled passivity can also be seen in these contracted gestures.

Body Building in Review

Body building can be a positive character builder for some people. It is a moderately social activity that develops qualities of control, self-confidence, and self-discipline. It can enhance your self-presence and assertiveness through body-image changes, as well as through the forcefulness of action required in weight training. It also can help increase your ability to focus or concentrate, at least for short periods of time.

From the muscle psychology side, body building may lessen feelings of vulnerability, but it could also decrease interpersonal sensitivity. The fact that lower-body muscles are strengthened adds to feelings of security and groundedness. Qualities of control, resoluteness, concentration, and deliberateness are emphasized in its required movements and, therefore, would become part of the character that this exercise form builds. In the more extreme addiction to body building, some of these traits might turn from assets to liabilities. For example, traits of stubbornness, insensitivity, rigidity, and extreme forcefulness could be overdeveloped.

Variations on Body Building

Before leaving body building, we need to examine a popular variation on the theme, namely, body building using stationary equipment such as the Nautilus, Keiser, or Polaris systems. Unlike more traditional approaches, these weight systems consist of individual machines arranged in a circuit so that the body builder progresses from one machine to the next until the circuit or sequence is completed. They are advertised as the modern, efficient way of obtaining a total body workout in the shortest time possible. As such, they are designed to fit into our fast-paced lifestyles, creating the least amount of pain and disruption. While these systems are used by serious body builders as adjuncts to their workouts, they would never comprise the full regimen. They tend to develop tone rather than muscle bulk, and, given the recommended frequency of three half-hour workouts per week, they are unlikely to produce dramatic change in body proportions.

Although many characterizations of body building would also apply to this form of weight lifting, there are some exceptions. For one, it is essentially a nonsocial activity that neither requires nor encourages social interactions. Theoretically, it is safer, in that your movements are controlled and there is no danger from falling weights. In some ways, it requires less discipline because you have a set circuit and you almost put yourself on a kind of exercise conveyor belt moving from one machine to the next with little thought demanded. This not only requires less self-motivation, but it also involves less focus. Once the machine is set, you just sit back and pump away. Supposedly, these machine systems allow for the development of muscle strength *and* flexibility, and if the machines are used correctly, flexibility is not seriously diminished. Few people, unless they are carefully supervised, use the machines correctly. The prescribed movements are shortened, with concomitant decreases in muscle extension and flexibility. These systems are convenient and make body building more palatable, but they certainly do not stir one's creative juices and may, in fact, add to one's sense of drudgery and ennui.

The Racquet Sports

Racquet sports include tennis, squash, and racquetball. Our analysis also applies to some other ball games, especially handball. Popular images of racquet players vary, depending on the game. Words most often associated with these sports are "competitive" and "aggressive." Reflecting another common theme are words like "energetic," "fast," and "tense." The word "sociable" occurs more frequently in reference to tennis players than to squash and racquetball players. We find few negative comments about these sports, so we assume they mostly carry a positive image for participants. In other words, playing these games is likely to give your image a boost.

In more formally analyzing racquet sports, we will treat them as a unit, recognizing that there are some appreciable differences in rules and settings, but that the underlying dynamics are largely similar.

PAD/Psychosocial Dimensions of Racquet Sports

Racquet games are played with just one partner (doubles in tennis being an exception) and for specific periods of time. Economic considerations may influence participation because membership in racquet clubs is often limited either by fees or club standards. With these qualifications in mind, let us turn to the dimensional analysis (Figure 8.13).

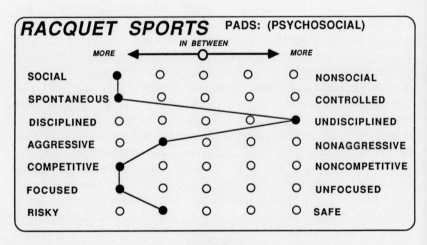

Figure 8.13

Social-Nonsocial: Rating — **Social**

You cannot play these games without a partner, and the inter-actions required are both verbal and nonverbal. Physical contact is likely in squash and racquetball even to the degree that protective equipment is advised. The nature of the interactions is, of course, critical in under-standing the effects it can have on your personality. Aside from the competitive aspect, there are many other bases for exchange, including social, playful, or even romantic ones. The constant presence of another person demands an *inter*personal as opposed to an *intra*personal focus.

Spontaneous-Controlled: Rating — **Spontaneous**

Racquet players often talk about strategy, for example, being an offensive rather than a defensive player, yet there is no way of predicting what will happen in the course of a game. Players have to be spontane-ous — they have to respond flexibly in the heat of a game, relying on an almost intuitive sense. There is little time for detailed rational analysis or conscious planning once the ball is in play.

Disciplined-Undisciplined: Rating — **Undisciplined**

Regular racquet players say they really enjoy, if not love, the game. They look forward to time on the court and most would not describe what they are doing as exercise. It's enjoyment, competition, a game, action, and, by the way, it happens to be good for you because you get some exercise. There is tension in games with particular partners, but more often than not this is interpreted as excitement. Rarely do you see racquet players dragging their bodies to the club, complaining about having to work out. There is an upbeat quality to the game and the players are drawn to it. It doesn't take a lot of self-discipline or internal pep talks to play regularly.

Aggressive-Nonaggressive: Rating — **Moderately Aggressive**

For most players, racquet games are about mastery and domination through forceful action. You smash the ball over the net or against the wall to defeat your opponent, to emerge on top. Players think of the game as a good way to blow off steam. It's a channel for pent-up feelings, for expressing frustration that builds through the day. Yet the game itself can be a source of frustration, in which case we see temper tantrums and racquets broken in anger. We believe an activity that is aggressive in nature reinforces the expression of aggression rather than reduces the frequency of aggressive reactions. This is not to deny that players get a release from emotional buildup. The game can give you this release while at the same time conditioning a quick, aggressive response pattern.

Competitive-Noncompetitive: Rating — **Competitive**

Points are won or lost. At the end there is one winner and one loser. The game is about rivalry, about competing, about winning and losing. The way players enact these roles may be individually determined, but in terms of what the game calls for, there is little doubt you are involved in a competitive match. There are friendly games and grudge matches, but in either case it's a match with one person's skills pitted against another's.

Focused-Unfocused: Rating — **Focused**

There are moments when you stoop to pick up the ball or when you are gasping for air between volleys. Then you can take your mind off the game. Otherwise, your attention is riveted to the ball, your opponent, your own readiness. It is an opportunity to get away from whatever is bothering you, to take a vacation from life's concerns. The game requires your concentration. It demands that you focus on the action and not on your plans for the evening. Even if you enter the game burdened with worries, you will have to leave these thoughts in the locker room. Having had a bad day will affect your game, but this does not detract from the game's power to make you switch mind-sets, to center in the present.

Risky-Safe: Rating — **Moderately Risky**

There are different medical maladies attributed to racquet sports. Probably the most popular is tennis elbow. These, however, do not constitute the major risk of racquet games. Your ego more than your body is on the line. The reputation of opponents modifies the stakes. Once you have advanced from the novice ranks and can no longer hide behind the "I'm just a beginner" excuse, winning and losing become closely aligned with your self-esteem. There are ways around this, of course. Defining yourself as an occasional player, not taking the game too seriously, or carefully choosing opponents can help manage ego risks. In team sports, responsibility for winning or losing is shared, but in individual sports it's all yours. One other aspect of risk in these games comes from the suddenness of movements. Not only do you have to duck balls or racquets, but sometimes you risk yourself in going for a difficult return. And although you can choose to play it safe, the game will always present you with opportunities to go beyond your limits.

BAD/Body Psychology for Racquet Sports

Racquet sports call for bursts of energy, for extreme flexibility in action, and for particular kinds of strength. People who regularly play racquet sports will be aware of the differences in muscular development in the playing arm and the nonplaying arm. This is probably the most obvious asymmetry, but surely not the only one. The body develops muscles that are strong, but that must be capable of full extension, as when a player serves or dives after a ball. The legs are highly stressed in racquet sports and the individual must learn how to use the ground for support. The crouched position, with knees flexed and torso low to the floor, readies the body for action. There is a fragile balance with the weight of the body leaning forward in an aggressive stance, easily knocked off center as it prepares for action. Hip and leg musculature must be able to respond with thrusting movements in any direction: forward, backward, sideways, and even circularly. As a result, all the leg's major muscle groups must be developed, including the flexors, extensors, abductors, adductors, and those that rotate the thigh. In the upper body the greatest development occurs on the side that controls the racquet, and this will include back, chest, shoulder, and arm muscles. While the opposite side does some work through the involvement of antagonists, synergists, and fixators, it does not undergo nearly the same kind or amount or stress. The torso must also have strength and flexibility. Racquet sports develop back muscles that curve and straighten the spine, and abdominal muscles that contract the stomach and twist the torso from side to side (Figure 8.14).

Psychologically, muscle development through racquet sports suggests an emphasis on both stability and movement through the grounding of the legs and their readiness for action. Yet, by the fact that the body is always preparing for action, there is greater emphasis on movement than on staying put. A kind of psychological flexibility is also implied by the development of muscles that enable the body to move in any direction. Racquet players learn to respond to threats or challenges from any side, but the nature of the response is more likely to be an advancing, aggressive one than a withdrawing or retreating gesture.

The upper body leans into the action and the dominant side is

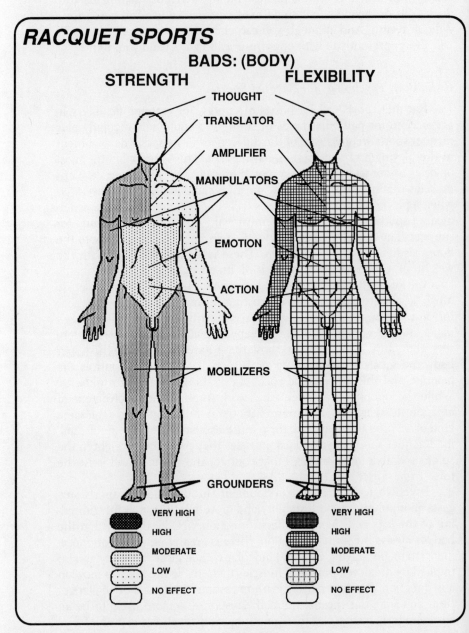

Figure 8.14

stressed in relation to the more passive side. Aggressive, controlling responses become more likely than do more receptive ones. This is further supported by muscle development in the dominant arm, which serves to directly manipulate and control interactions.

MAD/Movement Analysis for Racquet Sports

Racquet sports call for a wide range of movements. Not only are changes from one set of actions to another rapid, but there is great variation in types of movements: for example, twisting, bending, or stretching, and the way the body rises and lowers, or runs in straight, curving, circular, or zigzag patterns. These varied movements imply high levels of emotional and psychological functioning—if they are done well. More specific insights into what is potentially gained through practicing racquet sports can be seen in the analysis of the five motion factors (Figure 8.15).

Force: Rating—Range: Moderate to Very Strong

Racquet sports require moderate to very strong motions in both striking the ball and moving on the court. Such movements promote self-assertion and aggressive behavioral patterns. There is some balancing of this tendency through the variations of force applied, but the

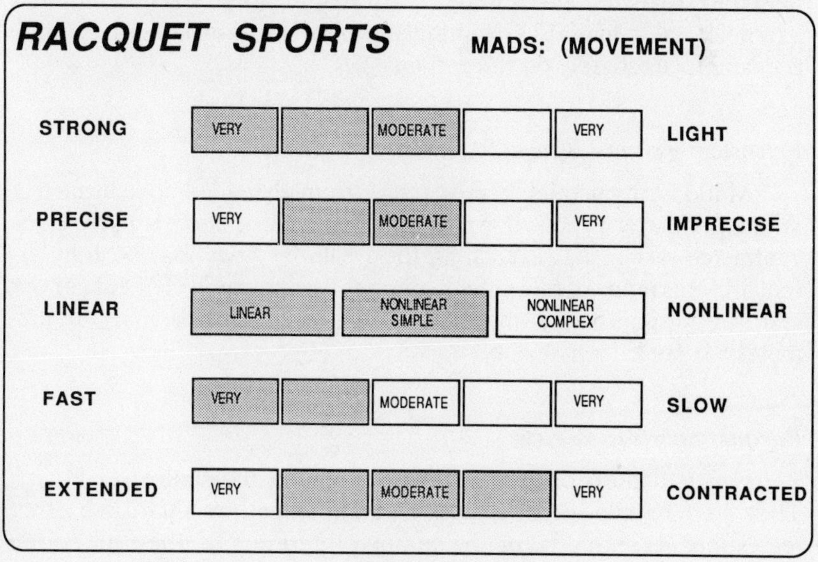

RACQUET SPORTS				MADS: (MOVEMENT)	
STRONG	VERY	MODERATE		VERY	LIGHT
PRECISE	VERY	MODERATE		VERY	IMPRECISE
LINEAR	LINEAR	NONLINEAR SIMPLE	NONLINEAR COMPLEX		NONLINEAR
FAST	VERY	MODERATE		VERY	SLOW
EXTENDED	VERY	MODERATE		VERY	CONTRACTED

Figure 8.15

majority of movements are more toward the strong than the light end of the scale.

Control: Rating—Range: Moderate to Precise

The game calls for precision. The better the player, the more precise the movements. As a player progresses up the ladder, body positioning and technique become crucial elements of the game. One can practice hitting a ball thousands of times before a serve is under control. To master the game you need to manage your actions with a resultant psychological emphasis on focus and control.

Linearity: Rating—Range: Linear to Non-linear (Simple)

Racquet games involve a mixture of linear and non-linear (simple) moves. The more advanced the player, the more intricate the movements. This suggests a balance in concentration and emotion, an ability to be flexible and to respond according to situational demands.

Speed: Rating—Range: Fast to Very Fast

Racquet games are fast to very fast; they are rarely slow. They require rapid changes in speed. Even when stationary, the player is poised to strike, to move quickly. This variable fast pacing encourages a psychological style of risky, spontaneous behavior. It makes us pay attention and focus sharply on the action.

Extension: Rating—Range: Extended to Contracted

Motions in racquet games range from extended to contracted. When the player is poised, waiting for a serve, the body is likely to be contracted. When he is reaching for a ball, his body may be fully extended. This range of movement contains psychological elements of risk and safety, spontaneity and control, aggression and passivity. It promotes a balanced personality.

Racquet Sports in Review

Racquet sports present a unique profile in the context of fitness. They are far more social, aggressive, and competitive than such other recreations as running or swimming. Interestingly, they are often thought of as something other than mere exercise. For this reason they require less self-discipline. They offer players a break from routine, an escape from daily worries. The price may be a potential roller coaster ride for the ego as competition creates its inevitable categories of winners and losers.

Although, muscularly, these sports emphasize lower-body development more than upper-body work, they gear the body (and the mind) more for action than for holding one's ground. The upper-body imbalance created by the greater development of the dominant side reinforces direct, aggressive tendencies. Movement analysis supports the view of racquet players as being high on flexibility but tending more toward action than toward passively sitting on things. The variety and range of movements required by racquet sports holds promise for an integration of emotional and mental life.

As is the case for all fitness activities, when carried to extremes, assets become liabilities and the racquet player overdevelops traits of aggressiveness, competitiveness, and impulsiveness. Yet, for people who need to develop skills in the social domain, who lack energy, who are overly rational, or who have even lost their sense of playfulness, racquet sports have much to offer.

What if you have never played? There is of course an initiation period, a time when you have to tolerate the awkwardness and embarrassment of a novice. This may be a hurdle you just don't want to jump. Take heart. There are lots of closet novices who would love to have an equally unskilled partner to share the miseries and triumphs of learning. And, there are always lessons. Mastering a racquet game can be a great ego trip. It can do wonders for your self-image. To say that you are a jogger is one thing, but to tell friends that you are a fair racquet player puts you in an entirely different league.

Aerobics

For a while it seemed everyone was taking aerobics. It was a fad—at least until injury rates began climbing. And before it faded, low-impact aerobics resurrected it and allowed devotees to resume with less fear of stress fractures, lower-back strain, and other popular diagnoses of sports medicine clinics.

Ten years ago, aerobics was the way women got in shape. It was a revival of the "phys ed" calisthenics class with a little modern dance thrown in. It was entertaining, colorful, and a total body workout to boot. Aerobic dancers were chic—they still are. Except now there are more men in the classes. Just as it has become okay for women to play men's games, so is it acceptable for men to put on tights and sweat to pop rock. Aerobic dancers don't fit a mold. They come for the singles scene, for glitter and fashion, but predominantly for fitness. In the extreme, aerobic dancers are labeled egotists and narcissists, as being obsessed with bodily perfection.

Most studios are mirrored. Looking at yourself becomes part of the workout. Bright lights and loud music mask the self-absorption. Sure, there are others to watch and compare, but it can become an intimate love/hate encounter with yourself and your body.

In a more structured way, what can we say about aerobic dance? Let's take it apart through our threefold analysis.

PAD/Psychosocial Dimensions of Aerobics

Let's be clear about this fitness option. It goes under such names as dancercize, aerobic dance, aerobics, low-impact aerobics, high-impact aerobics, stretch and tone, total workout, and no doubt a hundred others. It's a class in a club or private studio. It lasts for forty-five to ninety minutes, including a warm-up, an aerobics phase, and a cool-down. There's loud pop music and an instructor to take you through the paces. It's a little like dance and more like calisthenics. The class is structured, some might say choreographed, from start to finish. That's what we are calling "aerobics" (Figure 8.16).

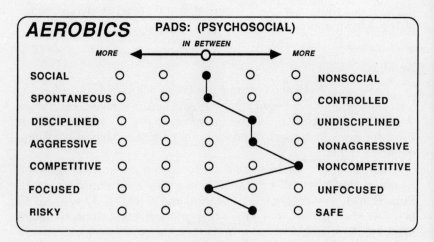

Figure 8.16

Social-Nonsocial: Rating — Intermediate

Aerobics classes do not require social interaction. You have to be aware of people around you and there is a definite "follow-the-leader" quality to classes, but if you want to remain anonymous, you can. Usually, when a person attends aerobics regularly, she will make a few acquaintances and small talk may be exchanged before and after class. But aside from promoting heavy breathing and occasional groans, the class itself does not call for social exchange. We rate it as intermediate only because it involves a group and opportunities for interaction exist.

Spontaneous-Controlled: Rating — Intermediate

Does this rating surprise you? You thought aerobics unleashed your creative, spontaneous urges. Far from it. From start to finish, you are part of the program. True, some movements may be novel and even a bit difficult. But the instructor leads, you follow. And there is a clear logic to the whole process. Warm up the muscles, stretch them out, and then burn in the aerobics section. Cool down, do some push-ups, sit-ups, and other calisthenics, and then a final stretch. It's all very routine, very predictable. What makes it intermediate is that you may not know what comes next. Just like responding to a racquet ball, you have to respond to the instructor's lead.

Disciplined-Undisciplined: Rating — Moderately Undisciplined

How is it undisciplined? Partly because it's fun: it's glittery, there's social support, and lots of mind-altering music. If you don't believe it, imagine a class without music, without mirrors, with everyone draped in grey sweatsuits and the instructor leading you through very traditional military calisthenics. It takes a lot less self-discipline to drag yourself to an aerobics class than it does to go out and run an hour a day — unless of course you have a serious body-image problem — or you are a man who wouldn't be seen dead in a Danskin.

Aggressive-Nonaggressive: Rating — Moderately Nonaggressive

Sure it takes energy and push to make it through an aerobics class, but just when you get tired of doing one thing, the instructor entertains you with another routine. There are some occasional forceful actions in aerobics, like overcoming the force of gravity as you leap around on the floor. But the atmosphere is light; the experience is mostly pleasing.

Perhaps the only way you are likely to feel very aggressive in an aerobics class is if you can't imitate the instructor's complicated moves. Men often complain about this and end up leaving early, or jogging defiantly in place while everyone else is dancing.

Competitive-Noncompetitive: Rating — Noncompetitive

Sure, you can try to kick higher, stretch farther, do better push-ups, and in every other way compete with your classmates, but aerobics doesn't ask you to do this. In fact, it mostly asks you to cooperate, to synchronize your movements with everyone else's. There are no winners or losers at the end of class — only survivors.

Focused-Unfocused: Rating — Intermediate

You have to pay attention because changes in movements come quickly, but, unfortunately, most aerobics routines are stagnant. Only the exceptional teacher makes efforts to regularly revise her choreography. After about three or four times in the same class you know what's coming and it doesn't take a lot of concentration to make the shift. Aerobics classes do little to make us focus better or learn how to concentrate.

Risky-Safe: Rating — Moderately Safe

There is some risk in an aerobics class, mostly to the ego. Those mirrors can be unflattering, and if you can't keep pace with the class, you may begin to feel as if everyone is watching. For men, the risk may be higher in that it isn't a traditionally masculine activity, and when a man compares himself to the majority of women he may feel pretty inadequate in terms of skill and stamina. For women, the issue may be more one of body image, of not matching up to the instructor's 12.4 percent body-fat rating. In other ways, however, it's a pretty tame activity. Aerobics has been around for a long enough time that it's a bona fide fitness outlet. You generally know what you are in for. Yes, there are more and more injuries attributed to aerobics, usually the result of poorly trained instructors, bad floors, or bad shoes. But with low-impact aerobics and more awareness about avoiding studios with concrete floors, this risk can be minimized.

BAD/Body Psychology for Aerobics

A good aerobics class has lots of body benefits. It strengthens and tones. It increases flexibility. It improves muscular endurance. And, in the low-impact variety, it lets you stay fit with less risk of injury (Figure 8.17).

What kind of body does it build? An aerobic dancer will develop adequately strong, flexible muscles. Exercises involve most major muscle groups. There are exercises for the upper and lower body, although they favor leg development over arm strengthening. Motions are to the side, front, and back, and sometimes circular. This means muscles on the side of the body (abductors and adductors) get worked, along with those in the front and back. All in all, it seems pretty balanced.

Problems in aerobics usually result from the instructor's qualifications and the lack of supervision in the classes. Some instructors have little idea of anatomy, physiology, or kinesiology, and at twenty-three years of age they may have little concept of the body limits of a forty-five-year-old novice. The second critical lack is that you can be doing everything wrong in an aerobics class and no one will tell you. Rarely will the instructor correct you. With thirty to forty sweating bodies to lead and motivate, who has time?

What this means is that we can rate aerobics pretty high in terms of body dynamics—if you go to a *good* class and if you do the exercises the way they should be done. Given these conditions, your body will not get overly muscled. It will develop increased range and flexibility. Each area will receive its due attention. And over time, with good coaching, your body alignment and balance will improve.

If it lacks anything, a good aerobics class will overemphasize mobility through all of the jumping movements and underemphasize stability through good grounding efforts. Even here, we can't knock aerobics too much because in many classes warm-up and cool-down exercises incorporate exercises to improve balance (standing on one leg while exercising the other), or grounding (varied exercises with legs bent at the knees, feet flat on the floor and spine erect).

In sum, aerobics scores high on body psychology, again keeping in mind the quality of instruction and coaching.

MAD/Movement Analysis of Aerobics

As we put this well-tuned aerobics body into motion, let's see how it rates on movement qualities (Figure 8.18).

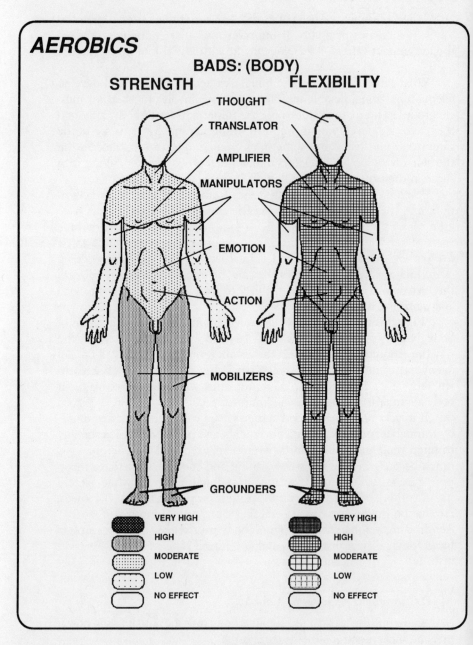

Figure 8.17

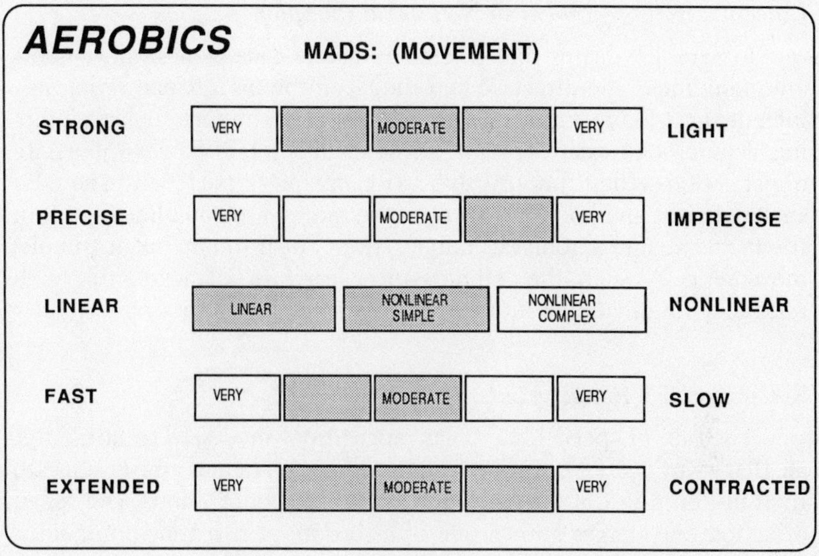

AEROBICS   MADS: (MOVEMENT)

STRONG	VERY		MODERATE		VERY	**LIGHT**
PRECISE	VERY		MODERATE		VERY	**IMPRECISE**
LINEAR	LINEAR		NONLINEAR SIMPLE	NONLINEAR COMPLEX		**NONLINEAR**
FAST	VERY		MODERATE		VERY	**SLOW**
EXTENDED	VERY		MODERATE		VERY	**CONTRACTED**

Figure 8.18

Force: Rating—*Range: Strong to Light*

Aerobics contains a range of forceful efforts, from push-ups to light dancing movements. So we rate it as having a breadth of force from strong to light. It never gets very strong or very light, but it does have a good balance between forceful and nonforceful actions. As we know, this promotes psychological balance in the use of force and in strength of determination. This balancing quality gives a person the option of having strength as well as delicacy to use as needed.

Control: Rating—*Imprecise*

In movement, control has to do with the precision of an action. Aerobics classes can improve precision by way of the mirror's constant feedback and the participant's efforts to mimic the motions of a good instructor. But without personal feedback, many aerobic dancers develop sloppy movement habits, and keep them for as long as they dance. We rate the actions of aerobics and participants' movements as imprecise. Motions don't have to be exact. They can be approximate or stylized, as the dancer wishes. The goal is more to get a good workout than to precisely mimic the instructor's actions. Some dancers are better than others and some instructors are more demanding of proper form.

*Linearity: Rating—**Linear to Non-linear (Simple)***

In aerobics classes that resemble upscale calisthenics, movements are more linear and direct. When they lean toward a dance style, they include more indirect movements. Exercises like running in place, jumping jacks, or leg kicks—common elements of aerobics classes—illustrate direct action. When the instructor choreographs a piece with shoulder shakes, twists, and body turns, you move more to the non-linear end. In the main, we rate aerobics as ranging from linear to non-linear (simple) movements. As such, the aerobic dancer learns to balance control with release, determination with flexibility, constraint with spontaneity.

*Speed: Rating—**Range: Moderate to Fast***

The rate of speed in aerobics ranges from moderate to fast. After all, that's why you feel so energized by aerobics. There is a brisk staccato rhythm—even in the warm-up. It demands response—now! The speed of action encourages an attitude of assertion, of risk and spontaneity. The faster the tempo, the more you throw yourself into the class, the more you abandon thought. Aerobics music pushes you along from a moderate pace at the outset to a rapid pace just before the cool-down.

*Extension: Rating—**Range: Extended to Contracted***

Reach out! Extend! Pull in! Push out! That's aerobics: a balance of contracted and extended movements. Depending on who teaches, you may have more of one than the other. Some instructors are big on push-ups, sit-ups, and running like a football player. Others want you to stretch and extend, to kick out and reach. Usually there's a balance. And that's good for teaching us to extend and withdraw, to take chances and to contain ourselves, to assert and to yield.

Aerobics in Review

How can aerobics help you change? You won't necessarily become more sociable, although the opportunity is there. In fact, there may even be a tendency toward self-absorption in the mirrored studio. It's a controlled activity, but its movements and body conditioning help you improve your flexibility in action, to be less rigid if that's a problem. It's easier to take than is a steady dose of running or weight lifting. You may even inject some upbeat rhythm into your life. On the downside, if you need to develop more self-discipline, a continued diet of aerobics can hook you on external support and the spell of the aerobics studio.

If you are a passive individual, it won't help. In fact, it could make matters worse. Remember, the instructor leads, you follow. On the other hand, if you have a tendency to be overly aggressive, it may tone you down. It brings out a cooperative spirit. But if you need to push yourself more competitively, look elsewhere.

It makes you concentrate and helps you focus your mind, but only in the early days. If you become a regular, the routine will be too repetitive to keep your attention, to take you away from pressing life problems or wishful fantasies. And maybe it's just a bit more adventurous an activity for men than for women. It challenges a lot of masculine concepts and may be helpful to males for just this reason.

Aerobics is pretty well-balanced, although it will do more for your feeling of support and mobility (lower body) than for your controlling/manipulating self (upper body). A good class can work wonders for releasing emotions, for energizing you and helping you feel connected all over. Its movements have a nice balance, too. It tends to be a bit speedy, but otherwise it will train your body to have good versatility. And if you take a class that pushes you physically, that makes you use strong movements as well as ones that stretch you out, you will counter some of the psychological passivity that an aerobics class might otherwise induce.

Cycling

Cycling has grown steadily in popularity over the past decade. And has it ever changed! Bikes used to be cumbersome beasts of burden used for short hauls and practical work. Now they are sleek and fast: mountain bikes, sport bikes, touring bikes, and some that look like they just came out of a science-fiction movie set.

What about the people who ride them? Cyclists are dedicated characters. They plot their routes with the strategies of a field marshal. They equip their bikes with mini-computers to gauge speed, mileage, cadence, and even pulse rate. They sheath their bodies in spandex and their feet in snug cycling shoes. When the weather is bad, they mount their bikes on stationary tracks that recreate wind and road resistance and pedal away in their living rooms.

You may say, "I thought cycling was my sport but I sure don't fit that description!" Remember, we're talking about people who cycle as a regular thing, maybe one hundred miles or more per week. It's their form of exercise—not just a recreational option like the annual fishing trip.

There are indoor and outdoor cycling tracks and there are special lanes on roadways. With the new mountain bikes there are also hilly off-road trails. When we talk about cycling, we are going to focus on the sport or touring cyclist who works out three or more times a week on roadways for periods of an hour or more. Our comments will be more or less applicable to other cyclists and even to those who regularly use stationary cycles.

PAD/Psychosocial Dimensions of Cycling

For the kind of sports enthusiast we are considering, cycling is her fitness choice. It isn't an activity undertaken for competition or strictly as a mode of transport. It's something the person does for the pleasure (and pain) of cycling (Figure 8.19).

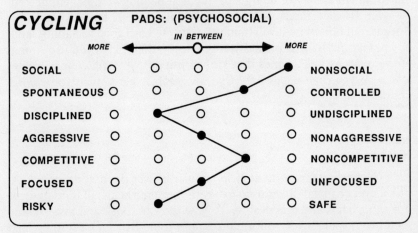

Figure 8.19

Social-Nonsocial: Rating—Nonsocial

Yes, there are cycling clubs and many cyclists ride together in packs. But what do you do while you are pedaling? You are alone with your bike and your thoughts. Most of the time you spend cycling will be spent alone in the privacy of your mind.

Spontaneous-Controlled: Rating—Moderately Controlled

Spontaneity involves a certain amount of impulsivity, of responding intuitively in the moment. Sound like cycling? Part of it does. When you have to make a quick judgment call on the road, you are moving too fast to think it through logically. You have to act! But how often does this happen? For the most part cycling represents a planned activity with routes and rates set for the workout.

Disciplined-Undisciplined: Rating — **Moderately Disciplined**

It takes commitment to get out on your bike day after day. Even after the saddle sores and aching thigh muscles subside, you have to make the workout happen. Nice scenery can help, but when you are burning up a hill, who sees it?

Aggressive-Nonaggressive: Rating — **Intermediate**

That you have to work so hard to get up hills, to keep the pedals spinning at 90 RPM, or to push on against strong head winds tells us you have to generate some aggressive feelings in cycling just to continue. Keeping your body hunched up for long periods of time and not giving in to the temptation to coast down hills means you have to forcefully dominate your body, the machine, the tortuous route you have chosen.

Competitive-Noncompetitive: Rating — **Moderately Noncompetitive**

Bear in mind that we are not talking about Olympic cyclists or transcontinental marathoners. The sports cyclist can be seen pacing himself against his computerized schedule or speeding along in the midst of a pack of cyclists. When alone, the race is against time, against oneself. With friends, the goal is to go as fast as possible while hanging together in a pack.

Focused-Unfocused: Rating — **Intermediate**

On a long ride your mind drifts. You feel the pain in your legs. Your stomach tells you to eat. Your back aches. You watch the passing scenery. Even so, you keep a keen eye on the road. There are potholes, rocks, pieces of glass, and four-wheeled demons spewing carbon monoxide. You glance and mentally record. Now it's internal time — check out the body works. Look at your gauges. Eyes back on the road. Where's your buddy? Change gears — going up a hill. There's still time to think about life. But if you are really moving, reality is far more demanding than thoughts past, present, and future.

Risky-Safe: Rating—Moderately Risky

When you are moving down a hill at about fifty miles per hour, you have to wonder what would happen if your tire blew, or you hit a pothole, or any of a number of other possibilities. Cycling is risky, mostly to the body, not as much to the mind. Yes, there are ego risks when you are cycling with some hotshots, but most cyclists are not out to embarrass you. Your risks will come more from passing cars and trucks and all those other things that might propel you from your seat, giving you a road rash or, more seriously, myriad fractures and abrasions.

BAD/Body Psychology for Cycling

There's little question about what gets developed in cycling: the lower body. Of course, cycling requires good abdominal and back strength and the arms are exercised, particularly in sprints and going up hills (Figure 8.20).

What's the nature of muscle development? For the most part, leg muscles become shortened through cycling. It isn't good cycling mechanics to have full extension of the leg when you are pedaling. This means the muscles of the thigh never fully extend. Also, most of the work gets done by the thigh muscles rather than the lower leg. The result is a bit of an imbalance—massive thighs on top of smaller calves.

Muscles along the back are held in contraction, as are the muscles that support the weight of the head. You need a good stretch before and after cycling to counter the restricting movements of this sport.

Psychologically, it's not very well balanced. Range of movement and flexibility may diminish unless the cyclist takes care to do flexibility exercises. The body is held in a bound position for most of the ride, which doesn't make for a graceful, fluid body. Your body will not feel very grounded through cycling. It simply does not teach you much about connecting yourself to the earth. And the leg musculature it develops is very limited and specific. So even though the main muscles worked in cycling are in the lower body, it doesn't do much for lower-body psychological functions—mobility and stability. As noted earlier, the upper body develops in a bound, contracted manner—not much help for developing one's capacity for articulate control and exploration.

MAD/Movement Analysis of Cycling

In analyzing body actions, we will just be considering the cyclist's movements, as if the cycle itself is invisible and we only observe the moving body (Figure 8.21).

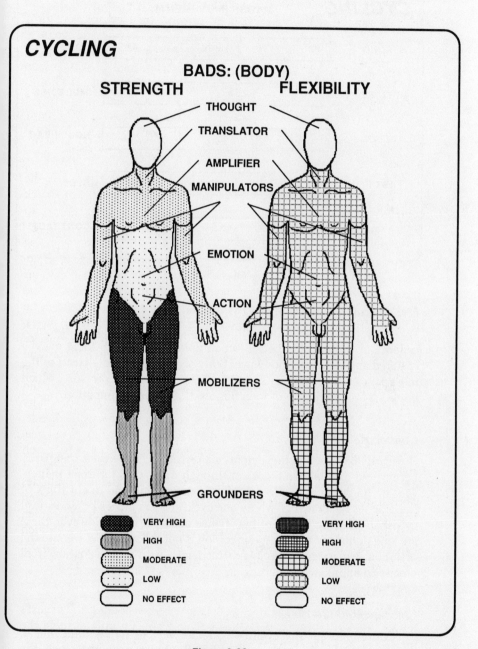

Figure 8.20

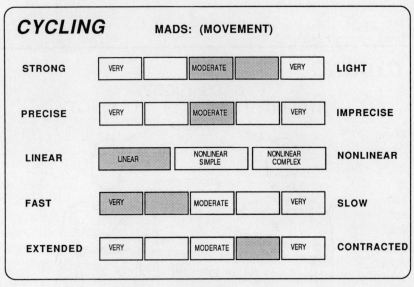

Figure 8.21

Force: Rating—*Range: Light to Moderate*

A cyclist uses relatively little pedal pressure and goes for high cadence or RPM of the pedal. On an uphill climb, more force may be required and the upper body may tense against the handlebars. For the most part, cycling requires a range of light-to-moderate pressure, which implies a limited degree of forceful assertion and determination.

Control: Rating—*Moderate*

Partly because the movements are restricted by the cycle and partly because riding a bike in a pack or through traffic calls for exact maneuvers, cycling requires some precision in movement. You might think of the practice of "drafting," where one cyclist hovers inches behind a lead cyclist at speeds in excess of twenty-five miles per hour. However, there are long periods of time when precision is not called for. So, we rate the precision demanded by cycling as moderate, with some variation from precise to imprecise depending on the cyclist's skill.

Linearity: Rating—*Linear*

Movements of the cyclist's body are very directional and linear. There may be some occasional wavy, flexible movements when the cyclist is trying to loosen up tight muscles, but these don't typify the actions of cycling. Linear motions go along with a psychological attitude of control, discipline, and mental focus. They also suggest a quality of self-assertion.

Speed: Rating — Range: Fast to Very Fast

Cycling ranges from fast to very fast. Remember, we are not talking about the speed of the bicycle, but about the speed of the cyclist's movements. To pedal at a rate of 80 to 100 RPM means you have to move your legs very fast. This isn't the pace of the recreational cyclist, who pedals at about 20 to 30 RPM. There are also moments where you have to respond instantly to road situations. High speed in action corresponds to traits of assertion, adventurousness, spontaneity, and mental focus.

Extension: Rating — Contracted

Movements in cycling are contracted. The cyclist's body is contained. It is bound to the machine in such a way that extension is impossible. This emphasizes development of emotional control and can help balance tendencies toward assertion and risk brought out by other MAD ratings.

Cycling in Review

If you picked up some contradictions in this analysis of cyclists, you got the message. Some of the body and movement dynamics of cycling counterbalance its psychological demands. For example, it's not a very aggressive activity, but the movement qualities of linearity, speed, and control foster a direct, assertive approach to life. It is a highly energizing activity when performed at the rate sports cyclists go. The result is a focused, active lifestyle.

Cyclists have a somewhat superior attitude. Even though our analysis depicts some of the drudgery of this sport, cyclists are exuberant about what they do. It thrills them. And that's understandable. It may be a grind pedaling up an 11,000-foot mountain, but what goes up must come down! Cyclists tell us they would never trade cycling shoes for running shoes. Running is "just too boring."

What about its social qualities? It won't improve your social skills and it won't help you feel more connected and grounded. It binds your body and reaching out is underdeveloped. Many cyclists may have good social skills, but they didn't develop them through cycling.

Cycling puts some restrictions on movement, body development, and personality dynamics. It's not well rounded. This is not to say it's bad. Along with other activities, it can be quite fulfilling. Alone, personality development may stagnate and movement qualities may become restrained.

Yoga

You may be turned off by the guru worship that seems to go along with yoga practice. Or maybe it's the burning incense, the chanting, or the cult-like atmosphere. Can you separate these aspects from the more physical practice of hatha yoga? The fact is you may have done many yoga stretches as part of aerobics or other exercise programs without even knowing it. Unlike most fitness activities, yoga is intentially a more integrated mind-body practice. Of course, the ultimate purpose of yoga is to add spirit to this equation, but that's an optional part of the package.

Let's get back to hatha yoga. What is it? In brief, it is a branch of yoga involving movement sequences and breathing practices aimed at physical and mental control. Yoga represents a quest for spiritual and mental perfection through mastery of the body. Yet, many people who practice yoga do so for more practical reasons, like feeling good or managing stress.

So much is written about yoga that it is impossible to summarize. We just want to be clear that this discussion is limited to hatha yoga exercises that a person may practice for any of a number of reasons, including health and physical fitness.

PAD/Psychosocial Dimensions of Yoga

When we examine yoga, we will be considering the period of time a person spends doing yoga postures, movements, and breathing exercises. This may range from thirty to ninety minutes or more per day. Our focus is on the person who practices yoga three or more times a week, not the occasional class attendee (Figure 8.22).

Social-Nonsocial: Rating—Nonsocial

Yoga can be practiced alone or in a group. Some prefer the social support of group sessions, but this is by no means an integral part of

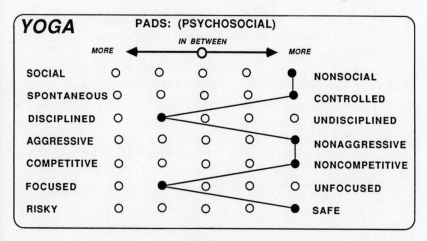

Figure 8.22

yoga practice. In fact, emphasis is on what goes on inside of you, not between you and someone else. If you happen to be in a class, the teacher is a guide helping you do the movements correctly. Surely in a class setting, opportunity for interactions are present before and after, and indeed the uniqueness of yoga eases friendship development. But this again is not an integral part of yoga practice.

Spontaneous-Controlled: Rating — *Controlled*

The practice of yoga is a very controlled activity. It emphasizes mind over matter and a very precise enactment of movement forms. Some believe that the effect of yoga may be to enhance spontaneity by releasing energy, and we think this may well be the case. But getting back to the practice, the student of yoga goes through a well-structured, highly planned routine of movements in each session. Spontaneous, intuitively guided movements are *not* part of yoga practice.

Disciplined-Undisciplined: Rating — *Moderately Disciplined*

A key to yoga practice is discipline — disciplining the body and the mind. Some students may use the crutch of a class to get themselves to practice regularly, but for those who live outside an ashram (a residential center for yoga students), you have to go it alone much of the time, and that takes discipline. We rate it as moderate in self-discipline mostly because there are a lot of immediate payoffs in yoga practice. You feel good when you go through particular movements. It gratifies you in the moment. You don't have to wait until you are finished in order to feel satisfaction.

Aggressive-Nonaggressive: Rating—**Nonaggressive**

There's no hedging on this one. Yoga pulls far away from the aggressive end of the continuum. It is a release into your body, not a fight against it. It is a process of trying to harmonize with yourself and eventually with others. You don't use force to master. That just messes things up. You need lots of patience and great sensitivity to what is happening inside.

Competitive-Noncompetitive: Rating—**Noncompetitive**

Yoga's emphasis on harmony stands in firm opposition to the spirit of competition. One does not beat the body into submission or try to do yoga better than others. It is an internal quest for peace and unity. People may nonetheless try to compete with others during yoga classes, but this is counter to yoga philosophy.

Focused-Unfocused: Rating—**Moderately Focused**

A purpose of yoga is to quiet the mind, to make it still. Yoga practice is an integrated mind-body activity. The mind is engaged in a special meditation while the body moves through the yoga postures. Unlike racquet sports where the mind *must* attend to the action, mental focusing in yoga comes from a conscious disciplining of thoughts. In essence, you teach your mind to concentrate. It's hard work and you may not always succeed.

Risky-Safe: Rating—**Safe**

If you have ever seen films of yoga masters twisting their bodies like pretzels, you might wonder how this activity could be safe. Bear in mind that these masters have been practicing yoga for decades. As a novice, your body flexibility will be far more restricted. Yet, with good supervision you will gradually advance in flexibility and to a lesser extent in strength. Even if you have a chronic medical problem, yoga can be practiced under advisement. Since the intention of yoga is to improve mental and physical functioning, we rate it as a safe outlet for a broad range of people. Probably the main risk in yoga comes from fears and preconceptions about its spiritual, cultic nature.

BAD/Body Psychology for Yoga

People who practice yoga are anything but muscle-bound. The practice of yoga mostly affects your flexibility and to a lesser extent your strength and endurance. It won't give you a highly muscled body or one that will necessarily perform well in endurance activities such as marathons (Figure 8.23).

A well-rounded yoga program works all areas of the body, developing adequate strength in both deep and superficial muscle layers. More critically, it massages internal body organs, assisting them in proper functioning. Body alignment is stressed, as is balance between different parts of the body.

A person who regularly practices yoga should manifest good emotional flow and a relative absence of body blockages. What this means is that there should be less chronic tension in different areas of the body. Yoga allows you to sense the flow of energy, to be aware of feelings, and to channel emotional energy, rather than store it in contracted muscles.

There are yoga movements that teach you balance and grounding so you experience more emotional support. But you have to be careful about creating a yoga exercise plan that is right for you. The tendency is to pick yoga exercises that you need least and avoid ones that would be most beneficial. A good teacher can help you get the most out of yoga.

The body psychology rating for yoga is high—with a few qualifications. It builds an adequately strong, balanced body with flexibility in joints and muscles. It enhances energy flow so that you can express your needs and still stay in grounded contact with your environment. How much you gain will depend on the quality of your instruction. A good teacher is a must!

MAD/Movement Analysis of Yoga

As we analyze hatha yoga, we will be considering the body's actions as you perform a typical sequence of movements over a thirty- to sixty-minute period (Figure 8.24).

Force: Rating—Range: Light to Strong

Yoga contains a wide range of force in its movements, from light to strong. Depending on the phase of a movement sequence, you may have to use pressure or, conversely, to emphasize lightness. We see this balanced emphasis on force as enhancing your ability to use strength or delicacy as the situation requires, to be assertive and strong when needed and passive and receptive as otherwise indicated.

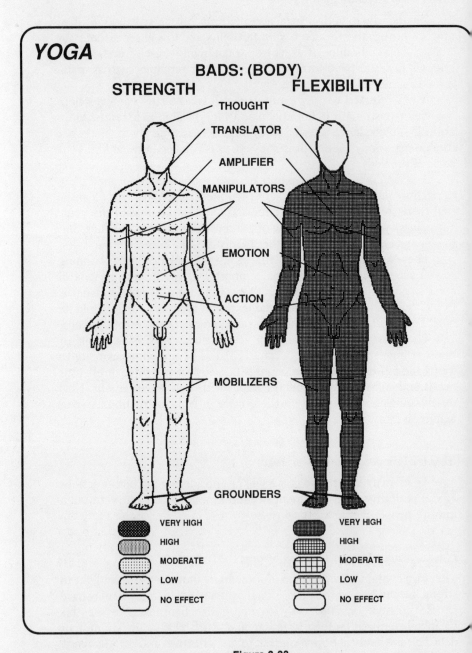

Figure 8.23

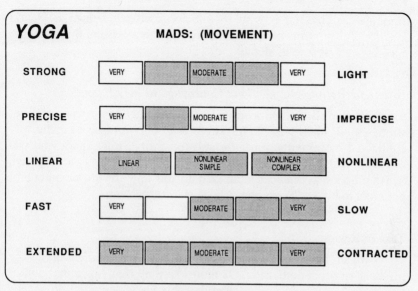

Figure 8.24

*Control: Rating—**Precise***

The emphasis is on precision in movement. You can do yoga sloppily, but if you do, you run the risk of injuring yourself or, at the least, not benefiting from it. Picking up a book and teaching yourself yoga is generally not a good idea. You need feedback about your yoga postures. And, as we know from our earlier discussion of precise movements, they help us develop psychological qualities of control, self-discipline, mental focus, and emphasize safety.

*Linearity: Rating—**Range: Linear to Non-linear** (**Simple and Complex**)*

The multitude of shapes and directions the body assumes throughout a yoga sequence ranges from linear to non-linear (simple and complex). This develops flexibility in how we approach life—being direct when we need to and using indirect accesses to life's predicaments on other occasions. It rounds out personality without stressing one quality over another.

*Speed: Rating—**Range: Very Slow to Moderate***

You are probably thinking that yoga is very slow. Well, some parts are, but others can be more dynamic. In fact, one recent modification combines aerobic dance with yoga to form what is known as *Dance-kinetics*. But in terms of the typical yoga practice session, our rating on speed is very slow to moderate.

Extension: Rating—Range: Very Contracted to Very Extended

The popular misconception of yoga practice is that you get stretched out like Plastic Man. That's true, but you also do some very contracted movements: you grow and you shrink, you expand and you contract. Our rating, therefore, is very extended to very contracted, which implies a balanced approach to life and the development of potential to be flexible in how we deal with situations.

Yoga in Review

With all this praise of yoga, why hasn't it caught on? Perhaps it's the mystical, spiritual dimension. Or, more likely, it's that yoga runs counter to our love of speed and excitement. No flashy leotards, no special equipment. Dull, dull, dull! These pseudocriticisms aside, there's no doubt yoga can be quite helpful to a wide range of people.

On a body level, yoga has much to recommend it. It develops balance and harmony between different areas of the body. It creates a flexible yet adequately strong musculature. And it shows you how to use the ground for emotional support. Its movements have good range and therefore help us balance our personal style so we don't emphasize one quality to the exclusion of another. It lacks the dynamic of speed, but a new westernized combination of yoga and aerobics, known as *Dance-kinetics*, offers this option to those who require more fast-paced activity.

This doesn't mean it's for everyone. Some people who are deeply involved in yoga complain that it is so otherworldly that they lose touch with the reality they live in. Others say that you get to be too flexible (mentally as well as physically) so that you end up accommodating everyone but yourself.

This means yoga's strengths can constitute weaknesses for certain people. It gives you private meditative time, but it does little to develop you socially. It is nonaggressive, noncompetitive, and very cautious. If you tend to be this way already, yoga may overdevelop a style of passive acceptance in a world that requires you to be assertive and even competitive, at least on occasion.

Overall, yoga deserves more consideration than most fitness buffs give it. Some health clubs are slipping yoga-like programs into their schedule under the guise of stretch and flex classes. This adaptation of yoga to our North American needs should have high payoffs in terms of rounding out fitness programs as well as aggressive, competitive psychological tendencies.

Martial Arts

There are so many schools of martial arts that it becomes difficult to discuss them as a single entity. What do we mean by martial arts? Basically, we are talking about different forms of self-defense, such as karate, judo, aikido, tae kwon do, kung fu, and tai chi chuan. Although each of these schools is supposedly a discipline of self-defense, some are far more aggressive than others. Most karate schools represent a "hard" approach to self-defense, meaning they rely upon aggressive training techniques. The approach of tai chi chuan typifies the "soft" approach, wherein students are taught evasion and a more passive, receptive self-defense process.

We might recognize from our own experience, or from films like *The Karate Kid*, how the master or don determines the quality of training. If the don is very aggressive, training resembles boxing, with its emphasis on being overly aggressive and even hurting your opponent. If the don takes a more philosophical view of the martial arts, the approach is likely to be more emotionally disciplined and tolerant.

How can we distinguish one from the other? Other than knowing that some schools such as tai chi chuan are typically soft, what we find will often be more a function of the instructor than of the school itself.

When we dissect the martial arts in this section, we will be analyzing a more optimistic view of how they function and what they instill. We will not be looking at the extreme schools where the emphasis is on inflicting injury and teaching technique without philosophy.

PAD/Psychosocial Dimensions of Martial Arts

We base this analysis on people who go to a club or school a minimum of three times per week. Lessons may last one hour or more and some individuals may practice on their own when classes are not scheduled (Figure 8.25).

Social-Nonsocial: Rating—Moderately Social

Why would this activity be rated as social? Because it requires interaction, mostly nonverbal, but interaction nonetheless. After the warm-up and the *katas* (precision movements in a prescribed sequence),

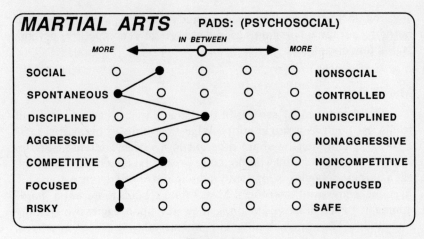

Figure 8.25

students learn by sparring with one another, practicing kicks, punches, throws, and falls. In practice, students give each other verbal feedback ranging from "Try it this way" to "Hey, take it easy!" You have to be attuned to your partner throughout the session. And if you stay with a group for a long period of time, you have to find ways to smooth over ruffled feathers from times when a kick accidentally connects.

Spontaneous-Controlled: Rating—*Spontaneous*

There is no program of events in martial arts. You do not have time to logically think through how you will react after catching a punch in the gut. Yes, there is strategy and it is also true that the spontaneity you see may be the result of years of practice. Martial arts training demands a balance between spontaneity and emotional control. But in the heat of the moment, you never know what is going to happen or how you will respond. This is spontaneity.

Disciplined-Undisciplined: Rating—*Intermediate*

Bet you're surprised. You might be saying that the core of martial arts is self-discipline. We have no argument with this. Yet when we talk about discipline in a psychosocial sense, we are considering how much you have to drive yourself versus how much you are pulled by qualities of the activity. Martial arts training occurs in groups with an instructor and with lots of interaction. You learn something new each day and what you do has a high degree of variety. There are special outfits and rituals. In a sense, it has glitter: it is attractive and inherently interesting. That it is not as playful as racquet sports or as personally undemanding as aerobics makes it more disciplined than these kinds of engagements and, therefore, the rating is intermediate.

Aggressive-Nonaggressive: Rating—**Aggressive**

It seems we can't evaluate martial arts on any dimension without qualifying comments. Aggression means the application of force to dominate or master. With the exception of schools like tai chi, martial arts demand forceful action. They develop the potential to apply force to dominate, even though the philosophical training helps you contain or channel aggressive tendencies in constructive ways. Research tells us that students of the martial arts gain higher levels of self-confidence and, as a result, are less likely to respond aggressively when provoked.[4] With good instruction we believe this will happen, but it doesn't change the fact that martial arts instill a capacity for aggressive action.

Competitive-Noncompetitive: Rating—**Moderately Competitive**

The purpose of martial arts training is not to compete, but to learn a system of self-defense. In doing so you have to practice with a partner. Enter the competitive element! Then, as you progress from yellow belt to black belt, you may find yourself in club-sponsored competitions where a point system defines winners and losers. We hold back on rating martial arts as highly competitive only because its purpose and philosophy are noncompetitive.

Focused-Unfocused: Rating—**Focused**

You have to pay attention in the martial arts, or you may not survive. It demands your attention. It makes you concentrate. If you are thinking about anything else, you may get injured. There is little time for extraneous thoughts, for daydreaming or worrying about life's concerns. Also, meditative training in the martial arts furthers this mental focus.

Risky-Safe: Rating—**Risky**

You can get hurt not only in the sparring and competitive activities of the martial arts, but also in practicing punches and kicks. Aside from physical injuries, the psychological side may be a bit easier. Sure, your ego might hurt as you go crashing to the floor, but it happens to everyone. And you don't have to wear spandex leotards that broadcast your percentage of body fat: your ego can hide comfortably beneath your *gi* (the outfit you wear in martial arts classes). Nonetheless, it's a risky activity that is exciting to participate in but that occasionally results in fatal injuries.

BAD/Body Psychology for Martial Arts

More than most popular fitness activities, martial arts training teaches grounding, balance, energy control, and release. It emphasizes muscle strengthening, endurance, *and* flexibility. There is relatively equal development of upper and lower body. And you learn to use your nondominant side, right or left, as well as your dominant one. A key to success in martial arts training is understanding and controlling your energy flow (Figure 8.26).

Martial arts training gets high ratings from the perspective of body psychology. If you stay in it long enough, you are likely to feel tremendous emotional grounding and support through the development of your lower body. No doubt, this is one of the reasons self-confidence improves so much. And your expressive side represented by upper-body strength and flexibility will also improve in quality and quantity. That is, your muscular development permits you to be delicate or strong, rigid or flexible. The choices are open. You are not bound to one way by virtue of how your body develops. Further, you learn a lot about balance, about how to use your weight, how to stand your ground, how to move from your center, and how to use your breath for expression. There are, of course, cautions that arise from excessive practice and use of force in the martial arts. But for the most part, body development through the martial arts will better enable you to satisfy psychological needs and desires for self-expression.

MAD/Movement Analysis of Martial Arts

The psychology of the martial arts can also be appreciated by examining its inherent movement patterns. Let's look at the five dimensions to see what characteristics are reinforced (Figure 8.27).

Force: Rating—Range: Very Strong to Very Light

When we think about the movement quality of force in martial arts,

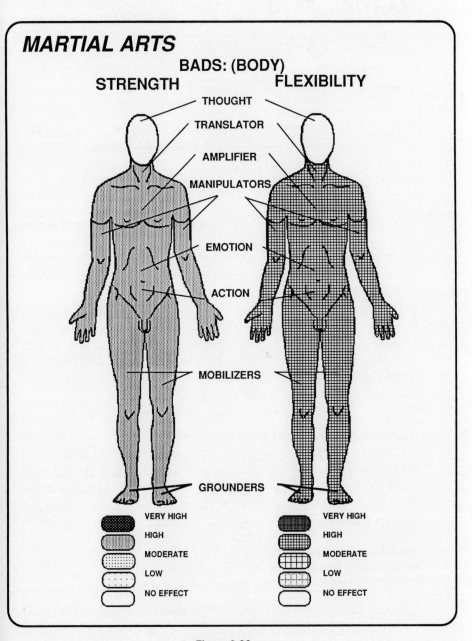

Figure 8.26

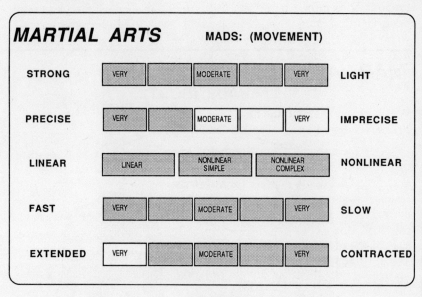

Figure 8.27

we may only focus on the strong movements of kicks and punches. But there are many other movements where training emphasizes a lightness of movement, such as walking on delicate rice paper without tearing it. You learn how to move with strength and with lightness, so our rating is the full range, from very light to very strong. This implies an excellent balance between aggressive and passive capabilities.

Control: Rating—*Range: Precise to Very Precise*

Martial arts training calls for precision in movement. Where you place your feet, how you move your arms, what you do with your torso are all part of a precise pattern. Of course, it takes a long time to learn these precision movements, so most trainees move with something less than exacting accuracy. Nonetheless, we would rate the emphasis of martial arts movements as precise to very precise. This tells us that martial arts training should help instill psychological qualities of discipline, control, mental focus, and an emphasis on safety.

Linearity: Rating—*Range: Linear to Non-linear (Simple and Complex)*

Movements in martial arts may be quite direct or they may require the body to assume varied shapes, patterns, and directions. We see linearity in a punch or a kick, but when you spar with a partner or perform ritual *katas*, movements are as likely to be non-linear as they are to be linear. Such range of movement from linear to non-linear (simple and complex) suggests the development of psychological balance in assertion, control, discipline, and focus. You learn to direct yourself as well as to know the value of indirection.

Speed: Rating — Range: Very Fast to Very Slow

Activities that have a wide range of speeds help us learn to pace ourselves in life. Martial arts training begins with slow, deliberate moves and then speeds up the action once the patterns become ingrained. Its range of speed runs the gamut from very slow to very fast. In the extremes, there are lightning-quick kicks and virtually motionless meditative moments. The psychological qualities that are reinforced through this action pattern are balanced between such opposites as aggressive and passive, focused and unfocused, risky and safe, controlled and spontaneous.

Extension: Rating — Range: Very Contracted to Extended

Martial arts movements encompass most of the range from very contracted to extended. The body may crouch or it may spring into extension. The arms may be tightly contracted before a punch and then extended when the punch is delivered. Through such training the body learns to appreciate the extremes and to know when to reach out and when to pull back. Since there is always a degree of tension in the body — for example, when a kick is delivered — we hold back on rating movements as fully extended.

Martial Arts in Review

Many people avoid martial arts training because of its seemingly harsh, aggressive movements. This is a limiting perspective. There's a whole lot more to martial arts than this. Perhaps its greatest liability is the risk involved in practice. This isn't limited to the danger of catching a stray kick, but also includes injuries incurred through overly zealous stretches and practice movements.

What will martial arts do for you? They can increase your self-confidence. Movements are assertive yet controlled. Your body learns to stand its ground and to feel centered. Psychologically, you are able to strike a balance between too much discipline and too little, as well as between too much spontaneity and too much emotional control. Your whole being learns to focus its energy. You do this through your breath, through the direction of your efforts, and through concentrating your attention.

It isn't just a body discipline. Probably the greatest complaints about martial arts training concern schools that teach body technique but omit the philosophical emphasis on mental and emotional control.

It rates high as a well-integrated mind-body training process, but it isn't for everyone. It may be too extreme for people who are overly passive as well as for people who tend to be too aggressive. Training involves some violent actions, and there is question about whether this reinforces similar thought processes. Research tells us that the more trained the person is, the less likely she is to respond to aggressive stimuli.[5] We would agree. But proper training takes a long time and, in the interim, violence-prone individuals may tend to act out their newly acquired skills.

Dance

Here's another case where great variety exists. There's ballet and jazz and modern dance and improvisational dance and on and on and on. So, what are we talking about?

Let's answer by considering our purpose. This book is about regular fitness activities. What do people who have an interest in dance do for fitness? They take classes. What kind of classes? For the most part, they either take something that is more toward ballet or more toward modern or jazz. To simplify, we are going to make two broad headings: *ballet* and *modern/jazz*. Of course, there are major schools that subdivide each of these dance concentrations, but for our purpose we will look primarily at the larger classifications of ballet and modern/jazz dance.

As you might know, there is a big difference between ballet training and modern or jazz dance training. Oftentimes, students cross-train in both approaches, but there are those who are strictly ballet dancers and those who are committed to modern or jazz dance. Since there is such a difference, we will point out in our threefold analysis where these two major styles diverge.

Before leaving this introduction, you might ask, "What about social dance?" This is also a popular activity, but it tends to be more of a once-a-week kind of program than something you might do seven days a week. It really doesn't fit our criteria for a regular fitness activity, even though some people may indeed practice social dance on a daily basis. If you are interested in this form of dance, you might apply some of the commentary about ballet and modern/jazz dance to social dance because it will be similar. Of course, a major point of difference is that it is *social* dance.

PAD/Psychosocial Dimensions of Dance

Many dancers first put on their tutus at an early age. After realizing they are not going to make a career out of dance, they continue dancing on a recreational level. Others start later in life, getting into the routine of taking classes three or four times a week. Dance in this context is something you do in a class with instruction. Classes are structured with a warm-up followed by combinations of movements in increasing complexity. There is work on the basics of movement followed by practice of a choreographed dance. Students imitate the instructor and receive frequent corrections throughout class. Here's how it can be described on our dimensions (Figures 8.28, 8.29):

Social-Nonsocial: Rating—*Intermediate*

Much as in other exercise activities that primarily take place in class settings, there are opportunities for interaction without the necessity of socializing. You may go to a class for a long period of time before you begin to develop relationships. There is little in the activity itself that causes you to talk to others or to have sustained nonverbal interactions.

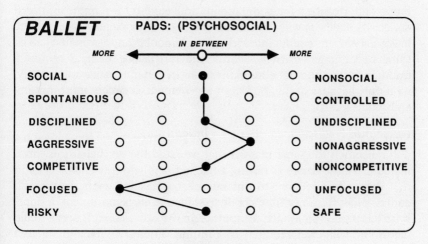

Figure 8.28

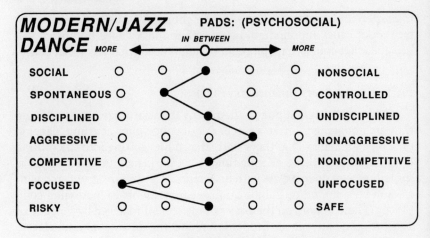

Figure 8.29

Spontaneous-Controlled: Ratings: Ballet — Intermediate;
Modern/Jazz — Moderately Spontaneous

Control, on a personal level, has to do with a logical, analytical process of organizing yourself. For activities, it concerns the logical, analytical process by which you determine what you do. A ballet class derives from a precise order of activities. One moves according to a formula. It may look spontaneous, but it isn't. A modern or jazz class may at times resemble the ordered character of ballet, but there are more opportunities for spontaneous movements, for improvisational dance. In reality it will depend on the teacher or ballet master. Some ballet classes are conducted with the regimentation of a military drill. Others encourage creativity. More characteristically, the modern dance tradition fosters spontaneous expression. In general, dance stirs creativity if only because of the intricacy of movements a dancer must imitate.

Disciplined-Undisciplined: Ratings — Intermediate

For much the same reasons that we rated the martial arts as intermediate, we see dance as having a magnetism that attracts dancers and that demands discipline to put oneself on the line each class, to do endless *pliés*, to subject one's body to someone else's movement designs. It isn't as much fun as racquet sports. On the other hand, it doesn't take nearly the willpower required by running. There's a group to support you and the movement itself may be its own reward.

*Aggressive-Nonaggressive: Rating — **Moderately Nonaggressive***

Dance training asks you to use the minimum amount of effort in order to effectively perform a movement. Ideally, there is no wasted energy. The dancer releases into a movement rather than forcing it. The more you try to make something happen in dance, the less successful you are. There are, of course, dance choreographies where you have to be forceful, but more often the emphasis is on a certain effortless quality. What makes dance contain an aggressive element is that some of its movements require full efforts, thereby instilling some appreciation of force. We see this when a dancer bounds off the floor or slashes through an angry choreography.

*Competitive-Noncompetitive: Rating — **Intermediate***

Remember, we are not talking about preprofessional dance programs, but about classes intended for a general audience. The idea is to do as well as you can in these classes — not to compete. Yet, it's hard not to feel some competitive urges in dance class. First of all, there are levels of classes, like beginning, intermediate, and advanced. Dancers try to get into as high a level as possible in order to challenge themselves. This means being better than others who may be trying for the same class. Second, when it comes to the part of the class where you line up for dance combinations that move across the floor, you want to be up toward the front of the line. You have to qualify for this position by being better than those behind you. Third, there's a certain status or pecking order that evolves in a dance class that is very much based on how well you dance. Again, the competitive juices are stirred. Yet, all of this occurs in an essentially noncompetitive activity where there are no explicit winners and losers. But is this really the case?

*Focused-Nonfocused: Rating — **Focused***

With the exception of the warm-up or routine at the dance bar, classes require your utmost concentration. You have to mentally and physically memorize dance combinations and, unless you are an advanced dancer in a beginner's class, you become completely immersed in the process. Unlike aerobics where the routine remains the same from week to week, dance combinations change daily. It's not going to be the same old thing that allows you to put your mind in neutral.

Risky-Safe: Rating—Intermediate

What's the risk in dance? From a physical perspective, dancers show the greatest respect for the workings of the body. They are careful to warm up each muscle and joint thoroughly before getting into high gear. And unless you are involved in acrobatic-like movements or dance with a lot of physical contact (contact improvisation, for example), you are unlikely to abuse your body. So, the risk is mostly psychological. It comes from the frustrations of trying to make your body do what the teacher's does or performing a dance that challenges you to the limit. It happens when you make a humiliating stumble or are forced to dance before an audience. Sometimes your ego is just not up to it. If you feel awkward and uncoordinated, dance can be extremely threatening. And even if you don't habitually bump into doors, your ego gets tested in a good class.

BAD/Body Psychology for Dance

In at least one way dance can be likened to running. The power-house for movement comes from the legs; the arms are along for the ride. The similarity stops here. The way in which dance and running develop musculature in the upper and lower body is quite opposite (Figure 8.30).

Lower-body development through dance stresses strength and flexibility. All the muscles, including the very small muscles of the feet, are extremely important. Painstaking care is given to working each muscle in the lower body both to strengthen it and to increase its flexibility. A rigid muscle is the dancer's enemy.

What about the upper body? The upper body is not strengthened to any degree unless you practice lifts with a partner. Most work on the upper body serves only to increase flexibility and range of motion. The psychological effect of dance training is to facilitate the expression of needs and emotions, to promote more fluid interactions with the environment, but not necessarily to increase the strength or powerfulness of these interactions.

Because the lower body is so well grounded and yet energized for motion, interactions through the upper body seem more potent. A dancer's image is bigger than life. Dancers do not necessarily have a lot of strength in their arms, but they have flexibility, which permits them to manipulate gracefully and without force. They project themselves through their arms. Their upper bodies are energized by a firm connection to strong, flexible legs.

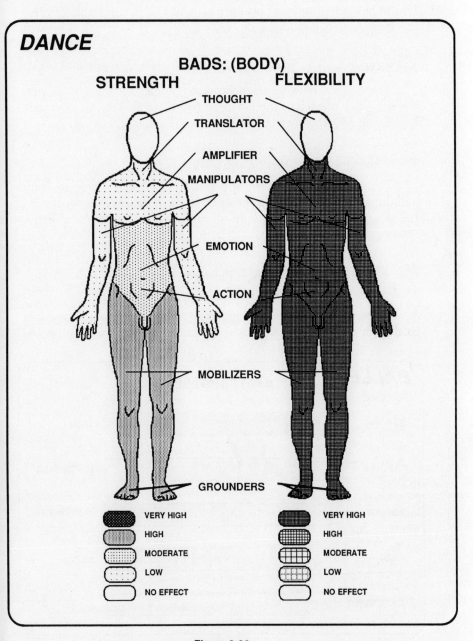

Figure 8.30

There is a high level of sensitivity in a dancer's body. This allows him to be acutely aware of his environment and to choose actions that are appropriately controlling or yielding, public or private, soft or hard.

MAD/Movement Analysis of Dance

The range of movements incorporated in dance training represents the full range of each of the five movement factors. For the most part, this is true of both ballet and modern/jazz (Figures 8.31, 8.32).

Force: Rating—Range: Very Strong to Very Light

There are light moves and strong moves in dance. There are leaps and thrusts as well as soft fluttering motions. A dancer experiences the full range of force from very light to very strong in the course of dance training.

Control: Ratings: Ballet—Range: Precise to Very Precise
Modern/Jazz—Range: Very Precise to Very Imprecise

Ballet tends to emphasize more precision in movement than does modern or jazz dance. In this sense we find more emotional control and

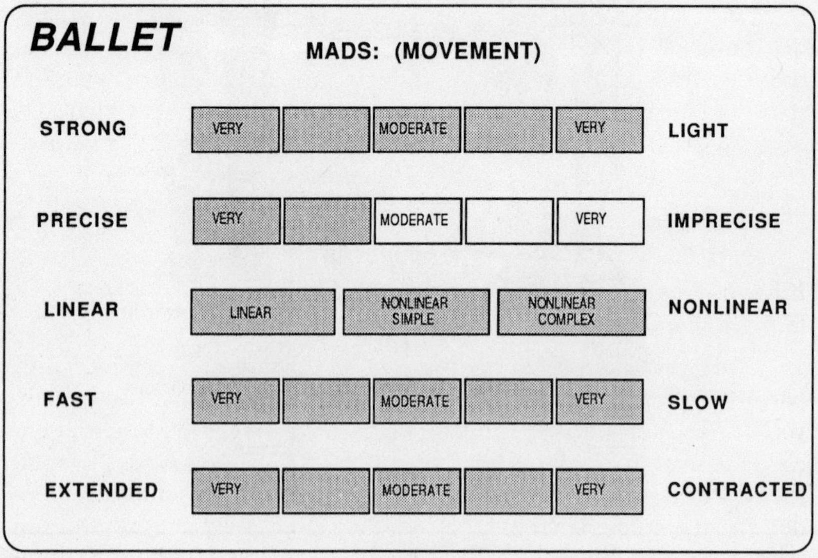

BALLET		MADS: (MOVEMENT)				
STRONG	VERY		MODERATE		VERY	LIGHT
PRECISE	VERY		MODERATE		VERY	IMPRECISE
LINEAR	LINEAR		NONLINEAR SIMPLE	NONLINEAR COMPLEX		NONLINEAR
FAST	VERY		MODERATE		VERY	SLOW
EXTENDED	VERY		MODERATE		VERY	CONTRACTED

Figure 8.31

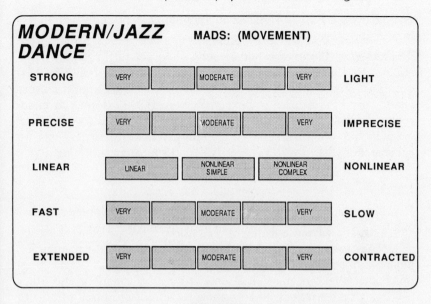

MODERN/JAZZ DANCE   MADS: (MOVEMENT)

STRONG	VERY		MODERATE		VERY	LIGHT
PRECISE	VERY		MODERATE		VERY	IMPRECISE
LINEAR	LINEAR		NONLINEAR SIMPLE	NONLINEAR COMPLEX		NONLINEAR
FAST	VERY		MODERATE		VERY	SLOW
EXTENDED	VERY		MODERATE		VERY	CONTRACTED

Figure 8.32

discipline in ballet than in many modern/jazz classes. Modern/jazz classes may incorporate free runs, leaps, and improvisational segments that call forth imprecise movements. This may also be found in some ballet classes where imprecise movements are used as a release from the strain of precision training. Our rating on this dimension distinguishes between ballet, where movements are precise to very precise, and modern/jazz, where we rate them in the full range from very precise to very imprecise.

*Linearity: Rating — **Range: Linear to Non-linear (Simple and Complex)***

A dance class makes you move in all directions, sometimes with parts of your body going in different directions. You jump, you crouch, you crawl, you glide. You run backwards and sideways and then in circles. You learn to focus out and focus in. You direct your attention and then contain it or let it wander. It balances between psychological tendencies. It develops abilities for assertion and receptivity, for control and release, for discipline and indulgence. We rate it the full range from linear to non-linear (simple and complex).

242 • Body Moves

Speed: Rating — *Range: Very Fast to Very Slow*

There are slow and fast movements in a dance class. Stretches are slow and so are pieces of a choreography where you might go from a full-out run to a lingering walk. You learn pacing and the transition that occurs as you accelerate or decelerate. Dance runs the gamut from very fast to very slow, helping you experience emotional extremes as in adventurous movements and those that are safe and secure. By experiencing both ends and the middle of different psychological dimensions, we become more fluent with varying styles and approaches to living.

Extension: Rating — *Range: Very Contracted to Very Extended*

A dancer will move with great extension when she leaps into space or reaches toward an imaginary horizon. And then she will contract, pulling into a ball as if in deep emotional pain. These physical expressions allow the dancer to experience a range of emotions and other psychological sensations, to know how to get out of herself or how to retreat into her shell. The movements, from very extended to very contracted, as represented throughout dance training, correspond not only to muscles and joints but to thoughts and emotions.

Dance in Review

Capturing the spirit of dance is difficult. In movement it brings out the full range of human expression. It rates as intermediate on a number of psychosocial scales, implying a certain balance in the lifestyle it encourages. And from a body angle it sets up a powerfully grounded base from which the individual can move or hold his ground as required. That upper-body strength is not greatly enhanced presents little problem because the body's fluid movements enable sufficient self-expression and control of the environment. Dance is unlikely to create an aggressive personality, but it does facilitate assertive behaviors.

Dancers appreciate the need for support and the concept of having a firm foundation. This comes through all the work on the lower body and its connection to the ground. As such, dance promotes a greater sense of personal security.

On the negative side, when dance training becomes too controlled, too emphatically precise, too rigidly disciplined, it fosters a character structure that becomes similarly rigid and controlled. Or when dance is too creative, too spontaneous, it promotes qualities of impulsivity, of flightiness that may impede a more pragmatic approach to living.

Overall, dance is a very positive body-mind training process. It may lack some on the physiological scorecard for aerobic activity, but psychologically it has lots of pluses.

Skiing

Unless you live in an alpine village, it's unlikely skiing will be a regular exercise. It's a seasonal outlet, and even at that, most people are limited to skiing on weekends or other days off. We include it not only for its popularity but also because many people identify themselves as skiers and make the transition from the slopes in winter to the waterways in summer. Skiers come in all sizes and skill levels, but if you have been skiing for a long enough time, you will tend to value many of the social and emotional qualities of the sport.

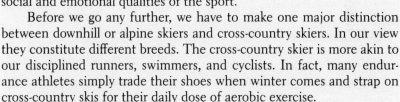

Before we go any further, we have to make one major distinction between downhill or alpine skiers and cross-country skiers. In our view they constitute different breeds. The cross-country skier is more akin to our disciplined runners, swimmers, and cyclists. In fact, many endurance athletes simply trade their shoes when winter comes and strap on cross-country skis for their daily dose of aerobic exercise.

Aerobic exercise? What does that mean to an alpine skier? Skiing isn't something you do for exercise. Sure, it taxes your muscles and you feel pleasantly exhausted after a day on the slopes, but to call it exercise? Please, let's distinguish between pleasure and masochism.

This is not to deny that regular skiers can be in great shape. But it's a question of means and ends. Many fitness fanatics exercise to get in shape. Skiers get in shape in order to ski—not to have a well-functioning cardiorespiratory system.

Excitement! Adventure! Romance! Fun! Oh, yes, DANGER! That's alpine skiing, more or less, for a lot of people. Would these words fit the experience of the cross-country skier? Highly unlikely. Maybe it's fun, but that comes through a lot of work getting up the hill that you are going to ski down.

So, let's see how skiing comes apart in our analyses. We are going to focus on both alpine and cross-country skiers. Be aware that commentaries about cross-country skiers may seem more related to runners than to alpine enthusiasts.

PAD/Psychosocial Dimensions of Skiing

Recognizing that few places in North America allow year-round skiing, we want to focus on the ski addicts, those who leave the office early on Friday afternoon and return exhausted on Monday morning after closing the slopes the night before. They may drive long distances to get to their ski chalets but excitement rises with each passing mile. They have season passes and the latest in ski technology. They are preparing for the slopes in September by doing their pre-ski-season exercises. Winter ski vacations are valued at least as much as summer vacations. These are the skiers. The rest of us are only dabblers, uncommitted dilettantes. For real skiers, what does the sport demand? What psychological processes does it reinforce (Figures 8.33, 8.34)?

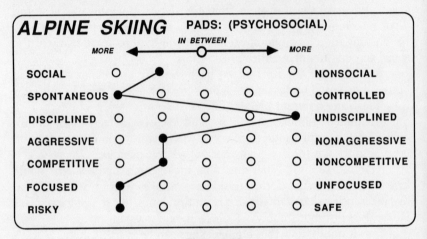

Figure 8.33

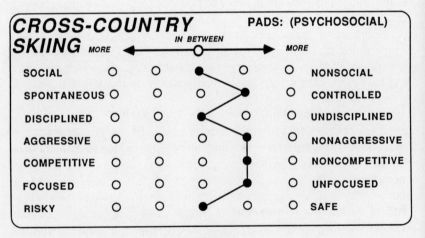

Figure 8.34

*Social-Nonsocial: Rating: Alpine — **Moderately Social**;*
*Cross-Country — **Intermediate***

While skiing down a slope does not involve social exchange, there are other features of this sport that make it social. Regular skiers usually ski with a friend or in a group. The drive to the mountains is typically long and company is appreciated. Staying over the weekend also involves being with others, for example, in a chalet rented by a group of friends. Then there is the trip up the slope on the chair lift. It's awkward to sit with someone for five to ten minutes without saying hello. For these reasons we see the activity as facilitating social interaction, giving people a common topic of conversation and large periods of time when they can share stories or massage aching muscles.

This pattern is less descriptive of cross-country skiing. Many cross-country skiers find a regular course close to home to do their solitary mileage. Yet, our rating for cross-country is intermediate. Even though the activity is solitary, the chances are greater than in running that you might want to go along with someone for safety's sake if for no other reason.

*Spontaneous-Controlled: Rating: Alpine — **Spontaneous**;*
*Cross-Country — **Moderately Controlled***

There is no set course or pattern that the alpine skier must follow. Instead, there is a high degree of freedom and spontaneity encouraged by the sport. By contrast, cross-country skiers follow marked trails making their way with rhythmic cadence and steady pace. The alpine skier responds almost instinctively to changes in conditions and terrain. The cross-country skier moves in tracks set by those who broke the trail. One activity calls for spontaneity, the other for staying in the groove.

*Disciplined-Undisciplined: Rating: Alpine — **Undisciplined**;*
*Cross-Country — **Intermediate***

An undisciplined sport naturally draws you. It is attractive and fun. By contrast, a disciplined sport is one that you have to work at. As we noted earlier, there is nothing inherently fun about lifting weights in body building. Cross-country skiing is work, but it also has elements of fun, so we rate it as intermediate. Some might say alpine skiing is work. For the most part, we just don't believe it. It's exciting, thrilling, and, yes, you might work up a bit of a sweat on occasion.

*Aggressive-Nonaggressive: Rating: Alpine — **Moderately Aggressive;***
*Cross-Country — **Moderately Nonaggressive***

You have to apply a lot of pressure to make slalom turns. You have to master the slope. It's raw courage against a mountain that wants to take you for a tumble. Not so in cross-country. You glide in a continuous effort. It's more akin to ice skating than to the pounding experience of running. Yet there is some push, at least to overcome inertia.

*Competitive-Noncompetitive: Rating: Alpine — **Moderately***
Competitive;** Cross-Country — **Moderately Noncompetitive

Not all downhill skiers are hot on competition, but if you ski every weekend throughout the season, there is a thrill that comes from doing it better and faster than anyone else. Cross-country is more of a cooperative venture. The goal is more to finish together if you are skiing in a group than to be the first one back.

*Focused-Unfocused: Rating: Alpine — **Focused;***
*Cross-Country — **Moderately Unfocused***

The contrast between these activities is clear. When you are moving slowly along a trail in cross-country, you don't have to pay attention every second. But when you are hurtling down a slope at speeds in excess of forty miles per hour, you better pay attention. That's the difference between an activity that demands your attention and one that allows you to daydream.

*Risky-Safe: Rating: Alpine — **Risky;** Cross-Country — **Intermediate***

There is little need for explanation here. Alpine skiing results in a number of fatalities each year and innumerable broken bones or other injuries. Ego risks also exist, but they pale by comparison to those of physical injury. Cross-country skiing also has its share of physical injuries, but far less than alpine skiing. For adventurous devils, alpine skiing delivers all that you ask for. Many alpine skiers don't even consider cross-country skiing to be in the same league as their sport.

BAD/Body Psychology for Skiing

You need a lot of lower-body strength in alpine skiing. Cross-country takes more endurance than strength. So, when we compare the two, we will be looking at quite different body development (Figures 8.35, 8.36).

The alpine skier needs to have strong legs with a certain explosive power to make it through a fast slalom or freestyle run. The hips and knees need to be flexible, as does the upper body and arms. It doesn't take much strength in the upper body to pole around turns. It has more to do with coordination. There is a lot that skiing will teach you about balance and weight transfer in the lower body. It's an excellent sport for learning how to ground yourself. When we say that you don't strengthen the upper body in alpine skiing, we don't mean to imply that the arms and torso are totally neglected. All of those weight shifts in the lower body are a lot easier if the upper body is tuned.

What are the effects of alpine training? Psychologically, you work on balance and, most of all, on grounding. You learn where your center of gravity is and how far you can extend yourself before you topple. That you have to be flexible means that energy flow throughout the body should be pretty good. You don't want to be stiff or tight in your joints if you ski regularly. Since the joints are thought of as psychosomatic crossroads, this reinforces the idea that a regular alpine skier will have reasonably good emotional flow.

On the negative side, muscles are held in a contracted state for long periods as you ski down the hill. Alpine skiers have to work on flexibility and stretching off the slope. Otherwise, muscles become tense and bound. This in turn can lead to problems in future ski performance as well as in the psychological arena.

The cross-country skier builds a different body. There is far greater need for endurance than for power. Champion cross-country skiers are usually lean and wiry, akin to marathon runners. There is an emphasis on upper-body strength, particularly in the deltoid and triceps muscles of the arms and shoulders, as well as on leg strength. Unlike alpine skiing, where ankle and foot movements are restricted by boots, the cross-country skier works through the entire leg and extensively employs foot muscles. The more advanced you are in cross-country, the more your whole body will be challenged to develop muscular endurance. Since the force required for movements in cross-country is less extreme than in alpine, muscular strength is not as important.

Cross-country skiing also develops flexibility and balance. The newer skis are extremely narrow and the skier must learn to balance while making long, gliding movements. These long extensions of arms and legs also help muscles develop range and flexibility.

The development of the arms and shoulders indicates that expressive, manipulative upper-body functions will be enhanced. And since

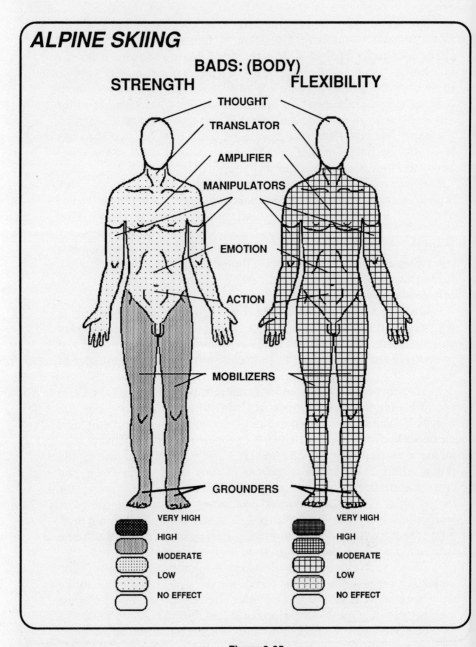

Figure 8.35

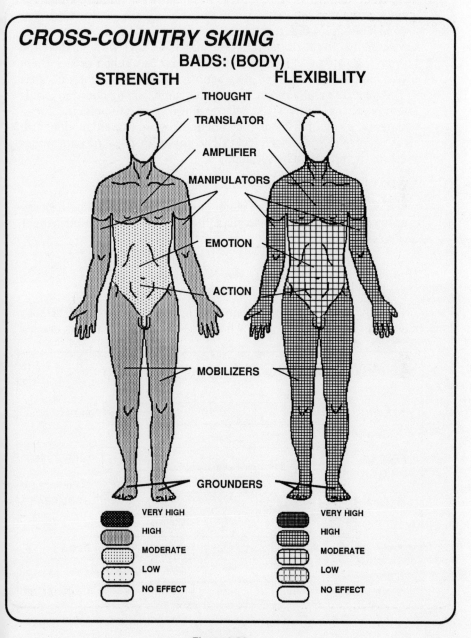

Figure 8.36

this upper-body development is adequately balanced by lower-body development, the cross-country skier's personality should have a high degree of symmetry.

To illustrate a difference between alpine and cross-country skiing development, think of one of those inflatable toys with sand in the bottom that is shaped like a bowling pin. You can punch or kick these toys as much as you like, but they bounce right back to center because of the weight in the bottom. That's what alpine skiing does for you. It grounds you and teaches you balance and response to pressure. Cross-country is less grounded and more oriented toward forward motion. The cross-country skier is more inclined to move, to press forward under pressure than to stand his ground.

MAD/Movement Analysis of Skiing

The contrasting styles of alpine and cross-country skiing become even more evident as we take apart these sports based on movement qualities (Figures 8.37, 8.38).

Force: Rating—Alpine: **Range: Very Strong to Very Light;**
Cross-Country: **Range: Strong to Light**

Alpine skiing requires strength and pressure in its movements, but it also uses light movements, as when you shift your weight from one leg

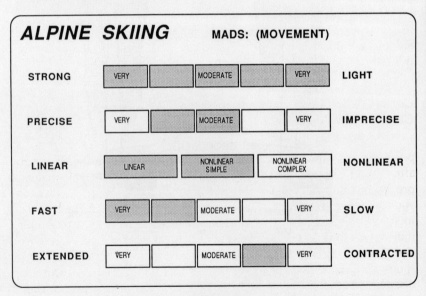

Figure 8.37

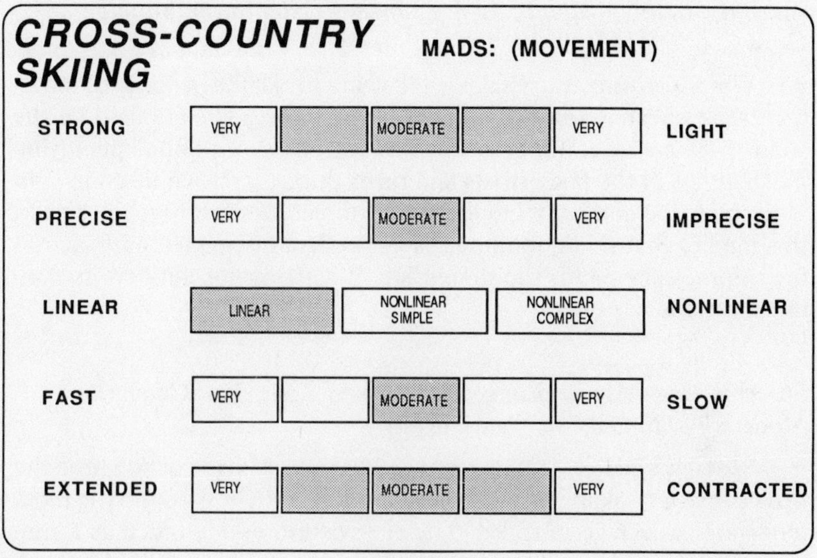

CROSS-COUNTRY SKIING   MADS: (MOVEMENT)

STRONG	VERY		MODERATE		VERY	LIGHT
PRECISE	VERY		MODERATE		VERY	IMPRECISE
LINEAR	LINEAR	NONLINEAR SIMPLE	NONLINEAR COMPLEX			NONLINEAR
FAST	VERY		MODERATE		VERY	SLOW
EXTENDED	VERY		MODERATE		VERY	CONTRACTED

Figure 8.38

to the other. Because of this constant shifting of weight and the alternating use of light and strong pressure, we rate downhill skiing as very strong to very light in its application of force. Psychologically, this suggests a balancing of assertive and receptive personality inclinations.

Cross-country skiing also uses variations in pressure, but tends to use more moderate pressures throughout. We rate it as strong to light, recognizing that the amounts of pressure applied in cross-country are not as extreme as in downhill.

Control: Rating—Alpine: *Range: Precise to Moderate;* Cross-Country: *Moderate*

Good cross-country skiers have relatively precise placements of poles and skis, but the sport does not demand great precision. Moreover, after skiing for an hour or so, fatigue may alter the skier's intended precision of movements. For this reason we rate it as moderate. Perhaps you can better understand this by comparing it to the precision required in slalom skiing. The degree of control that the skier must exert in his movements far exceeds that called for in cross-country. Our rating for alpine incorporates more of a range from precise to moderate. Both sports emphasize psychological qualities of emotional control and self-discipline, but alpine reinforces mental focus or concentration more so than does cross-country training.

Linearity: Rating—Alpine: **Range: Linear to Non-linear (Simple);** *Cross-Country:* **Linear**

When a cross-country skier is following a trail, the majority of movements are linear. There are few non-linear movements required by the sport. Alpine skiing, however, involves both linear and non-linear (simple) motions as the body twists and turns through a downhill course. In both sports the dominant emphasis is on directed effort. Psychologically, this implies that skiing reinforces a controlled, disciplined approach to life. Alpine skiing adds the dimension of spontaneity through its non-linear actions.

Speed: Rating—Alpine: **Range: Fast to Very Fast;** *Cross-Country:* **Moderate** *(with range from slow to fast)*

Speed is typically fast to very fast in alpine skiing. That's where the thrill comes in—skiing a course better *and* faster. Cross-country is more moderate or average in speed. The cross-country skier, much as a runner, tries to keep up a steady pace over a long period of time. And as is the case with other endurance athletes, some cross-country skiers will be faster or slower than others. The difference in speed in the two sports contributes to one (cross-country) being more oriented toward conservatism and safety, while the other (alpine) promoting an adventurous, risky approach to life.

Extension: Rating—Alpine: **Contracted;** *Cross-Country:* **Range: Contracted to Extended**

Alpine skiers have to hold their bodies in tight control, keeping their center of gravity low to the ground. This means there is a lot of emphasis on contracted movements. By contrast, the cross-country skier needs to extend and contract in order to get a good push-off with poles and skis. The ratings, then, are contracted for alpine and extended to contracted for cross-country. Although this would imply that the alpine skier has less development in extending herself socially or that she has a more cautious approach to life than the cross-country skier, other MADs and PADs factors serve to counter this interpretation.

Skiing in Review

Now that we have contrasted alpine and cross-country skiing through the avenues of movement, body development, and psychosocial demands, we can better understand why they seem to attract different people and why they reinforce different characteristics. The most dominant feature of alpine skiing is its sense of risk and adventure. It feeds your need for excitement. It also promotes a certain spontaneity and aggressiveness in relationships. Because of its emphasis on lower-body strength and control, you learn to keep balanced even if you do push aggressively forward. While it is a dangerous sport, we have to recognize how it nonetheless teaches us to be controlled and focused in our actions, to extend but not beyond our reach.

Cross-country skiing is not nearly as aggressive, although its linear motions and emphasis on forward progression imply that training in this sport will bring out a kind of persistence, if not stubbornness, in addressing life's problems. It's likely to be a more social activity than running, but not quite as social as alpine skiing. Its body development rates higher than alpine skiing mostly because of its equal emphasis on upper- and lower-body development.

Both sports can be exciting and can add to our sense of adventure. Alpine teaches us a bit more about variation and dealing with the unexpected than does cross-country, but both call forth an emphasis on balance in movement. They inform us about the costs of too much speed or too little control or not paying attention. They teach us how to use our weight or our strength to get through difficult turns on the course—and in life.

Golf

Golf is another kind of addiction. You may not get those endorphins from playing golf, but people get hooked on other things. That's if you can get beyond all the frustrations of the game. Aside from the expense, there are other factors that might hold you back from playing regularly. It takes a lot of time to get around 18 holes, even if you ride in a golf cart. Then there's the question of finding a partner whose schedule meshes with yours.

Let's assume you meet the prerequisites for becoming a regular golfer. You live in a sunny climate, you have lots of time and a reasonable amount of money, and you can find a partner or two whenever you want. Then what? What will the sport do for you? Forgetting about the debate over how much exercise you get from golf when you ride around in a cart, there are some important psychological characteristics you can reinforce in golf.

Let's look at our threefold analysis of golf and see what it tells us about the way it develops a person.

PAD/Psychosocial Dimensions of Golf

If you go out onto the golf course a couple of times or more a week, what kinds of psychological traits will be reinforced (Figure 8.39)?

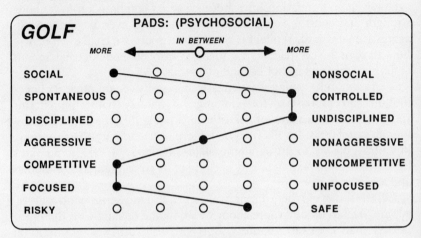

Figure 8.39

Social-Nonsocial: Rating—Social

Of all the activities we have reviewed, golf is clearly the most social. You start off with at least one partner who will be with you throughout the 18 holes. It offers long periods of time centered around a game. Conversations can range as far as you wish because you will have plenty of time to pursue mutual interests.

Spontaneous-Controlled: Rating—Controlled

The game calls for control, for analyzing and planning your actions. If your emotions sneak into a shot, you may veer off at a forty-five-degree angle. You have to be in control of yourself, of your feelings. You have to direct your attention. You cannot allow impulsive reactions to guide your behavior. It's a great game for teaching you how to be patient and in control of your emotions. Of course, this depends on whether you are receptive to its lessons. Another way in which it is controlled is in how it makes you plan your drives and putts. You have to recall all of those laws of physics, calculating wind resistance, angles, and velocities to get the ball where you want it to go. It's not something you estimate intuitively although you may say "it's intuitive" after a dozen years of play.

*Disciplined-Undisciplined: Rating — **Undisciplined***

Remember that when we talk about discipline, we are describing how much an activity draws you to it by virtue of its inherent attraction. Ask a golfer whether he would trade a round of golf for jogging five miles, and the hearty belly laugh you'll hear will give you a key to understanding. Golfers enjoy themselves. They look forward to getting up at five o'clock A.M. to be the first to tee off. The 19th hole is only one of the many rewards they experience. And perhaps play is another key to understanding. It's a game that allows you to get away from whatever else is bothering you. (Of course, it could give you another kind of headache.)

*Aggressive-Nonaggressive: Rating — **Intermediate***

Too much force and you have blown it. Too little and the ball dribbles down the fairway. You have to use just the right amount of force when you hit the ball. This is one of the biggest lessons of the game. You have to judge the situation with exceptional accuracy.

*Competitive-Noncompetitive: Rating — **Competitive***

Many golfers would say that all they are interested in is improving their game. But when you play with someone else and keep score on each hole using handicaps for the game, you have all of the elements necessary to stir those competitive feelings. So, how do you react? You compete. It's not necessarily as competitive as a game of racquetball because you and your partner can play more against yourselves than against each other. That's a choice you will make based on how well matched you are and your general inclination toward competition.

*Focused-Unfocused: Rating — **Focused***

Golfing makes you concentrate. If your attention drifts, if you allow yourself a momentary distraction as you are preparing to swing, you will pay for it. That's another way in which golf tames the spirit. It's mind over matter. When you are walking or riding between strokes, you can unleash your mind. But even then, the game offers you a substitute set of thoughts.

BAD/Body Psychology for Golf

This is a place where we can get into a bit of trouble. What kind of body does golf build? Certainly, we have seen all sizes and shapes on the golf course and even championship players don't conform to any particular mold, as they do in many other sports (Figure 8.40).

We know there is a lot of attention paid to placement and alignment in golf. Also, the motion of the body has to permit the swing of the club to be made in a smooth and utterly controlled arc. There can be no distortions in the energy flow as the force of the club is delivered to the ball.

What this means is that you have to be keenly aware of your body, to know where your weight is distributed, to sense your center of gravity. You have to deliver a force to the ball that is appropriate to the distance you want it to travel. This means knowing your strength and how to apply it.

Golfers have a lateral preference, swinging from the right side or the left. This means the body develops more on one side than the other. Just as in tennis, this implies an overdevelopment of our aggressive capacity. Would this mean that golfers emphasize assertion over passive-receptive behaviors? Yes, we think so. But since the assertiveness is highly controlled and directed, golf teaches you how to use assertion carefully and without emotional distortion. This is an important lesson.

Golf may not be a well-rounded sport in terms of body development. On the positive side, swinging a club does call into play all of the major muscle groups and it requires a good comprehension of balance and grounding. Further, you have to know how strong you are and how to apply your strength. You have to be flexible, particularly in shoulder and arm joints. And you have to know exactly where your center is.

On the negative, you build up muscles on one side of the body more than on the other. Also, muscles in the upper body, particularly those in the shoulders, back, and arms, will be overemphasized compared to those in the lower body. This implies a slightly imbalanced development of upper body functions (manipulation, control, self-expression) compared to lower body ones (stability and mobility). This imbalance is not likely to be great because golfing makes us learn how to use the ground for support and balance. The limited activity in a game of golf, particularly if you ride around in a golf cart, means you will have to work on maintaining strength and flexibility off the green, because golf itself won't do it for you.

MAD/Movement Analysis of Golf

Some of the questions about how golf affects us through its required body work will be better understood in this section on movement

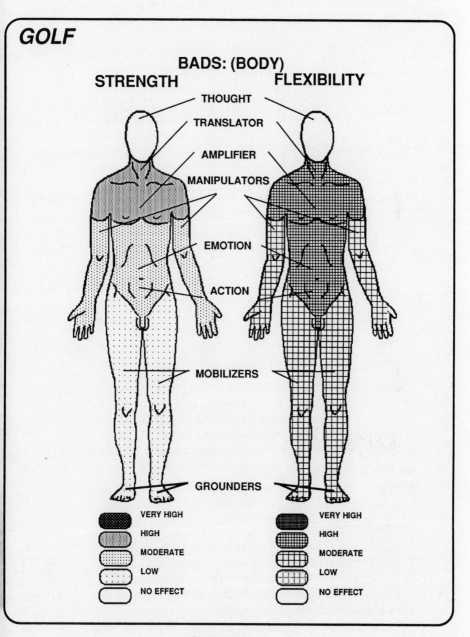

GOLF

BADS: (BODY)

STRENGTH   FLEXIBILITY

THOUGHT
TRANSLATOR
AMPLIFIER
MANIPULATORS
EMOTION
ACTION
MOBILIZERS
GROUNDERS

VERY HIGH
HIGH
MODERATE
LOW
NO EFFECT

VERY HIGH
HIGH
MODERATE
LOW
NO EFFECT

Figure 8.40

analysis. The basis for these remarks comes from an analysis of the golfer as she moves to strike the ball, not what happens at other times on the course (Figure 8.41).

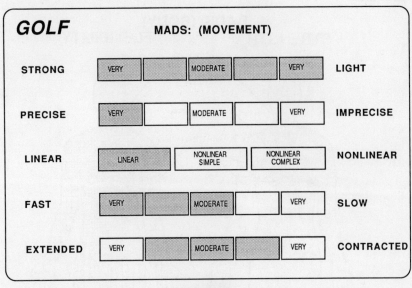

Figure 8.41

*Force: Rating—**Range: Very Strong to Very Light***

Golfers have to learn to vary the pressure required to deliver the ball to its destination. In our analysis, this means that force will vary from very strong to very light depending on whether the golfer is trying to drive the ball a few hundred yards or putt it a few inches. The psychological lesson is one of balancing efforts, of being appropriately aggressive, of using the right amount of strength to accomplish one's goals.

*Control: Rating—**Very Precise***

If you are a fraction of an inch off when your driver strikes the ball, it could land you in one of the many traps on the course. That's the fun and frustration of the game. If you stick with it, you will learn to control your movements, to be very precise. Psychologically, this means that golf will ask you to discipline yourself, to monitor your emotions, and to focus your attention. It will emphasize calculated behavior rather than a risky, impulsive style of living.

*Linearity: Rating — **Linear***

There isn't much about golf that is indirect unless we consider the meanderings across the fairway or the search for a lost ball. In terms of the principal activity of golf — driving the golf ball to the hole — the motions are linear and at least intentionally direct. This form of motion calls for psychological qualities of control, discipline, focus, and assertion.

*Speed: Rating — **Range: Very Fast to Moderate***

Sometimes the swing of your club is swift, other times it may move with measured slowness. Our assessment of movement speeds required by the game ranges from very fast to moderate, depending on where the ball is and where you want it to go. This relative emphasis on speed appropriate to the situation suggests a psychological process of assessing one's rate of progress or need for restraint in action.

*Extension: Rating — **Range: Extended to Contracted***

The golfer will contract certain muscles, particularly those in the upper body, as she prepares to swing, but the real emphasis in golf is on the extension of the body as the ball is driven to its destination. The golfer must contract just enough to release properly into her swing. In putts the contraction is maintained throughout. Our rating of extended to contracted takes into account the importance of both actions of the muscles to effective delivery.

Golf in Review

Many people think of golf as a mental game, a contest of will. We know from this analysis that it teaches you patience and control, that it shows you how to assert yourself without getting carried away, and that it makes you focus your attention in the moment. Maybe, if you are too impulsive and impatient, you will never stick with the game. If you have a hard time getting yourself to organize and plan before you act, you will find the game too controlled. But if, for whatever reasons, you stay with it, golf will demand a particular psychological stance. In time, this stance will become part of your response pattern, an acquired style if you didn't have it at the beginning.

A golfer understands how to stand her ground and how to apply force. There is a strategy to the game, one that asks you to monitor your spontaneous, impulsive inclinations. While we can see a lot of stress on assertion and directed activity in golf, we also have to see how carefully considered your actions must be in order to succeed. You learn to think through your behavior, to rehearse your swing, before you translate thought into action.

We noted earlier that golf is not a well-rounded activity in terms of developing us into multipurpose beings. And that's perfectly fine. It plays a limited but important role in development. In some ways it can be likened to racquet games with their lopsided emphasis on direct, aggressive action, but the planfulness of golf is something quite unique. When the ball is delivered in tennis, the timing of response is determined by someone else and we have no choice but to respond instantly. In golf we move at our own pace, according to a delicate sensing of our internal readiness and an exacting calculation of how to behave. It almost seems like controlled spontaneity or some other contradiction in terms. And, perhaps for this reason, the game is known for its power to make us or break us.

9

Choosing Your Exercise Program

Now What?

You have looked at yourself inside and out. And you have read all about the psychology of different exercise programs. How do you put this information together? Where do you start?

Let's begin with a simple premise: No one is perfect! We can all stand a little improvement. This doesn't mean radical psychosurgery, but maybe a few minor adjustments. What we will do in this chapter is outline a strategy for identifying what's important to change and matching your needs to the best moves for you.

Before outlining a step-by-step procedure, let's look at the big picture. If you were totally honest with yourself going through the three-fold evaluations of personality, body structure, and movement habits, the answer you are searching for is right in front of you. You can look at your profiles and pick out your number-one enemy — your biggest problem. This is something that bothers you a lot. It may even get you into trouble with others, or at the very least it makes you unhappy. Probably it shows up most clearly on your PADs scores. The MADs and BADs profiles help complete its identity.

In the last chapter you examined the characteristics of different exercise programs and you probably paid close attention to the one you do most often. You may have quibbled with some of the ratings of your favorite fitness routine, but no doubt you recognized more than a grain of truth in the profile. If you ventured beyond your favorite to read about activities you have avoided, you might have understood why you steered away from these fitness outlets.

The hard question is, how much do you really want to change? Are you motivated enough to try something new and put yourself in a potentially uncomfortable position for a while? You may want guarantees that it won't be too hard and that the promised results won't take too long. Well, you can have them. If you go about your change sensibly, you may hardly even notice that something different is happening. And if you are a regular fitness fan, you will reap your usual exercise rewards while adding new benefits from your personality transformation.

Of course, you can always choose shock treatment. In this case, that means doing something that is so foreign to your makeup that pain and failure are inevitable. It would be like an avid tennis player deciding to take up yoga. It just might be too large of a leap.

The big picture is something you are aware of, something you probably knew intuitively before you read this book, but you didn't know how to label it or what to do about it. Having read this far means the image is in focus; all the knobs have been adjusted and you can see yourself without distortion. You also can see what it is you have to do.

Even though you might have the answer in mind, why not complete the process systematically? In the next section, we will outline a procedure and give you a few more tools to work with.

Step by Step

There are four questions you need to ask yourself to determine the best way to bring about long-lasting gains in your lifestyle:

1. What do I need to change?
2. What am I doing now?
3. What is my new plan?
4. How do I get going?

As we go through these questions, we will use a case study to illustrate how the process works. First we will describe what the step is and then we will apply it to a real person. There is a worksheet for your use in Figure 9.1.

WORKSHEET FOR EXERCISE PRESCRIPTION

STEP 1A: Your description of a problem or area you need to change.

STEP 1B: How does it show in your profiles?

PADS?

BADS?

MADS?

STEP 2: What is your present exercise plan?

STEP 3: What changes should you make?

STEP 4: What, when, where, and how will you get started?

Figure 9.1

Question 1. *What Do I Need to Change?*

Notice the question says *need*, not *want*, to change. This is a real test of courage. There is an axiom in psychology that says "people always want more of what they already have." Beautiful people want to be more beautiful. Rich people want to be richer. And fit people want to be fitter.

We have become who we are because it rewards us. We get some goodies from our style. Changing means giving up some of these goodies. It means mourning. Fritz Perls, a renowned psychotherapist, said it more poignantly: "To suffer one's death and be reborn again is not easy!"

Hey! We're only talking about exercise, not life and death. If you think this is true, then why all the fuss about "My sport is better than yours" or "I would never be caught *dead* a) in running shoes, b) at Gold's Gym, c) on a golf course, d) in a tutu." Caught dead? Commitment to particular sports may be more deeply based in our personalities than we care to admit. And changing from one sport to another could involve a great deal more than going to a sports shop and buying a new outfit.

Back to need. What you need to change is something that gives you trouble, something that gets you in trouble. A little self-reflection can help. You may think of it as a habit. Like you continually run into the same kinds of difficulties on the job, in romance, or at home. Some examples?

— You always date people who take advantage of your good nature.
— You get into trouble because you act before you think.
— You can't relax because you feel people will get the edge on you.
— You like sensitive people but they shy away from you.
— You feel horribly tense at parties.
— You can't regulate the power dial—you come on too strong all the time.
— Your ego feels like a pin cushion.
— You can never stick to anything long enough to get the benefits.
— You are a forty-year-old daredevil and your body is complaining.

The list is endless. If you don't find yourself in these examples, you can surely write your own.

Step 1a in the procedure is to write down a simple statement of what bothers you about your style. It should be a statement similar to the ones above, but in your own words.

PADs, BADs and MADs: Having reflected on what kind of trouble you get yourself into regularly or perhaps on what you just don't like about your style, it might be time to turn back to those profiles you developed earlier.

PADs is probably the best one to start with. It should pinpoint reasons for your difficulties. As you look over your scores, you may find ratings that are pretty high or low, but they don't bother you. You like being this way. Fine—no problem. If you rate yourself as being nonsocial and you enjoy your private time, you may feel no need to become more sociable. And no one is saying you have to. You have to make this judgment call based on your own experience. There are perfectly good reasons why people should be exactly the way they are even though their style may seem extreme to others.

On the other hand, if you are experiencing some personal difficulties or just don't think you are well-rounded enough for your own tastes, one or more of the PADs scores should indicate this. It will likely be a *very high* or a *very low* score.

Step 1b is to write down the PADs dimension that indicates the problem. Rather than write down the score, you can use words like, "too aggressive," "compulsively social," "too cautious," or "overly impulsive."

What about BADs and MADs? Review these scores, too. Look for indications of how your problem shows itself in your body shape and in your movement habits. As part of Step 1b, write down any body characteristics or patterns of movement that go along with the PADs results.

It is important to look at the problem from all angles. If you leave out body dynamics or movement qualities, you may end up picking an exercise program that is not as helpful as it could be. For example, if you are too passive and lacking in self-confidence, maybe body building would be a good choice. But if your movements tend to be habitually slow, you may need something that is fast-paced to energize you and get you moving in your world. In this case, body building would be less than ideal. Maybe something like martial arts or even running would be better to start.

The Case Study—Step 1. "Susan" is twenty-six years old and in her third year of work as a real estate agent. She surprised friends and family with her career choice as well as by her success on the job. She was going to be a ballerina, but turned off somewhere along the road and went into the real estate business. After a year of transition, she was in full stride. For the past nine months she had the best sales record in the agency. She felt a lot of pressure to keep it up.

At work she was highly aggressive—a real take-charge woman. She got things done. Her performance was impressive, especially since she was still learning the business. But she had trouble getting out of fifth gear. She was fast paced, demanding, and just push, push, push. Off the job, she felt friends backing off from her. They told her she came on "real strong." And she didn't like that feedback.

She just couldn't let things pass. She couldn't let other people take care of things. She had to do it because then it would get done. Tell Susan about a problem and she would be on the case. She would solve it—now! No waiting, no hesitating. Surprisingly, her rewards were meager. By the time she had solved the problem, she had ruffled so many feathers that no one thanked her.

Step 1a: How did she see the problem? She thought she was too aggressive, too forceful in all her interactions. Sometimes it was okay to be pushy, but with friends and family she had to learn to back off a bit. And she worried whether, in years to come, she would end up alienating all of her coworkers.

Step 1b: Her profiles as described in Figure 9.2 verify Susan's concern with aggression. In PADs the aggressive score is her highest. Her body shape was not a problem, but she experienced a great deal of tension in her back and chest. In movement she found that her style had changed since her years as a dancer. She had become more extreme. Her pattern was to move very fast and directly. Her movements were strong and exact, rarely light and easy. For all that she had gained in flexibility through dance, she rated her extension as only moderate, believing that under pressure her body felt very compacted.

Question 2. What Am I Doing Now?

There are many ways to answer this question, but our interest is in fitness and exercise. So, a good hard look at your exercise program is what is called for here. This means looking at such factors as the *frequency, intensity,* and *duration* of your activities. If you dabble, then you better make note of this too.

Step 2 of the procedure involves making a few notes about your present exercise plan. It helps to record the pattern over the past year, including activities that you have engaged in with some regularity. So the two-day canoe trip last summer doesn't count, but the weekly round of golf over the summer months would.

Why is it important to make note of this? We have talked about the dangers of throwing out the baby with the bath water before. There may be some helpful components of your present program. Maybe what you need is a modification of *how* you exercise rather than changing *what* you do. Perhaps you need to add an activity on a regular basis to supplement what you are doing, thereby keeping the old and adding the new.

SUSAN'S PRESCRIPTION

WORKSHEET FOR EXERCISE PRESCRIPTION

STEP 1A: Your description of a problem or area you need to change.

Being too aggressive. My friends tell me I'm a bit too pushy.
Also, I just can't seem to back off. I have to take charge of everything.

STEP 1B: How does it show in your profiles?

PADS?
My highest score was on the aggression scale.
My other scores were pretty reasonable.

BADS?
My body seems okay except for a lot of tension in my back and chest.
I also seem to be stronger in my upper body than in my lower.

MADS?
My movements are mostly strong - they are rarely light.
They are also pretty bound or contracted, especially when
I am under pressure.

STEP 2: What is your present exercise plan?

3x per week I do weight training and I do 20 minutes each
or running on a treadmill, a stationary bike and swimming.
3x per week I do two long aerobic workouts of about one hour each.
I work out in the morning and then after work, alternating swimming
biking and running.

STEP 3: What changes should you make?

I want to learn how to do tai chi chuan. I think it will help me.
I plan to include it in my daily routine as a warm-up or as a way
of cooling down. I would do it for abouta 20 minutes each day and
cut back on some of my other workouts.

STEP 4: What, when, where, and how will you get started?

I found a place where I can take tai chi lessons twice a week.
I'll eliminate one of my morning workouts and cut back on my
Saturday training so I can take classes. I will get started in
two weeks when the new session begins at the tai chi school.

Figure 9.2

We will see how this works in the next step. For the moment, let's return to Susan.

The Case Study—Step 2.   Susan trained in dance up through her early twenties and then took up running at the same time that she began her career. Running wasn't entirely new to her. She had trained for short periods during her late teens as her infatuation with dance began to wane. It fit her schedule better than dance class and she felt she got more out of it.

She was a born athlete. Five feet seven inches, 122 pounds, 12.7 percent body fat, VO_2 Max in the ninety-ninth percentile, and what a mover. She was running eight-minute miles the first month, seven-minute miles the second month, and at the six-month mark she ran a 10K in under forty minutes. She was ecstatic and her boyfriend said she should become a triathlete. She took him up on it.

She got a program at her health club from a trainer who had done the Ironman twice. It was tough sticking with it, but she did. It took a lot of time, yet it had payoffs in helping her blow off steam at the end of the day. Or sometimes it got her rolling in the morning. There was nothing like swimming five thousand yards to wake her up for that nine o'clock sales meeting.

She liked the training, but she also felt it made her more aggressive. She told a friend, "When I was dancing, I never felt very strong. Now, if some guy hassles me, I just feel like punching him out." She could, and she began to fear that she would.

Step 2: What was her program? She trained six days a week. Endurance workouts with weights three times a week. This meant moderate weights with high repetitions at a fast pace. On weight-training days her aerobic workouts were light: twenty minutes apiece for biking and running on stationary equipment and then twenty minutes in the pool. On the other three days, she would do a long run or swim in the morning and then another aerobic workout after work. She felt stronger all the time, but she really had to drive herself hard.

Question 3. What Is My New Plan?

Knowing what you need to change and what you are presently doing prepares you for the next step: developing an alternative plan. In order to make your first move wisely, you have to guard against dramatic changes. This means choosing something that you can handle mentally and physically. How will you know what's too big and what's just right?

A few extra tools may help. Figures 9.3 to 9.9 summarize the PADs ratings of all the fitness activities we looked at in Chapter 8. For each of the seven Psychosocial Activity Dimensions, fitness programs are ordered from one end of the scale to the other. You can see, for example, how all the sports and exercise programs compare on the *Social-Nonsocial Scale*. If you want to improve your sociability score, you might not want to jump completely from the nonsocial end of the scale to the social end. You may want to move more gradually. In terms of activities, this may mean choosing an intermediate activity like aerobics rather than activities that are fully social. Or it could mean changing *how* you exercise. Example: If you are a nonsocial runner, always running alone, make it a point to ask a friend to run with you once or twice a week.

A momentary digression. One of the reasons that sports and exercise are such good change agents is that they take care of some of your emotional discomfort while you are blazing new trails. If you are shy and have trouble making friends, it's really difficult to muster up the courage to talk to people at social gatherings or, worse, to walk up to a stranger in a bar. But it's not too difficult to find people who like running and to join them. Health clubs usually post notices of group runs or in the office some of your coworkers may have regular noontime runs.

Now, what happens to all of that social anxiety when you are running? It's amazing but you don't notice it as much. You might notice how hard it is to breathe or how much your muscles ache—but social anxiety? Besides, when people go running together, they don't necessarily chat the entire way, especially if they run up and down hills. So, you don't have to talk very much—just an occasional grunt or acknowledgment of points of interest along the way.

What else happens when you do fitness activities with other people? Surprisingly, relationships build faster. It's not just that you have a common interest, but the physical ordeal that you share as you grind out the miles or struggle through the classes can bring you closer than dozens of hours spent over lunch or evening socials. There is a kinship that grows with the shared agonies and ecstasies of sports and fitness pursuits.

Back to the question: How do you pick that first step wisely? The PADs summaries in Figures 9.3 to 9.9 will give you an idea of how to move gradually and not take on more than you can handle. You might refer back to the BADs profiles in Chapter 8 to help you choose an activity that is right for your body and for your mind. The body profiles will tell you whether an activity emphasizes upper body, lower body, or total body development. And you can identify the nature of this development. Is it more for strength or for flexibility?

What about movement? Refer back to the MADs profiles in Chapter 8. Remember, some activities have broad range. They condition movement patterns across the entire scale, such as dance or the martial arts. Others are more specific, such as running or body building. There may be a tendency to say activities with a broader range are better overall, but this really depends on what you need. If you need more focus, more direction, more charging ahead in life, then you don't want to get your directions all confused by mixing up your movements. An activity such as dance would be less helpful than one such as running, which is more direct and unidimensional.

Step 3 of the procedure involves writing down an activity that suits your needs for change. Using all three activity profiles (PADs, BADs, MADs) will give you a more complete picture of this activity's potential, as well as identify dimensions that may bring about unwanted change.

The Case Study—Step 3. Susan's program involved four activities: running, cycling, swimming, and weight work. Since she was in training for competition, there was a driving edge to all four. She pushed hard and thereby reinforced her aggressive tendencies. Although swimming isn't rated as being as aggressive as running, the fact that Susan was going for faster and faster times and ever stronger movements would give even this activity a more aggressive cast.

She needed to back off, to slow down, to be more in tune with her environment rather than always racing ahead of it. She didn't need aerobic dance and she wasn't inclined to go back to ballet classes. Bear in mind, she needed her aggressive style for work—it just had to be balanced.

Two possibilities came out of her search. Yoga and tai chi. Why these? Yoga may be more evident. We have seen how it works. And as a nonaggressive, noncompetitive, slow-moving, mind-centering activity, it makes good sense for her. Except for one thing. Susan thought people who practiced yoga were just flabby middle-aged ladies who couldn't muster up the energy to take aerobics. "Forget it! No way! Yoga—maybe when I'm 80!" So much for this option.

What about tai chi? It intrigued her. It is kind of a martial art, but it's also something different. And it represents a dance form, which means it couldn't be too bad. As she investigated tai chi she discovered that part of the training involves learning a ten-to-fifteen-minute ritual movement pattern that is like a moving meditation. It is done very slowly and you have to concentrate throughout. It really helps open up the muscles and improve the body's flexibility. And once you learn it, you can practice it wherever and whenever. It would mean an investment of a year learning it properly, but then she would have it for life.

Another attraction was that it would be a good way to cool down after a workout or even to warm up those stiff muscles in the morning.

Question 4. How Do I Get Going?

Now we confront reality. It has been fun doing all these analyses, but here comes the hard part: making it happen.

Rule Number 1 — Be Realistic!   Be practical in your planning. Look at your resources and what you want to accomplish. Choosing something that requires large investments of time, money, or emotional energy will make it difficult, especially if you are lacking in any of these precious resources.

Rule Number 2 — Go Slowly!   Take it easy at the beginning. Don't make a complete change from what you are doing. Gradually introduce your new activity into your life. Instead of running five days a week (old plan), you may try running four days and taking a racquetball lesson on the fifth day (new plan). In time you might switch to a three-to-two ratio of three days running to two days of racquetball. At some point, you will feel the balance that is right for you.

Rule Number 3 — Be Patient!   Remember, we are talking about long-term gains, about changes in personality and lifestyle. This isn't easy stuff. It may even be uncomfortable at times. Expect that there could be some rough spots and think about how you might handle them — in advance. Don't allow discouragement to creep in. If you find your resolve flagging, look at what you are doing and your expectations. Maybe you are pushing yourself too hard and too fast. Maybe your expectations for overnight change are out of line with reality. It takes a long time to change your somatotype from an endomorph's to that of a mesomorph, but it can be done. The quick cures are not likely to last. The ones you work for and are patient with are more likely to give you the rewards and satisfactions you seek.

Step 4 involves putting it down in writing: when, where, and how. If you anticipate obstacles, try to identify them. If you can't do it all at once, figure out what you need to do now and what you might be able to do later.

The Case Study — Step 4.   Susan figured she needed to do something quickly. She didn't want to burn out or to alienate all her friends. At the same time, she wasn't willing to let go of her training program.

She felt good about becoming a triathlete. Maybe a minor adjustment could be made, like slowing down her program a bit. After all, it was just her first year and she would feel content with finishing some of the races, never mind leading the pack.

She found a local studio that offered tai chi classes at different hours of the day. Even though they were group classes, instruction was on an individual basis. It didn't matter which class she went to. She discovered that with a little bit of juggling she could take two classes a week. Her triathlon training would get cut back a little, as in dropping one of her runs in exchange for an early morning tai chi class.

It didn't seem like a big inconvenience. In fact, she was looking forward to learning "the form," as they called it. It would help her quiet her mind and, she hoped, take a more receptive stance at times.

It's Up To You!

You have a lot of information and tools at your disposal. It's up to you how you use them. You may need some creativity in finding a plan that works well for you. It isn't a simple formula that you plug your psyche into and get the programmed results. It takes thought and commitment.

It's very possible that what you need to change is minor. Just as in Susan's case, there was no dramatic transformation, no major upheaval in lifestyle. Even so, we can expect that with commitment, the plan will pay off in the long run. Susan's learning of this "moving meditation," tai chi, will give her an outlet. It may be something she does first thing in the morning. Built into her life structure, it will add balance to her aggressive tendencies. And it doesn't take away from all the drive that she gets through other activities.

If you think you need a major overhaul, be sure to go slowly. Recognize that sports and fitness activities can give you access to parts of yourself you didn't think existed. You may find that coordination the high school basketball coach said you didn't have as he crossed your name off the try-out sheets. You may find there is a sleeping lion inside and that you are not such a pushover. You may discover a potential to direct your energy and get things accomplished like you never have before. It won't come overnight. It also won't come if all you do is think about it.

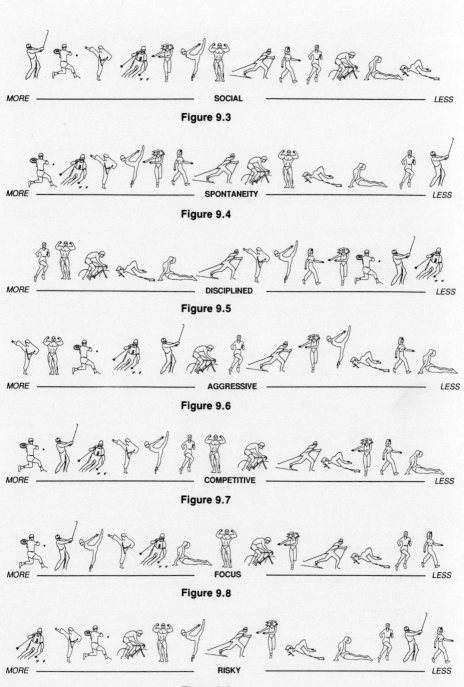

MORE ——————————— SOCIAL ——————————— LESS

Figure 9.3

MORE ——————————— SPONTANEITY ——————————— LESS

Figure 9.4

MORE ——————————— DISCIPLINED ——————————— LESS

Figure 9.5

MORE ——————————— AGGRESSIVE ——————————— LESS

Figure 9.6

MORE ——————————— COMPETITIVE ——————————— LESS

Figure 9.7

MORE ——————————— FOCUS ——————————— LESS

Figure 9.8

MORE ——————————— RISKY ——————————— LESS

Figure 9.9

10

Fitness and Lifestyle Changes

Ignorance Is Bliss

Sometimes, when you read a book, there is one good idea that you can hold onto for life. We hope that will be the case here. There is much to digest from your self-evaluations and the information about sports and fitness. Whether or not you agree with all you have read, the truth is, if you have come this far, you can't return. You will never be able to see the world the way you once did. When you are out running, you will begin looking at the body types of your fellow joggers. You will watch to see where they are tight and rigid, or whether their brows are creased with inner worry. If you go to a health club, you will make mental note of who files into the aerobics room and who heads for the racquetball courts. When friends talk to you about their fitness programs, you will find yourself slipping in little questions about their personality and you will try to size them up physically.

A psychiatrist who studied fitness fanatics commented that the odds were better than seventy-five percent that if a married man suddenly took up running with a passion, he was contemplating or involved in a divorce.[1] If you read this on page one, you might have scoffed. Now, you might be trying to figure out why this is so. The link between physical and psychological activity is a lot more real.

Ignorance is bliss and knowledge is power. Knowledge is also responsibility. Once you know something, you can't play naive anymore. Healthy people use knowledge to improve their lives, even though it may be difficult. They stop smoking, they alter their diets, and they exercise. Now we are asking you to make another change based on new information. How necessary is this change? How much do you have to change?

The necessity of change is based in your experience. You are the judge of whether to change and how much. Bear in mind that if you are committed to lifelong fitness, you have lots of years ahead when you will be training your body, and your mind. Small changes now can vector your life in a new direction even though the change may be imperceptible for years.

Variations

Small change is a smart way to start. You take on something too big and you get discouraged or lose interest. What you have learned in this book can be divided into two major categories: self-knowledge, and information about sports and fitness. If you focus on what you have learned about yourself, you have a fund of information that can guide you toward change. And since we want to look at small change, what can you do with this knowledge?

Changing How You Exercise

When we analyzed sports and fitness programs in Chapter 8, we had to make some assumptions based on the typical way an activity is performed. Talking about "typical" is like describing the average American family with 2.3 children. It's not something you can deal with on a practical level—we're all a bit different.

To illustrate, let's look at a woman who called herself a swimmer. She complained about feeling depressed at times, of bouts of anxiety, and of having trouble sticking to things. She took on too many projects and then became overwhelmed. She was about forty pounds overweight and had little strength in her muscles. Her movements were heavy, slow, and contracted. Remember, she was a swimmer. Doesn't this sound inconsistent? It does and with good reason. When she swam, she trudged through the water with slow, heavy arm movements. Occasionally, she became panicked about drowning, as if her body would just sink. It seemed reasonable, too, if you watched her.

Changing How. There were better exercise programs for her than swimming, but she was stubborn. She didn't want to do anything else. She said she had tried. She felt embarrassed in aerobics, couldn't play tennis, was too fat to run, and was afraid of yoga. Would she consider changing how she swam? Well, yes, she would do that. She went for swimming lessons with a good coach who taught her proper breathing technique, arm placement, and kicking. When she had all of this down, she got the new program: Lap sprints—interval training. No more plodding through the water. Fast-paced swims. A thousand-yard warm-up and then fifty-yard sprints. Did she like it? Not at all—at first. Then she began to feel better, stronger. Her endurance improved. And her mood swings decreased. She felt more focused. She couldn't daydream as much when she was sprinting. And she never worried about drowning again.

This is a change in *how*, not *what*. Was it effective? Yes. Was it difficult? A little.

How did we know what to change? It came out of her profiles. Endurance activities like swimming, running, and cycling tend to be *unfocused* because your body actions become mechanical. They don't require your attention. But when you are doing interval training, like wind sprints, your whole being is involved. And afterward, you are too tired to think. Also, endurance activities can settle into a slow pace that feels sluggish and certainly not very energizing. When this happens, it's a good idea to vary the pace. You see runners do this when they sprint the last quarter-mile of their five-mile run. A key to success for this woman was coaching. We will return to this later. For now, just note the difference between what a person does and how she does it. There are over 23 million runners in the States. How many of them run with proper technique?

To recap, small changes in your program can come out of a careful look at your profiles. If you rate yourself as having a controlled personality, maybe you can introduce some variety into your exercise program. *Retro-running* is "in" now,[2] so you can try running backward through the park or even running zigzag grapevine steps. Try swinging your arms, singing, skipping, or leaping. You might want to take along a friend just in case you need some emotional support or testimony to your sanity.

If you move in a slow, rigid manner, do some good stretching and then try interval work. Push yourself to extend, to reach out—go for the brass ring. If you need to become more sociable, make it a point to find a partner. If you are always with people, use your exercise period as private time; give yourself the pleasure of your own company for a change.

You can use your profiles to change how you exercise without making major life adjustments. Try it—you might like it.

Other Minor Variations

One of the nice things about your new knowledge is that it gives you three distinct angles to work with. We have a good idea about exercise prescription from the personality side and we just illustrated how movement plays into prescription. But we haven't said too much about the body angle, so let's look at its role in reshaping your personality.

In Chapter 6 we took apart the body limb by limb, muscle by muscle. And you did the same with your body as you rated your strength, flexibility, and shape. How can you make small changes based on these ratings? If specific parts of your body are weak, inflexible, or shaped in ways suggesting chronic emotional blockage, can you change them? The answer is yes. Any weight trainer can tell you what exercises to do to strengthen your pectoral muscles, abdominal muscles, thighs, calves, arms, or neck. If your head juts forward, there are exercises to help you realign it. If your lower back is weak, there are exercises to strengthen it. If your shoulders sag, there are exercises to build them up.

But it's not just strengthening. You may have to loosen certain muscles. You may need to learn some good stretches to increase your flexibility in different regions. You may need to open up your breathing by working on the flexibility of your chest. You may need to free your arms by stretching out muscles in your back and shoulders. You may need to unleash the energy in your hands by increasing the flexibility around all of the finger and wrist joints.

How effective can this be? A brief story gives part of the answer. A movement therapist was working with a group of adults in a course entitled "Fundamentals of Movement." The work was based on well-established principles of human physiology and psychological development. Participants were lying on their backs with arms out to the side in the position of a cross. As the therapist introduced the next movement, she commented to an observer that the upcoming exercise often resulted in emotional release, whereby some participants would suddenly begin crying. The exercise involved reaching one arm over the body to touch the other arm and then slowly dragging it across the chest and back to the floor. The exercise worked on releasing tension in the chest. It seemed a simple enough movement and the observer was skeptical about this having any kind of emotional impact. But within minutes, as the participants repeated the exercise, tears streamed down the cheeks of two class members. The therapist calmly said to the observer, "It always seems to happen with this exercise."

What does this prove? Perhaps it illustrates more than proves that releasing tension in specific regions of the body can have emotional side effects. This is certainly one of the reasons that some people are as addicted to their yoga classes as runners are to their routes.

When you reshape yourself physically, you also influence your psychology. At the very least, the feedback you get when your body changes will cause you to feel differently about yourself. If you once looked like a scrawny wimp and now your muscular frame intimidates people, the feedback has got to change the way you perceive yourself. Of course, we think it goes much deeper than this. Changing the strength, flexibility, and shape of different regions of your body will have corresponding effects on psychological processes. As your arms feel stronger, it won't be as difficult for you to take hold of your world. As your legs give you greater support and power to stride into life, your self-confidence and assertiveness will improve.

Acknowledging that you weren't born with stooped shoulders or that your arms are not genetically weak may strip you of excuses, but it could help you take responsibility for your body shape — with all that this implies.

Alternatives

You may feel overwhelmed with information, but the fact is we have only scratched the surface. In one way or another, we touched on about twenty fitness activities — a narrow slice of fitness outlets. There is Frisbee, Hackey Sack, skateboarding, roller skating, surfing, scuba diving, rugby, mountaineering, canoeing, water ballet, volleyball, softball, and all the new creations. The list is endless. How do we rate them? The problem is we can't. That's work we will leave to you.

Ideally, finding the right exercises for you would involve going to a list and looking up an activity's ratings. But, as we have just seen, how you perform an activity may have as much bearing on its psychological impact as what it is you are doing. You need to think through your profiles and determine activities that best fit your needs. A little brainstorming could help.

Let's take an example. "Arnie" was a creative artist for an advertising company. He liked aerobics so much that he took class at least five times a week. He stood out in class not because he was male but because of the way he moved. He jumped around like a rag doll. His arms flapped wildly and his head bobbed on his shoulders as if it was attached by a rubber band. Once the aerobics started, his heels never touched the ground. He looked at times like he was going to take off. In life it was the same. He didn't have a whole lot of control, and although his airy quality made him a good artist, it had its downside as well. What would you prescribe? It's not in the list of Chapter 8. Are you ready? *Fencing!*

Why fencing? Think about it for a minute. You are standing with your feet firmly planted on the ground, your center of gravity right under you, your arm poised with foil in hand, your back erect, and your head squarely on your shoulders. Lots of control, lots of balance, lots of dexterity. Is this what Arnie needed? You bet it is. If more were told about his lifestyle, you would see how right this exercise was for him. And guess what? He liked it. It challenged him. It gave him direction he never got in aerobics. And he felt sturdier. (He looked sturdier, too.)

A year later Arnie was able to see the humor in a story about the first few weeks in fencing class. He had an old Polish Count as an instructor who got so frustrated with Arnie's flighty movements that for half the class the count crawled around on his knees holding Arnie's ankles down and pressing his feet into the floor. The next class he rigged up some heavy ankle weights for Arnie to wear during the session. Get the picture?

Fencing is not one of the popular fitness activities, but there are classes in most cities. And if fencing isn't right, there are all kinds of alternatives you can look into. The point is not to restrict yourself to the traditional or the popular. What you need may be something very special or even something you invent for yourself. Who knows—you may originate the next fitness fad!

Transitions

A transition is a passage from one state of being to another, a period of change. It can be abrupt, as in a sudden job change or accident, or more prolonged, such as in the infamous midlife crisis. When we are going through these periods of change, our needs are different. Perhaps what once worked for us no longer helps. Old methods of maintaining equilibrium only add to the confusion.

Transitions are thought of as crises of opportunity. They are moments in life when we can choose a new way of relating to the world, or we can refuse to change and in so doing perpetuate behaviors that are no longer productive. A little child may cry to get his way with his parents but as an adult this pattern is seen as puerile. A person who keeps getting fired for being too independent can find other jobs or she can start her own company.

One of the things about transitional periods is that we feel as if we are spinning—sometimes out of control. The old ways aren't working and we haven't figured out what the new ways should be. How can exercise help or hinder?

A short example. "Becky" was going through a not-so-merry go round of separations and reconciliations with her husband of seven years. He had a girlfriend and then he didn't and then he did. She felt she was going out of her mind. She loved him and couldn't figure out what to do. She took up running, half a mile at first and then gradually more. She began setting goals for herself and at the end of the year was running in local 10K races. Meanwhile, the merry-go-round continued. Surprisingly, she could see it more objectively. She wasn't spinning any more. She knew what her conditions were and made them clear to her husband. But he wanted his cake and his sweetie, too. In the end he got neither. Becky didn't feel great about getting divorced, but she did feel good about herself. She said at least she was moving ahead and not just doing endless pirouettes.

Depending on what you need, exercise can be a process that helps you reorient yourself. Just as there are right moves and wrong moves in the long run, so too in transitional periods there are activities that can facilitate or impede growth. Let's look at the downside.

"Bill" was big on yoga. He practiced regularly and felt it really helped when he was under pressure. He meditated and tried to breathe his problems away. He released the tension in his body with long stretches. After an hour of yoga, nothing seemed to matter. Problems just weren't as monumental as they had seemed before. He was cool; he was like the river flowing along. Except that people around him didn't function that way. In fact, his boss thought Bill was aloof and disengaged. The company was in trouble—everyone's job was on the line and Bill was reciting his mantra. When his wife complained about having to take care of the two kids and not having time to finish her degree, he breathed in relaxation and breathed out tension. He seemed unaffected. After the dam burst, leaving him unemployed and separated, he stepped up his practice by going to a yoga center each morning and night, and occasionally at noon. He thought it helped.

Transitions. Sometimes we need a sense of direction in periods of change. Sometimes we have to take a stand. Sometimes we have to become more flexible. Exercise programs that contain elements we need will help. Those that perpetuate the old style will keep us where we were, or worse. A time of change at home, on the job, or elsewhere may

282 • *Body Moves*

mean a change in how we exercise—at least for the present. It shouldn't mean dropping our fitness pursuits, but rather altering them to suit the situation's needs and to help us cope.

Coaching

It's funny how when we were in school there were all these people called coaches wandering through the high school corridors and locker rooms. Whatever happened to them? In health clubs there are instructors, trainers, and fitness appraisers, but where are the coaches? Instructors usually lead classes like aerobics. Trainers walk around and make sure the equipment is working and occasionally help someone with a workout routine. But who coaches you? Who stands by and watches how you are doing your workout? Who screams in your ear telling you to try harder?

Sure, we're too old for coaches. That's high school and collegiate stuff. That's for when you are on a team or competing. This is the adult world. We're not out to beat anyone, just to stay in shape, fight off midriff bulge, keep the old ticker tocking. Tennis players might not agree, and certainly golfers sneak visits to the pro shop. Skiers also sign up for clinics. But the majority of fitness buffs don't feel the need for coaching. They are not out to win the Boston Marathon, maybe just to complete it. And there are plenty of books that tell you how you should train.

Who needs a coach? We all do. To frame it differently, we all need feedback on how we move, our technique, our training program. We need consultation about what we do. And we need people to watch us, to tell us about our body alignment, about our movement qualities. We need someone to coach us from time to time, to stop us when we are doing it wrong and show us how to do it right.

Not every coach or trainer understands what is best for us. Some coaches operate out of quasi-sadistic training philosophies. Others think all bodies should be molded the same way. We need coaches who can look at us and understand our unique makeup—who can take us where we are and give us sensible and sensitive feedback.

Who are these coaches and where do we find them? Sometimes they are people working in clubs or recreation centers. They may be retired jocks who have a keen eye for good form and proper technique. They may be classmates who mesmerize us when they move. We have to look for them. And having found them, we have to swallow our pride and ask for their help. We will be surprised how willingly it is offered.

A rose is a rose is a rose, but are all runners alike? More to the point, just because you say you are a: bodybuilder, swimmer, dancer, or bowler doesn't mean we all do it the same, or that we *should* all do it the same. Ask the coach—she'll tell you how to do it the way that's best for you.

Commitment

Last point. Ron Hill, a three-time Olympian and a Boston Marathon winner, has completed at least one run a day for more than eight thousand days in a row—that's over twenty-two-and-a-half years! And that's commitment. We're not all Olympians, or even marathon runners, but at heart the question we need to ask is, "How committed am I?"

Bodies change slowly. The average American gains one pound per year between ages twenty-five and fifty-five. That's gradual change, but at age fifty-five, when we are thirty pounds heavier, we might notice the difference. A nineteen-year-old who smokes a pack a day hardly notices the effects, but at age sixty with obstructive lung disease, each rasping breath is noticeable. Psychological change is also slow, but, just as with the pound-per-year phenomenon, it does happen.

If you exercise regularly, and particularly if you do the same thing all the time, you know you are shaping your body in a specific fashion, and now you also know you are reinforcing personality traits. Which traits you choose to reinforce is up to you. At least you are aware of the choice.

If you don't exercise regularly but want to get the most out of your program, you might recognize by now that you have to increase your investment in order to reap the benefits. Personality gains are part of the benefit package. But we're talking about slow gains.

It's an investment in yourself, just like putting money away each paycheck for your retirement. A recent study informs us that for every hour we spend exercising we get two back in terms of additional lifetime.[4] This means that if you count up all the hours you spent exercising over your lifetime and it comes out to about one year, you can expect to get *two more years of lifetime* on top of all those joyous hours you spent sweating. That's the physical side.

Psychologically, if we invest in our creativity through exercise, what might we reap at age seventy-five? If we invest in our isolation, how will that pay off in the long run? There is little question that exercise can help us change directions psychologically; it may be only a one- or two-degree shift, but over the long haul what a difference that can make.

Notes

Chapter 1

1. Johnson, W. O. Marching to euphoria. *Sports Illustrated*, 1980, *53* (3), 72–76, 78–79, 81–82.
2. Sheldon, W. H. *The varieties of human temperament*. New York: Harper and Row, 1942; Sheldon, W. H. *The varieties of human physique*. New York: Harper and Row, 1940.
3. Friedman, M., and Rosenman, R. H. *Type A behavior and your heart*. New York: Alfred A. Knopf, 1974; Kraiuhin, C. et al. The Type A behaviour pattern and physique. *Journal of Psychosomatic Research*, 1983, *27* (6), 479–483.
4. Murphy, M., and White, R. *The psychic side of sport*. New York: Addison-Wesley, 1978.

Chapter 2

1. The ten cases represent composites derived from the life experiences of a large number of athletes and fitness addicts. In this regard, the "stories" are not about specific people, rather they are about patterns observed in people devoted to exercise.

Chapter 3

1. Sheehan, G. Body and soul. In M. H. Sacks and M. L. Sachs (Eds.), *Psychology of running*. Champaign, Ill.: Human Kinetics, 1981, 189–190.
2. Hughes, J. R. Psychological effects of habitual aerobic exercise: A critical review. *Preventive Medicine*, 1984, *13* (1), 66–78.
3. Armstrong, H. E. Jr., and Armstrong, D. C. Relation of physical fitness to a dimension of body image. *Perceptual and Motor Skills*, 1968, *26*, 1173–1174;

Bahrke, M. S., and Morgan, W. P. Anxiety reduction following exercise and meditation. In M. H. Sacks and M. L. Sachs (Eds.), *Psychology of running*. Champaign, Ill.: Human Kinetics, 1981, 57–66; Buffone, G. W. Future directions: the potential for exercise as therapy. In M. L. Sachs and G. W. Buffone (Eds.), *Running as therapy*. Lincoln, Neb.: University of Nebraska Press, 1984, 215–226; Cooper, L. Athletics, activity and personality: a review of the literature. *Research Quarterly*, 1969, *40* (1), 17–22; Flippin, R. Are runners better lovers? *The Runner*, 1987, *9* (6), 32–35; Folkins, C. H. Effects of physical training on mood. *Journal of Clinical Psychology*, 1976, *32* (2), 385–388; Folkins, C. H., and Sime, W. E. Physical fitness training and mental health. *American Psychologist*, 1981, *36* (4), 373–389; Haskell, W. L. Overview: Health benefits of exercise. In J. D. Matarazzo, S. M. Weiss, N. E. Miller, and S. M. Weiss (Eds.), *Behavioral health: a handbook of health enhancement and disease prevention*. New York: Wiley, 1984, 409–423; Jasnoski, M. L., and Holmes, D. S. Influence of initial aerobic fitness, aerobic training and changes in aerobic fitness on personality functioning. *Journal of Psychosomatic Research*, 1981, *25* (6), 553–556; Joesting, J. Comparison of students who exercise with those who do not. *Perceptual and Motor Skills*, 1981, *53* (2), 426; Kostrubala, T. *The joy of running*. New York: Lippincott, 1976; Morgan, W. P., and Roberts, J. Psychological effects of chronic physical activity. *Medicine and Science in Sports and Exercise*, 1970, *2*, 213–218; Perri, T., and Templer, D. I. The effects of an aerobic exercise program on psychological variables in older adults. *International Journal of Aging and Human Development*, 1985, *20*, 167–172; Powell, R. R. Psychological effects of exercise therapy upon institutionalized geriatric mental patients. *Journal of Gerontology*, 1974, *29*, 157–161; Powell, R. R., and Pohndorf, R. H. Comparison of adult exercisers and nonexercisers on fluid intelligence and selected physiological variables. *Research Quarterly*, 1971, *42* (1), 70–77; Sacks, M. H., and Sachs, M. L. *The psychology of running*. Champaign, Ill.: Human Kinetics, 1981; Sharp, M. W., and Reilley, R. R. The relationship of aerobic physical fitness to selected personality traits. *Journal of Clinical Psychology*, 1975, *31* (3), 428–430; Sime, W. E. Psychological benefits of exercise training in the healthy individual. In J. D. Matarazzo, S. M. Weiss, N. E. Miller, and S. M. Weiss (Eds.), *Behavioral health: a handbook of health enhancement and disease prevention*. New York: Wiley, 1984, 488–507; Slusher, H. Personality and intelligence characteristics of selected high school athletes and non-athletes. *Research Quarterly*, 1964, *35*, 539–543; Solomon, E. G., and Bumpus, A. K. The running meditation response: an adjunct to psychotherapy. In M. H. Sacks and M. L. Sachs (Eds.), *Psychology of running*. Champaign, Ill.: Human Kinetics, 1981; Sonstroem, R. J. Exercise and self-esteem. In R. Terjung (Ed.), *Exercise and sport science reviews*. (Volume 12). Lexington, Mass.: D. C. Heath, 1984, 123–155; Sutton, R. *Body worry*. New York: Viking, 1987; Dishman, R. K. Exercise compliance: A new view for public health. *The Physician and Sportsmedicine*, 1986, *14* (5), 127–145. See Bibliography for additional references.

4. Altshul, V. A. Should we advise our depressed patients to run? In M. H. Sacks and M. L. Sachs (Eds.), *Psychology of running*. Champaign, Ill.: Human Kinetics, 1981, 50–56; Blue, F. R. Aerobic running as a treatment for moderate depression. *Perceptual and Motor Skills*, 1979, *48*, 228; Blumenthal, J. A., Williams, R. S., Williams, R. B. Jr., and Wallace, A. G. Effects of

exercise on the Type A (coronary prone) behavior pattern. *Psychosomatic Medicine,* 1980, 42 (2), 289–296; Buffone, G. W. *Running and depression.* In M. L. Sachs and G. W. Buffone (Eds.), *Running as therapy.* Lincoln, Neb.: University of Nebraska Press, 1984, 6–22; Dishman, "Medical psychology"; Driscoll, R. Anxiety reduction using physical exertion and positive images. *Psychological Records,* 1979, 26, 87–94; Gal, R., and Lazarus, R. S. The role of activity in anticipating and confronting stressful situations. *Journal of Human Stress,* 1975, 7, 4–20; Griest, J. H., et al. Running through your mind. *Journal of Psychosomatic Research,* 1978, 22, 259–294; Griest, J. H., et al. Running as a treatment for depression. *Comprehensive Psychiatry,* 1979, 20, 41–54; Haskell, "Health benefits"; Hughes, "Psychological effects"; Kobasa, S. C., Maddi, S. R., and Puccetti, M. C. Personality and exercise as buffers in the stress-illness relationship. *Journal of Behavioral Medicine,* 1982, 5 (4), 391–404; Kostrubala, T. Running and therapy. In M. L. Sachs and G. W. Buffone (Eds.), *Running as therapy.* Lincoln, Neb.: University of Nebraska Press, 1984, 112–124; Lake, B. M., et al. The Type A behavior pattern, physical fitness, and psychophysical reactivity. *Health Psychology,* 1985, 4 (2), 169–187; Lion, L. S. Psychological effects of jogging: a preliminary study. *Perceptual and Motor Skills,* 1978, 47 (3, Pt. 2), 1215–1218; Martin, J. E., and Dubbert, P. M. Exercise in hypertension. *Annals of Behavioral Medicine,* 1985, 7, 13–18; Monahan, T. Exercise and depression: Swapping sweat for serenity. *The Physician and Sports Medicine,* 1986, 14 (9), 192–197; Orwin, A. Treatment of a situational phobia—A case for running. *British Journal of Psychiatry,* 1974, 125, 95–98; Orwin, A. "The running treatment": a preliminary communication on a new use for an old therapy (physical activity) in the agoraphobia syndrome. In M. H. Sacks and M. L. Sachs (Eds.), *Psychology of running.* Champaign, Ill.: Human Kinetics, 1981, 32–39; Price, W. A., Dimarzio, and Gardner, P. R. Biopsychosocial approach to premenstrual syndrome. *American Family Physician,* 1986, 33 (6), 117–122; Roth, D. L., and Holmes, D. S. Influence of physical fitness in determining the impact of stressful life events on physical and psychologic health. *Psychosomatic Medicine,* 1985, 47 (2), 164–173; Sime, "Psychological benefits"; Simons, A. D., Epstein, L. H., McGowan, C. R., and Kupfer, D. J. Exercise as a treatment for depression: an update. *Clinical Psychology Review,* 1985, 5, 553–568; Williams, J. M., and Getty, D. Effect of levels of exercise on psychological mood states, physical fitness, and plasma betaendorphin. *Perceptual and Motor Skills,* 1986, 63 (3), 1099–1105; Young, R. J., and Ismail, A. H. Personality differences of adult men before and after a physical fitness program. *Research Quarterly,* 1976, 47 (3), 513–519; Young, R. J., and Ismail, A. H. Ability of biochemical and personality variables in discriminating between high and low physical fitness levels. *Journal of Psychosomatic Research,* 1978, 22, 193–199.

5. Colt, E. W., Dunner, D. L., Hall, K., and Fieve, R. R. A high prevalence of affective disorders in runners. In M. H. Sacks and M. L. Sachs (Eds.), *Psychology of running.* Champaign, Ill.: Human Kinetics, 1981, 234–248; Cooper, A. M. Masochism and long-distance running. In M. H. Sacks and M. L. Sachs (Eds.), *Psychology of running.* Champaign, Ill.: Human Kinetics, 1981, 267–273; Dickhoff, G. M. Running amok: Injuries in compulsive runners. *Journal of Sport Behavior,* 1984, 7 (3), 120–129; Dielens, S. Narcissism and fashionable physical activities: psychological profiles of aerobic

dancers, joggers and bodybuilders. *Revue de l'Education Physique*, 1984, *24* (1), 21–25; Little, J. C. Neurotic illness in fitness fanatics. *Psychiatric Annals*, 1979, *9* (3), 49–56; Morgan, W. P. Negative addiction in runners. *The Physician and Sports Medicine*, 1979, *7*, 57–70; Sachs, M. L. Running addiction. In M. H. Sacks and M. L. Sachs (Eds.), *Psychology of running*. Champaign, Ill.: Human Kinetics, 1981, 116–126; Sachs, M. L., and Pargman, D. Running addiction. In M. L. Sachs and G. W. Buffone (Eds.), *Running as therapy*. Lincoln, Neb.: University of Nebraska Press, 1984, 231–252; Sacks, M. H. Running addiction: a clinical report. In M. H. Sacks and M. L. Sachs (Eds.), *Psychology of running*. Champaign, Ill.: Human Kinetics, 1981, 127–130; Sours, J. A. Running, anorexia nervosa and perfection. In M. H. Sacks and M. L. Sachs (Eds.), *Psychology of running*. Champaign, Ill.: Human Kinetics, 1981, 80–91; Valliant, P. M. Personality and injury in competitive runners. *Perceptual and Motor Skills*, 1981, *53* (1), 251–253; Wrenn, M. Running to extremes. *Life*, 1987, *10* (2), 46–53; Yates, A., Leehey, K., and Shisslak, C. M. Running—An analogue of anorexia? *New England Journal of Medicine*, 1983, *308* (5), 251–255.

6. American College of Sports Medicine. *Guidelines for exercise testing and prescription*. Philadelphia: Lea and Febiger, 1986; ACSM, *Guidelines*.

7. American Psychiatric Association, A *psychiatric glossary* (Fourth Edition). New York: Basic Books, 1975.

8. Spielberger, C. D. *Anxiety and behavior*. New York: Academic Press, 1966.

9. Schwartz, G. E., Davidson, R. J., and Goleman, D. J. Patterning of cognitive and somatic processes in the self-regulation of anxiety: effects of medication versus exercise. *Psychosomatic Medicine*, 1978, *40*, 321–328.

10. Dishman, "Medical psychology."

11. Bahrke and Morgan, "Anxiety reduction"; Dishman, "Medical psychology"; Morgan, W. P. Anxiety reduction following acute physical activity. *Psychiatric Annals*, 1979, *9*, 141–147.

12. Bahrke and Morgan, "Anxiety reduction."

13. Buffone, "Running and depression"; Dishman, "Medical psychology"; Monahan, "Swapping sweat"; Simons, et al., "Exercise as a treatment"; Sime, "Psychological benefits."

14. Griest, et al., "Running as a treatment."

15. Dishman, "Medical psychology"; Buffone, "Running and depression"; Simons, et al., "Exercise as a treatment"; Sime, "Psychological benefits."

16. Monahan, "Swapping sweat"; Griest, et al., "Running through mind"; Simons, et al., "Exercise as a treatment."

17. Eischens, R. R., and Griest, J. H. Beginning and continuing running: steps to psychological well-being. In M. L. Sachs and G. W. Buffone (Eds.), *Running as therapy*. Lincoln, Neb.: University of Nebraska Press, 1984, 63–82; Griest, et al., "Running through mind"; Griest, et al., "Running as treatment."

18. Simons, et al., "Exercise as a treatment."

19. Morgan, "Negative addiction."

20. Selye, H. *The stress of life*. New York: McGraw Hill, 1956.

21. American College of Sports Medicine. *Position stands and opinion state-*

ments. Sixth Edition. Indianapolis, Ind.: ACSM, April 1987; Cooper, K. H., Gallman, J. S., and McDonald, J. L. Jr. Role of aerobic exercise in reduction of stress. *Dental Clinics of North America,* 1986, *30* (4), S133–142; Diensbier, R. A., et al. Exercise and stress tolerance. In M. H. Sacks and M. L. Sachs (Eds.), *Psychology of running.* Champaign, Ill.: Human Kinetics, 1981, 192–210; McMahon, M., and Palmer, R. M. Exercise and hypertension. *Medical Clinics of North America,* 1985, *69* (1), 57–70; Paffenbarger, R. A., and Hyde, R. T. Exercise in the prevention of coronary heart disease. *Preventive Medicine,* 1984, *13,* 3–22; Paffenbarger, R. A., et al. A natural history of athleticism and cardiovascular disease. *Journal of the American Medical Association,* 1984, *252,* 491–495; Paffenbarger, R. A. Physical activity, coronary heart disease and longevity. *Proceedings of the American College of Sports Medicine,* Las Vegas: May 1987; Sharkey, B. J. *Physiology of fitness* (second edition). Champaign, Ill.: Human Kinetics, 1984; Hammond, H. K., and Froelicher, V. F. The physiologic sequelae of chronic dynamic exercise. *Medical Clinics of North America,* 1985, *69* (1), 21–39; Leon, A. S. Physical activity levels and coronary heart disease: analysis of epidemiologic and supporting studies. *Medical Clinics of North America,* 1985, *69* (1), 3–20.

22. Goldberg, L., and Elliot, D. L. The effect of physical activity on lipid and lipoprotein levels. *Medical Clinics of North America,* 1985, *69* (1), 41–55; McCunny, R. J. Fitness, heart disease, and high-density lipoproteins: a look at the relationships. *The Physician and Sportsmedicine,* 1987, *15* (2), 67–79.

23. Driscoll, "Anxiety reduction"; Gal and Lazarus, "Role of activity"; Dishman, "Medical psychology"; Martin and Dubbert, "Exercise and hypertension."

24. Bahrke and Morgan, "Anxiety reduction."

25. Rosenberg, M. *Conceiving the self.* New York: Basic Books, 1979.

26. Sonstroem, "Exercise and self-esteem."

27. Folkins and Sime, "Physical fitness."

28. Grossman, A. Endorphins: "opiates for the masses." *Medicine and Science in Sports and Exercise,* 1985, *17* (1), 101–105; Grossman, A., and Sutton, J. R. Endorphins: What are they? How are they measured? What is their role in exercise? *Medicine and Science in Sports and Exercise,* 1985, *17* (1), 74–81; Bulbulian, R., and Darabos, B. L. Motor neuron excitability: the Hoffman reflex following exercise of low and high intensity. *Medicine and Science in Sports and Exercise,* 1986, *18* (6), 697–702; Heller, G. V., et al. Plasma beta-endorphin levels in silent myocardial ishemia induced by exercise. *American Journal of Cardiology,* 1987, *59* (8), 735–739.

29. Markoff, R. A., Ryan, P., and Young, T. Endorphins and mood changes in long distance running. *Medicine and Science in Sports and Exercise,* 1982, *14,* 11–15.

30. Lilliefors, J. *The running mind.* Mountain View, Calif.: World Publications, 1978; Sachs, M. L. The runner's high. In M. L. Sachs and G. W. Buffone (Eds.), *Running as therapy.* Lincoln, Neb.: University of Nebraska Press, 1984, 273–287; Dishman, "Medical psychology."

31. Sachs. "The runner's high."

32. Ateyo, O. *Blood and guts: violence in sports.* New York: Paddington Press, 1979; Bredemeier, B. J., and Shields, D. L. Values and violence in sports today. *Psychology Today,* 1985, *19* (10), 22–25; 28–32; McCutcheon, L. E.

290 • *Body Moves*

Does running make people more creative? *Journal of Sport Behavior, 1982, 5* (4), 202–206; McCutcheon, L. E., and Yoakum, M. E. Personality attributes of ultramarathoners. *Journal of Personality Assessment*, 1983, 47 (2), 178–180; Rummele, E. Sexuality in marathon runners. *Leitungssport*, 1985, 15 (5), 23–26. See Note 5 for additional references.

33. Glasser, W. *Positive addiction.* New York: Harper and Row, 1976; Morgan, "Negative addiction"; Sachs, "Running addiction"; Sachs and Pargman, "Running addiction"; Sacks, "Running addiction."

34. Glasser, *Positive addiction.*

35. Dishman. "Medical psychology"; Glasser, *Positive addiction*; Morgan, "Negative addiction"; Sachs, "Running addiction"; Sachs and Pargman, "Running addiction"; Sacks, "Running addiction."

36. Grossman, "Endorphins"; Grossman and Sutton, "Endorphins."

37. Morgan, "Negative addiction"; Sachs, "Running addiction"; Glasser, *Positive addiction.*

38. Morgan, "Negative addiction"; Glasser, *Positive addiction.*

39. Morgan, "Negative addiction."

Chapter 4

1. Solomon, H. A. *The exercise myth.* New York: Harcourt Brace Jovanovich, 1984.

2. Haskell, W. L. Overview: Health benefits of exercise. In J. D. Matarazzo, S. M. Weiss, N. E. Miller, and S. M. Weiss (Eds.), *Behavioral health: a handbook of health enhancement and disease prevention.* New York: Wiley, 1984, 409–423.

3. Weltman, A. Exercise and diet to optimize body composition. In J. D. Matarazzo, S. M. Weiss, N. E. Miller, and S. M. Weiss (Eds.), *Behavioral health: a handbook of health enhancement and disease prevention.* New York: Wiley, 1984, 509–523.

4. Toufexis, A. Getting an F for flabby. *Time,* January 26, 1987, 54–56.

5. American College of Sports Medicine. *Position stands and opinion statements.* Sixth Edition. Indianapolis, Ind.: ACSM, April 1987; Elliot, D. L., and Goldberg, L. Nutrition and exercise. *Medical Clinics of North America,* 1985, 69 (1), 71–82; Nieman, D. C. *The sports medicine fitness course.* Palo Alto, Calif.: Bull Publishing, 1986.

6. ACSM, *Position stands*; American College of Sports Medicine. *Guidelines for exercise testing and prescription.* Philadelphia: Lea and Febiger, 1986.

7. Weltman, "Exercise and diet"; Elliot, D. L., and Goldberg, L. Nutrition and exercise. In J. D. Matarazzo, S. M. Weiss, N. E. Miller, and S. M. Weiss (Eds.), *Behavioral health: a handbook of health enhancement and disease prevention.* New York: Wiley, 1984; Golding, L. A., Myers, C. R., and Sinning, W. E. *The Y's way to physical fitness.* Champaign, Ill.: Human Kinetics, 1982.

8. Leon, A. S. Physical activity levels and coronary heart disease: analysis of epidemiologic and supporting studies. *Medical Clinics of North America,* 1985, 69 (1), 3–20; Levy, R. I., and Feinleib, M. Risk factors for coronary artery disease and their management. In E. Braunwald (Ed.), *Heart disease: a*

textbook of cardiovascular medicine (volume 2). Second Edition. Philadelphia: W. B. Saunders, 1984, 1205–1234; LaPorte, R. The relationship of physical activity and physical fitness to cardiovascular disease and health. *Proceedings of the American College of Sports Medicine,* Las Vegas: May 1987; Nieman, *Sports medicine;* Paffenbarger, R. A., and Hyde, R. T. Exercise in the prevention of coronary heart disease. *Preventive Medicine,* 1984, *13,* 3–22; Paffenbarger, R. A. Physical activity, coronary heart disease and longevity. *Proceedings of the American College of Sports Medicine,* Las Vegas: May 1987; Paffenbarger, R. A. Physical activity and cancer in college alumni. *Proceedings of the American College of Sports Medicine,* Las Vegas: May 1987.

  9. Hammond, H. K., and Froelicher, V. F. The physiologic sequelae of chronic dynamic exercise. *Medical Clinics of North America,* 1985, *69* (1), 21–39; Martin, J. E., and Dubbert, P. M. Exercise in hypertension. *Annals of Behavioral Medicine,* 1985, *7,* 13–18; Nieman, *Sports medicine;* Golding, et al., *Y's way;* Perkins, K. A., Dubbert, P. M., Martin, J. E., Faulstich, M. E., and Harris, J. K. Cardiovascular reactivity to psychological stress in aerobically trained versus untrained mild hypertensives and normotensives. *Health Psychology,* 1986, *5,* 407–421; Stone, M. H., and Wilson, G. D. Resistive training and selected effects. *Medical Clinics of North America,* 1985, *69* (1), 109–122.

10. American Heart Association Subcommittee on Exercise/Cardiac Rehabilitation. Statement on exercise. *Circulation,* 1981, *64,* 1302–1304.

11. Nieman, *Sports medicine;* Leon, "Activity and CHD"; Levy and Feinleib. "Risk factors"; LaPorte, "Cardiovascular disease"; Paffenbarger, R. A., et al. A natural history of athleticism and cardiovascular disease. *Journal of the American Medical Association,* 1984, *252,* 491–495.

12. Dishman, R. K. Exercise compliance: A new view for public health. *The Physician and Sportsmedicine,* 1986, *14* (5), 127–145; Dishman, R. K. *Exercise adherence: Its impact on public health.* Champaign, Ill.: Human Kinetics, 1987.

13. Reid, J. G., and Thomson, J. M. *Exercise prescription for fitness.* Englewood Cliffs, N.J.: Prentice Hall, 1985.

14. Fixx, J. G. *The complete book of running.* New York: Random House, 1977.

15. Reid and Thomson, *Exercise prescription.*

16. Reid and Thomson, *Exercise prescription;* ACSM, *Guidelines;* Nieman, *Sports medicine;* Golding et al., *Y's way.*

17. Normative data taken from: *Standardized test of fitness: Operations manual.* (Second Edition). Ottawa: Fitness and Amateur Sport Canada, 1981.

18. Weltman, "Exercise and diet."

19. Cohen, M. *The Marine Corps 3X fitness program.* New York: Little, Brown and Co., 1986.

20. Nieman, *Sports medicine.*

21. Reid and Thomson, *Exercise prescription.*

22. *Canadian standardized test of fitness (CSTF): Operations manual* (Third Edition). Ottawa: Fitness and Amateur Sport Canada, 1986; Golding et al., *Y's way;* Nieman, *Sports medicine;* Reid and Thomson, *Exercise prescription;* ACSM, *Guidelines;* Ribisl, P. M. Developing an exercise prescription for

health. In J. D. Matarazzo, S. M. Weiss, N. E. Miller, and S. M. Weiss (Eds.), *Behavioral health: a handbook of health enhancement and disease prevention.* New York: Wiley, 1984, 448–465; Sharkey, B. J. *Physiology of fitness* (second edition). Champaign, Ill.: Human Kinetics, 1984.

23. Golding et al., *Y's way*; Nieman, *Sports medicine*; Reid and Thomson, *Exercise prescription.*

24. Normative data taken from: *Canadian Standardized Test of Fitness: Operations Manual* (Third Edition).

25. Normative data taken from: *Canadian Standardized Test of Fitness: Operations Manual* (Third Edition).

26. Spence, A. P. *Basic human anatomy.* Menlo Park, Calif.: Benjamin/Cummings, 1982.

27. Cooper, K. H. *The aerobics way.* New York: Bantam, 1977.

28. ACSM, *Guidelines.*

29. Kline, G. M., et al. Estimation of VO_2 max from a one-mile track walk, gender, age, and body weight. *Medicine and Science in Sports and Exercise,* 1987, *19* (3), 253–259. Normative data taken from: *Canadian Standardized Test of Fitness: Operations Manual* (Third Edition).

30. Reid and Thomson, *Exercise prescription.*

31. ACSM, *Guidelines*, p. 31.

32. Arnot, R. B., and Gaines, C. L. *Sportselection.* New York: Viking Press, 1984.

33. Pesman, C. Five athletic body types. *Esquire*, 1986, *105* (5), 109–118.

34. ACSM, *Position stands*; ACSM, *Guidelines.*

Chapter 5

1. Dishman, R. D. Contemporary sport psychology. *Exercise and Sport Science Reviews*, 1982, *10*, 120–159; Bird, A. M. and Cripe, B. K. *Psychology and sport behavior.* Toronto: Times Mirror/Mosby, 1986; Wiggins, D. K. The history of sport psychology in North America. In Silva, J. M., and Weinberg, R. S. (Eds.), *Psychological foundations of sport.* Champaign, Ill.: Human Kinetics, 1984, 9–34.

2. Henry, F. M. Personality differences in athletes, physical education and aviation students. *Psychological Bulletin*, 1941, *38*, 745.

3. Aamodt, M. G., Alexander, C. J., and Kimbrough, W. W. Personality characteristics of college non-athletes and baseball, football, and track team members. *Perceptual and Motor Skills*, 1983, *57* (1), 143–146; Buffone, G. W. Running and depression. In M. L. Sachs and G. W. Buffone (Eds.), *Running as therapy.* Lincoln, Neb.: University of Nebraska Press, 1984, 6–22; Canada Fitness Survey. *Fitness and lifestyle in Canada.* Ottawa: Government of Canada, 1983; Cooper, L. Athletics, activity and personality: a review of the literature. *Research Quarterly*, 1969, *40* (1), 17–22; Diensbier, R. A., et al. Exercise and stress tolerance. In M. H. Sacks and M. L. Sachs (Eds.), *Psychology of running.* Champaign, Ill.: Human Kinetics, 1981, 192–210; Eysenck, H. J. Sport and personality. *Advances in Behavior Research and Therapy*, 1982, *4* (1), 1–56; Folkins, C. H. Effects of physical training on mood. *Journal of Clinical Psychology*, 1976, *32* (2), 385–388; Folkins, C. H., and Sime, W. E. Physical fitness training and mental health. *American*

Psychologist, 1981, 36 (4), 373–389; Griest, J. H., et al. Running as a treatment for depression. *Comprehensive Psychiatry*, 1979, 20, 41–54; Hughes, J. R. Psychological effects of habitual aerobic exercise: A critical review. *Preventive Medicine*, 1984, 13 (1), 66–78; Morgan, W. P. The trait psychology controversy. *Research Quarterly*, 1980, 51 (1), 50–76; Morgan, W. P., and Roberts, J. Psychological effects of chronic physical activity. *Medicine and Science in Sports and Exercise*, 1970, 2, 213–218; Murphy, M., and White, R. *The psychic side of sport*. New York: Addison-Wesley, 1978; Nideffer, R. M. *The inner athlete*. New York: Thomas Crowell, 1976; Sime, W. E. Psychological benefits of exercise training in the healthy individual. In J. D. Matarazzo, S. M. Weiss, N. E. Miller, and S. M. Weiss (Eds.), *Behavioral health: a handbook of health enhancement and disease prevention*. New York: Wiley, 1984, 488–507; Simons, A. D., Epstein, L. H., McGowan, C. R., and Kupfer, D. J. Exercise as a treatment for depression: an update. *Clinical Psychology Review*, 1985, 5, 553–568; Sonstoem, R. J. Exercise and self-esteem. In R. Terjung (Ed.), *Exercise and sport science reviews*. (Volume 12). Lexington, Mass.: D. C. Heath, 1984, 123–155; Valliant, P. M., Simpson-Housley, P., and McKelvie, S. J. Personality in athletic and non-athletic college groups. *Perceptual and Motor Skills*, 1981, 52 (3), 963–966; Zuckerman, M. Sensation seeking and sports. *Personality and Individual Differences*, 1983, 52 (2), 511–516.

4. Eysenck, "Sport and personality."
5. Dielens, S. Narcissism and fashionable physical activities: psychological profiles of aerobic dancers, joggers and bodybuilders. *Revue de l'Education Physique*, 1984, 24 (1), 21–25.
6. Eysenck, "Sport and personality."
7. Slusher, H. Personality and intelligence characteristics of selected high school athletes and non-athletes. *Research Quarterly*, 1964, 35, 539–543.
8. Cattell, R., Eber, H., and Tatzucka, M. *Handbook of the sixteen Personality Factor Questionnaire*. Champaign, Ill.: Institute for Personality and Ability Testing, 1970.
9. Gabler, H. *Leistungsmotivation im hockleistungs sport*. Hofmann, Schorndorf, 1972.
10. Ogilvie, B. Psychological consistencies within the personalities of high level competitors. *Journal of the American Medical Association*, 1968, 205, 156–202.
11. Slusher, "Personality and intelligence."
12. Hendry, L. Assessment in personality traits in the coach-swimmer relationship. *Research Quarterly*, 1968, 39, 543–551.
13. Rushall, B. S. Personality profiles and a theory of behavior modification for swimmers. *Swimming Techniques*, 1967, 4, 66–71.
14. Dickhoff, G. M. Running amok: Injuries in compulsive runners. *Journal of Sport Behavior*, 1984, 7 (3), 120–129.
15. Yates, A., Leehey, K., and Shisslak, C. M. Running—an analogue of anorexia? *New England Journal of Medicine*, 1983, 308 (5), 251–255.
16. Mikel, K. V. Extraversion in adult runners. *Perceptual and Motor Skills*, 1983, 57 (1), 143–146.

17. Dolphin, C., O'Brien, M., Cahill, N., and Cullen, J. Personality factors and some physiological correlates in athletes. *Journal of Psychosomatic Research*, 1980, 24 (5), 281–285.

18. Kostrubala, T. *The joy of running*. New York: Lippincott, 1976; Sachs, M. L., and Buffone, G. W. (Eds.), *Running as therapy*. Lincoln, Neb.: University of Nebraska Press, 1984; Dielens, "Narcissism."

19. Flippin, R. Are runners better lovers? *The Runner*, 1987, 9 (6), 32–35.

20. Zarski, J. J., West, J. D., and Bubenzer, D. L. Social interest, running and life adjustment. *Personnel and Guidance Journal*, 1982, 61 (3), 146–149.

21. Hall, C. S., and Lindzey, G. *Theories of personality* (Second Edition). New York: John Wiley, 1970.

22. Morgan, "Trait psychology"; Martens, R. The paradigmatic crisis in American sport personology. *Sportwissenschaft*, 1975, 5, 9–24.

23. Allport, G. W. *Personality: a psychological interpretation*. New York: Holt, 1937.

Chapter 6

1. Hall, E. T. *The silent language*. Greenwich, Conn.: Fawcett, 1959.

2. Fast, J. *Body language*. New York: M. Evans and Company, 1970.

3. Morris, D. *Bodywatching: a field guide to the human species*. London: Jonathon Cape, 1985.

4. Selye, H. *The stress of life*. New York: McGraw Hill, 1956.

5. Kobasa, S. C., Maddi, S. R., and Puccetti, M. C. Personality and exercise as buffers in the stress-illness relationship. *Journal of Behavioral Medicine*, 1982, 5 (4), 391–404; Levy, R. I., and Feinleib, M. Risk factors for coronary artery disease and their management. In E. Braunwald (Ed.), *Heart disease: a textbook of cardiovascular medicine (volume 2)*. Second Edition. Philadelphia: W. B. Saunders, 1984, 1205–1234; Rice, P. L. *Stress and health*. Monterey, Calif.: Brooks/Cole, 1987.

6. Siegel, B. S. *Love, medicine and miracles*. New York: Harper and Row, 1986.

7. Cassileth, B. R., et al. Psychosocial correlates of survival in advanced malignant disease? *New England Journal of Medicine*, 1985, 312, 1551–1555; Teshima, H., et al. Psychosomatic aspects of skin diseases from the standpoint of immunology. *Psychotherapy and Psychosomatics*, 1982, 37, 165–175; Gliner, J. A., Bedi, J. F., and Horvath, S. M. Somatic and non-somatic influences on the heart: hemodynamic changes. *Psychophysiology*, 1979, 16, 358–362.

8. Granville-Grossman, K. Mind and body. In Millon, T., et al. (Eds), *Handbook of clinical health psychology*. New York: Plenum Press, 1982, 5–13.

9. World Health Organization. *World Health Organization's Expert Committee on Mental Health*. (Report No. 13). New York: WHO, 1964.

10. Sheldon, W. H. *The varieties of human temperament*. New York: Harper and Row, 1942; Sheldon, W. H. *The varieties of human physique*. New York: Harper and Row, 1940.

11. Sheldon, *Varieties of temperament*; Sheldon, *Varieties of physique*.

12. Sheldon, *Varieties of temperament*; Sheldon, *Varieties of physique*; Smith, E. W. *The body in psychotherapy*. London: McFarland, 1985.

13. Reich, W. *Character analysis*. New York: Farrar, Strauss, and Giroux, 1949.
14. Lowen, A. *The language of the body*. New York: Collier Books, 1958.
15. Lowen, A. *The betrayal of the body*. New York: Collier Books, 1972.
16. Lowen, A. *Bioenergetics*. New York: Coward, McCann, and Geoghegan, 1975.
17. Lowen, *Body reveals*; Lowen, *Bioenergetics*; Lowen, A. The body in personality theory: Wilhelm Reich and Alexander Lowen. In A. Burton (Ed.), *Operational theories of personality*. New York: Brunner/Mazel, 1974.
18. Kurz, R., and Prestera, H. *The body reveals: An illustrated guide to the psychology of the body*. New York: Harper and Row, 1976.
19. Lowen, *Betrayal of body*.
20. Lowen, *Language of body*; Lowen, *Betrayal of body*; Lowen, *Bioenergetics*; Lowen, "Personality theory." Also see Smith, *Body in psychotherapy*.
21. Dychtwald, K. *Bodymind*. New York: Pantheon Books, 1977.
22. See Note 21.
23. See Note 21.
24. See Note 21.
25. Bertherat, T., and Bernstein, C. *The body has its reasons*. New York: Random House, 1977; Espenak, L. *Dance therapy: theory and application*. Springfield, Ill.: Charles C. Thomas, 1981; Fisher, S. *Body consciousness: You are what you feel*. Englewood Cliffs, N.J.: Prentice-Hall, 1973; Harrison, R. P. *Beyond words: An introduction to nonverbal communication*. Englewood Cliffs, N.J.: Prentice-Hall, 1974; Morris, D. *Bodywatching: a field guide to the human species*. London: Jonathon Cape, 1985; Prestera, H., and Kurz, R. *The body reveals*. New York: Harper and Row, 1976; Todd, M. E. *The thinking body*. New York: Dance Horizons, 1972; Vaughan, B. L. *Body talk*. Allen, Tex.: Argus Communications, 1982; Dychtwald, *Bodymind*; Smith, *Body in psychotherapy*; North, M. *Personality assessment through movement*. Boston: Plays, 1972; Lowen, *Bioenergetics*; Lowen, *Betrayal of body*.
26. Dychtwald, *Bodymind*.
27. Espenak, *Dance therapy*; Todd, *Thinking body*; Kurz and Prestera, *Body reveals*; Dychtwald, *Bodymind*; North, *Personality assessment*.
28. Dychtwald, *Bodymind*; Lowen, *Betrayal of body*; Lowen, *Bioenergetics*; Espenak, *Dance therapy*.
29. Dychtwald, *Bodymind*.
30. Espenak, *Dance therapy*; Dychtwald, *Bodymind*.
31. Dychtwald, *Bodymind*.
32. See Note 31.
33. Lowen, *Bioenergetics*.
34. Espenak, *Dance therapy*; Dychtwald, *Bodymind*.
35. Espenak, *Dance therapy*.
36. Dychtwald, *Bodymind*.
37. Lowen, *Betrayal of the body*; Lowen, *Bioenergetics*; Espenak, *Dance therapy*; Todd, *Thinking body*; Morris, *Bodywatching*; Dychtwald, *Bodymind*; Kurz and Prestera, *Body reveals*.
38. See Note 37.

Chapter 7

1. North, M. *Personality assessment through movement*. Boston: Plays, 1972.

2. Birdwhistle, R. *Introduction to kinesics*. Louisville, Ken.: University of Louisville Press, 1952; also, Birdwhistle, R. *Kinesics and context: essays on body motion communication*. Philadelphia: University of Pennsylvania Press, 1970.

3. Goffman, E. *Interaction ritual*. New York: Anchor, 1967.

4. Goffman, E. *Behavior in public places*. New York: Free Press, 1963.

5. Morris, D. *The naked ape*. London: Jonathon Cape, 1967.

6. Morris, D. *Manwatching: a field guide to human behavior*. New York: Harry N. Abrams, 1977.

7. Morris, D. *Bodywatching: a field guide to the human species*. London: Jonathon Cape, 1985.

8. Fast, J. *Body language*. New York: M. Evans and Company, 1970.

9. Vaughan, B. L. *Body talk*. Allen, Tex.: Argus Communications, 1982.

10. Laban, R., and Lawrence, F. C. *Effort*. London: MacDonald and Evans, 1947; Laban, R. *The mastery of movement*. Boston: Plays, 1971; Laban, R. *The language of movement*. Boston: Plays, 1974; Laban, R. *Modern educational dance*. Boston: Plays, 1975.

11. Bartenieff, I., Davis, M., and Paulay, F. *Four adaptations of effort theory in research and teaching*. New York: Dance Notation Bureau, 1970; Bartenieff, I. *Body movement: coping with the environment*. New York: Gordon and Breach, 1980; Bertherat, T., and Bernstein, C. *The body has its reasons*. New York: Random House, 1977; Bruya, L. D. Effect of selected movement skills on positive self-concept. *Perceptual and Motor Skills*, 1977, *45*, 252–254; Christiansen, B. *Thus speaks the body: attempts toward a personology from the point of view of respiration and posture*. Oslo, Norway: Institute for Social Research, 1963; Condon, W. S., and Ogston, W. D. Sound-film analysis of normal and pathological behavior patterns. *Journal of Nervous and Mental Disease*, 1966, *143*, 338–347; Dosamantes-Alperson, E., and Merrill, N. Growth effects of experiential movement psychotherapy. *Psychotherapy: Theory, Research and Practice*, 1980, 17 (1), 63–68; Espenak, L. *Dance therapy: theory and application*. Springfield, Ill.: Charles C. Thomas, 1981; Preston, V. *A handbook for modern educational dance*. London: MacDonald and Evans, 1963; Pritchard, O. H. Movement and personality: a component analysis and descriptive model. *Momentum*, 1980, *5* (3), 23–32; Puretz, S. L. Modern dance's effect on the body image. *International Journal of Sport Psychology*, 1982, *13* (3), 176–186; Redfern, H. B. *Concepts in modern educational dance*. London: Henry Kimpton, 1973; Rosenthal, M. M., and Beutell, N. J. Movement and body image: a preliminary study. *Perceptual and Motor Skills*, 1981, *53* (3), 758; Sweigard, L. E. *Human movement potential*. New York: Harper and Row, 1974; Todd, M. E. *The thinking body*. New York: Dance Horizons, 1972.

12. North, *Personality assessment*; Dell, C. *A primer for movement description using effort-shape and supplementary concepts*. New York: Dance Notation Bureau, 1970; Lamb, W. *Body code*. London: Routledge and Kegan Paul, 1979. Also see Note 11.

13. North, *Personality assessment*.

Chapter 8

1. Flippin, R. Are runners better lovers? *The Runner,* 1987, 9 (6), 32–35; Hughes, J. R. Psychological effects of habitual aerobic exercise: A critical review. *Preventive Medicine,* 1984, 13 (1), 66–78; Monahan, T. Exercise and depression: Swapping sweat for serenity. *The Physician and Sports Medicine,* 1986, 14 (9), 192–197; Sachs, M. L., and Buffone, G. W. (Eds.), *Running as therapy.* Lincoln, Neb.: University of Nebraska Press, 1984; Sacks, M. H., and Sachs, M. L. *The psychology of running.* Champaign, Ill.: Human Kinetics, 1981; Zarski, J. J., West, J. D., and Bubenzer, D. L. Social interest, running and life adjustment. *Personnel and Guidance Journal,* 1982, 61 (3), 146–149.

2. *USA Today,* Walkers outpacing joggers. May 28, 1987.

3. Harlow, R. G. Masculine inadequacy and compensatory development on physique. In W. P. Morgan (Ed.), *Contemporary readings in sport psychology.* Springfield, Ill.: Thomas, 1970, 271–283; Thune, J. B. Personality of weightlifters. *Research Quarterly,* 1949, 20, 296–306; Tucker, L. A. Weight training experience and psychological well-being. *Perceptual and Motor Skills,* 1982, 55 (2), 553–554; Tucker, L. A. Muscular strength and mental health. *Journal of Personality and Social Psychology,* 1983, 45 (6), 1355–1360; Darden, E. A comparison of body image and self-concept variables among various sport groups. *Research Quarterly,* 1972, 43 (1), 7–15.

4. Konzak, B., and Boudreau, F. Martial arts training and mental health: an exercise in self-help. *Canada's Mental Health,* 1984, 32 (4), 2–8; Pyecha, J. Comparative effects of judo and selected physical education activities on male university freshman personality traits. *Research Quarterly,* 1970, 41 (3), 425–431; Rothpearl, A. Personality traits in martial artists: a descriptive approach. *Perceptual and Motor Skills,* 1980, 50 (2), 395–401.

5. See Note 4.

Chapter 10

1. Altshul, V. A. Should we advise our depressed patients to run? In M. H. Sacks and M. L. Sachs (Eds.), *Psychology of running.* Champaign, Ill.: Human Kinetics, 1981, 50–56.

2. Miller, P. Forward thinking. *Runner's World,* 1986, 21 (7), 74–75.

3. Gambaccini, P. Get in gear. *Runner's World,* 1987, 22 (5), 85–94.

4. Paffenbarger, R. A. Physical activity, coronary heart disease and longevity. *Proceedings of the American College of Sports Medicine,* Las Vegas: May 1987.

Bibliography

Aamodt, M. G., Alexander, C. J., and Kimbrough, W. W. Personality characteristics of college non-athletes and baseball, football, and track team members. *Perceptual and Motor Skills*, 1983, 57 (1), 143–146.

Allport, G. W. *Personality: a psychological interpretation*. New York: Holt, 1937.

Alter, J. B. Creativity profile of university and conservatory dance students. *Journal of Personality Assessment*, 1984, 48 (2), 153–158.

Altshul, V. A. Should we advise our depressed patients to run? In M. H. Sacks and M. L. Sachs (Eds.), *Psychology of running*. Champaign, Ill.: Human Kinetics, 1981. Pp. 50–56.

American College of Sports Medicine. *Guidelines for exercise testing and prescription*. Philadelphia: Lea and Febiger, 1986.

American College of Sports Medicine. *Position stands and opinion statements*. Sixth Edition. Indianapolis, Ind.: ACSM, April 1987.

American Heart Association Subcommittee on Exercise/Cardiac Rehabilitation. Statement on exercise. *Circulation*, 1981, 64, 1302–1304.

American Psychiatric Association. *A psychiatric glossary* (Fourth Edition). New York: Basic Books, 1975.

Armstrong, H. E. Jr., and Armstrong, D. C. Relation of physical fitness to a dimension of body image. *Perceptual and Motor Skills*, 1968, 26, 1173–1174.

Arnot, R. B., and Gaines, C. L. *Sportselection*. New York: Viking Press, 1984.

299

Ateyo, O. *Blood and guts: violence in sports.* New York: Paddington Press, 1979.

Bahrke, M. S., and Morgan, W. P. Anxiety reduction following exercise and meditation. In M. H. Sacks and M. L. Sachs (Eds.), *Psychology of running.* Champaign, Ill.: Human Kinetics, 1981. Pp. 57–66.

Bartenieff, I., Davis, M., and Paulay, F. *Four adaptations of effort theory in research and teaching.* New York: Dance Notation Bureau, 1970.

Bartenieff, I. *Body movement: coping with the environment.* New York: Gordon and Breach, 1980.

Berger, B. B. Effect of uncertainty, physical harm, and competition upon selected characteristics of athletes. *International Journal of Sports Psychology,* 1977, *8* (3), 198–209.

Bertherat, T., and Bernstein, C. *The body has its reasons.* New York: Random House, 1977.

Bird, A. M., and Cripe, B. K. *Psychology and sport behavior.* Toronto: Times Mirror/Mosby, 1986.

Birdwhistle, R. *Introduction to kinesics.* Louisville, Ken.: University of Louisville Press, 1952.

Birdwhistle, R. *Kinesics and context: essays on body motion communication.* Philadelphia: University of Pennsylvania Press, 1970.

Blair, S. N. How to assess exercise habits and physical fitness. In J. D. Matarazzo, S. M. Weiss, N. E. Miller, and S. M. Weiss (Eds.), *Behavioral health: a handbook of health enhancement and disease prevention.* New York: Wiley, 1984. Pp. 424–447.

Blue, F. R. Aerobic running as a treatment for moderate depression. *Perceptual and Motor Skills,* 1979, *48,* 228.

Blumenthal, J. A., Williams, R. S., Williams, R. B. Jr., and Wallace, A. G. Effects of exercise on the Type A (coronary prone) behavior pattern. *Psychosomatic Medicine,* 1980, *42* (2), 289–296.

Brant, J. And the word was aerobics. *Runner's World,* 1987, *22* (5), 68–76.

Bredemeier, B. J., and Shields, D. L. Values and violence in sports today. *Psychology Today,* 1985, *19* (10), 22–25; 28–32.

Brooks, C. M. Adult participation in physical activities requiring moderate to high levels of energy expenditure. *The Physician and Sportsmedicine.* 1987, *15* (4), 119–121; 124–132.

Bruya, L. D. Effect of selected movement skills on positive self-concept. *Perceptual and Motor Skills,* 1977, *45,* 252–254.

Buffone, G. W. Running and depression. In M. L. Sachs and G. W. Buffone (Eds.), *Running as therapy.* Lincoln, Neb.: University of Nebraska Press, 1984. Pp. 6–22.

Buffone, G. W. Future directions: the potential for exercise as therapy. In M. L. Sachs and G. W. Buffone (Eds.), *Running as therapy.* Lincoln, Neb.: University of Nebraska Press, 1984. Pp. 215–226.

Bulbulian, R., and Darabos, B. L. Motor neuron excitability: the Hoffman reflex following exercise of low and high intensity. *Medicine and Science in Sports and Exercise,* 1986, *18* (6), 697–702.

Canada Fitness Survey. *Fitness and lifestyle in Canada.* Ottawa: Government of Canada, 1983.

Canadian standardized test of fitness (CSTF): Operations manual (Third Edition). Ottawa: Fitness and Amateur Sport Canada, 1986.

Cassileth, B. R., et al. Psychosocial correlates of survival in advanced malignant disease? *New England Journal of Medicine,* 1985, *312,* 1551–1555.

Cattell, R., Eber, H., and Tatzucka, M. *Handbook of the sixteen Personality Factor Questionnaire.* Champaign, Ill.: Institute for Personality and Ability Testing, 1970.

Chelladurai, P. and Saleh, S. D. Person-task congruence in sports. *Canadian Journal of Applied Sports Sciences,* 1979, *4* (2), 172–177.

Christiansen, B. *Thus speaks the body: attempts toward a personology from the point of view of respiration and posture.* Oslo, Norway: Institute for Social Research, 1963.

Cohen, M. *The Marine Corps 3X fitness program.* New York: Little, Brown and Co., 1986.

Colt, E. W., Dunner, D. L., Hall, K., and Fieve, R. R. A high prevalence of affective disorders in runners. In M. H. Sacks and M. L. Sachs (Eds.), *Psychology of running.* Champaign, Ill.: Human Kinetics, 1981. Pp. 234–248.

Condon, W. S., and Ogston, W. D. Sound-film analysis of normal and pathological behavior patterns. *Journal of Nervous and Mental Disease,* 1966, *143,* 338–347.

Conforto, C. and Marcenaro, M. Psychometric and psychodynamic investigation of the personality of tennis players. *International Journal of Sport Psychology,* 1979, *10* (4), 217–230.

Cooper, A. M. Masochism and long-distance running. In M. H. Sacks and M. L. Sachs (Eds.), *Psychology of running.* Champaign, Ill.: Human Kinetics, 1981. Pp. 267–273.

Cooper, K. H. *The aerobics way.* New York: Bantam, 1977.

Cooper, K. H., Gallman, J. S., and McDonald, J. L. Jr. Role of aerobic exercise in reduction of stress. *Dental Clinics of North America,* 1986, *30* (4), S133–142.

Cooper, L. Athletics, activity and personality: a review of the literature. *Research Quarterly,* 1969, *40* (1), 17–22.

Darden, E. A comparison of body image and self-concept variables among various sport groups. *Research Quarterly,* 1972, *43* (1), 7–15.

Darden, E. Sixteen personality factor profiles of competitive body builders and weightlifters. *Research Quarterly,* 1972, *43* (2), 142–147.

Delk, J. L. Some personality characteristics of skydivers. *Life-Threatening Behavior,* 1973, *3* (1), 51–57.

Dell, C. *A primer for movement description using effort-shape and supplementary concepts.* New York: Dance Notation Bureau, 1970.

DeMan, A. F., and Blais, G. Relationship between preference for a type of sport and two aspects of personality: social alienation and self-esteem. *Perceptual and Motor Skills,* 1982, *54* (1), 11–14.

DeMan, A. F., and Blais, G. Relationship between preference for a type of sport and two aspects of personality: revised data. *Perceptual and Motor Skills,* 1982, *55* (3), 982.

Dickhoff, G. M. Running amok: Injuries in compulsive runners. *Journal of Sport Behavior*, 1984, 7 (3), 120–129.

Dielens, S. Narcissism and fashionable physical activities: psychological profiles of aerobic dancers, joggers and bodybuilders. *Revue de l'Education Physique*, 1984, 24 (1), 21–25.

Diener, E. Subjective well-being. *Psychological Bulletin*, 1984, 95 (3), 542–575.

Diensbier, R. A., et al. Exercise and stress tolerance. In M. H. Sacks and M. L. Sachs (Eds.), *Psychology of running*. Champaign, Ill.: Human Kinetics, 1981. Pp. 192–210.

Dishman, R. K. Contemporary sport psychology. *Exercise and Sport Sciences Reviews*, 1982, 10, 120–159.

Dishman, R. K. Medical psychology in exercise and sport. *Medical Clinics of North America*, 1985, 69 (1), 123–143.

Dishman, R. K. Exercise compliance: A new view for public health. *The Physician and Sportsmedicine*, 1986, 14 (5), 127–145.

Dishman, R. K. *Exercise adherence: Its impact on public health*. Champaign, Ill.: Human Kinetics, 1987.

Dishman, R. K., Sallis, J. F., and Orenstein, D. R. The determinants of physical activity and exercise. *Public Health Reports*, 1985, 100 (2), 158–171.

Dolphin, C., O'Brien, M., Cahill, N., and Cullen, J. Personality factors and some physiological correlates in athletes. *Journal of Psychosomatic Research*, 1980, 24 (5), 281–285.

Dosamantes-Alperson, E., and Merrill, N. Growth effects of experiential movement psychotherapy. *Psychotherapy: Theory, Research and Practice*, 1980, 17 (1), 63–68.

Dowd, R., and Innes, J. M. Sport and personality: effects of type of sport and level of competition. *Perceptual and Motor Skills*, 1981, 53 (1), 79–89.

Driscoll, R. Anxiety reduction using physical exertion and positive images. *Psychological Records*, 1979, 26, 87–94.

Dychtwald, K. *Bodymind*. New York: Pantheon Books, 1977.

Eischens, R. R., and Griest, J. H. Beginning and continuing running: steps to psychological well-being. In M. L. Sachs and G. W. Buffone (Eds.), *Running as therapy*. Lincoln, Neb.: University of Nebraska Press, 1984. Pp. 63–82.

Elliot, D. L., and Goldberg, L. Nutrition and exercise. *Medical Clinics of North America*, 1985, 69 (1), 71–82.

Engleman, S. R., Clance, P. R., and Imes, S. Self and body-cathexis change in therapy and yoga groups. *Journal of the American Society of Psychosomatic Dentistry and Medicine*, 1982, 29 (3), 77–88.

Espenak, L. *Dance therapy: theory and application*. Springfield, Ill.: Charles C. Thomas, 1981.

Eysenck, H. J. Sport and personality. *Advances in Behavior Research and Therapy*, 1982, 4 (1), 1–56.

Fast, J. *Body language*. New York: M. Evans and Company, 1970.

Fisher, S. *Body consciousness: You are what you feel*. Englewood Cliffs, N.J.: Prentice-Hall, 1973.

Fixx, J. G. *The complete book of running*. New York: Random House, 1977.

Flippin, R. Are runners better lovers? *The Runner*, 1987, 9 (6), 32–35.

Folkins, C. H. Effects of physical training on mood. *Journal of Clinical Psychology*, 1976, 32 (2), 385–388.

Folkins, C. H., and Sime, W. E. Physical fitness training and mental health. *American Psychologist*, 1981, 36 (4), 373–389.

Friedman, M., and Rosenman, R. H. *Type A behavior and your heart*. New York: Alfred A. Knopf, 1974.

Gabler, H. *Leistungsmotivation im hockleistungs sport*. Hofmann, Schorndorf, 1972.

Gal, R., and Lazarus, R. S. The role of activity in anticipating and confronting stressful situations. *Journal of Human Stress*, 1975, 7, 4–20.

Gambaccini, P. Get in gear. *Runner's World*, 1987, 22 (5), 85–94.

Gavin, J. *Psychosocial activity dimensions: Toward the development of an instrument for the measurement of sports/fitness activities and their participants*. Technical manuscript. Montreal: Concordia University, 1986.

Gavin, J. Psychotherapeutic dimensions of exercise. *Proceedings: Canadian Association of Sports Sciences*. Ottawa, 1986.

Glasser, W. *Positive addiction*. New York: Harper and Row, 1976.

Gliner, J. A., Bedi, J. F., and Horvath, S. M. Somatic and non-somatic influences on the heart: hemodynamic changes. *Psychophysiology*, 1979, 16, 358–362.

Goffman, E. *Behavior in public places*. New York: Free Press, 1963.

Goffman, E. *Interaction ritual*. New York: Anchor, 1967.

Goldberg, L., and Elliot, D. L. The effect of physical activity on lipid and lipoprotein levels. *Medical Clinics of North America*, 1985, 69 (1), 41–55.

Goldfarb, L. A., and Plante, T. G. Fear of fat in runners: an examination of the connection between anorexia nervosa and distance running. *Psychological Reports*, 1984, 55 (1), 296.

Golding, L. A., Myers, C. R., and Sinning, W. E. *The Y's way to physical fitness*. Champaign, Ill.: Human Kinetics, 1982.

Granville-Grossman, K. Mind and body. In Millon, T., et al. (Eds), *Handbook of clinical health psychology*. New York: Plenum Press, 1982. Pp. 5–13.

Grossman, A. Endorphins: "opiates for the masses." *Medicine and Science in Sports and Exercise*, 1985, 17 (1), 101–105.

Griest, J. H., et al. Running through your mind. *Journal of Psychosomatic Research*, 1978, 22, 259–294.

Griest, J. H., et al. Running as a treatment for depression. *Comprehensive Psychiatry*, 1979, 20, 41–54.

Grossman, A., and Sutton, J. R. Endorphins: What are they? How are they measured? What is their role in exercise? *Medicine and Science in Sports and Exercise*, 1985, 17 (1), 74–81.

Hall, C. S., and Lindzey, G. *Theories of personality* (Second Edition). New York: John Wiley, 1970.

Hall, E. T. *The silent language*. Greenwich, Conn.: Fawcett, 1959.

Hammond, H. K., and Froelicher, V. F. The physiologic sequelae of chronic dynamic exercise. *Medical Clinics of North America*, 1985, 69 (1), 21–39.

Harlow, R. G. Masculine inadequacy and compensatory development on physique. In W. P. Morgan (Ed.), *Contemporary readings in sport psychology.* Springfield, Ill.: Thomas, 1970. Pp. 271–283.

Harris, D. V. *Involvement in sport: a somatopsychic rationale for physical activity.* Philadelphia: Lea and Febiger, 1973.

Harrison, R. P. *Beyond words: An introduction to nonverbal communication.* Englewood Cliffs, N.J.: Prentice-Hall, 1974.

Haskell, W. L., Overview: Health benefits of exercise. In J. D. Matarazzo, S. M. Weiss, N. E. Miller, and S. M. Weiss (Eds.), *Behavioral health: a handbook of health enhancement and disease prevention.* New York: Wiley, 1984. Pp. 409–423.

Heller, G. V., et al. Plasma beta-endorphin levels in silent myocardial ishemia induced by exercise. *American Journal of Cardiology,* 1987, *59* (8), 735–739.

Hendry, L. Assessment in personality traits in the coach-swimmer relationship. *Research Quarterly,* 1968, *39,* 543–551.

Henry, F. M. Personality differences in athletes, physical education and aviation students. *Psychological Bulletin,* 1941, *38,* 745.

Highlen, P. S., and Bennett, B. B. Elite divers and wrestlers: a comparison between open- and closed-skill athletes. *Journal of Sport Psychology,* 1983, *5* (4), 390–409.

Hughes, J. R. Psychological effects of habitual aerobic exercise: A critical review. *Preventive Medicine,* 1984, *13* (1), 66–78.

Janssen, B., and Whiting, H. T. Sheldon's physical-psychical typology revisited. *Journal of Research in Personality,* 1984, *18* (4), 432–441.

Jasnoski, M. L., and Holmes, D. S. Influence of initial aerobic fitness, aerobic training and changes in aerobic fitness on personality functioning. *Journal of Psychosomatic Research,* 1981, *25* (6), 553–556.

Jerome, W. C., and Valliant, P. M. Comparison of personalities between marathon runners and cross-country skiers. *Perceptual and Motor Skills,* 1983, *56* (1), 35–38.

Joesting, J. Comparison of students who exercise with those who do not. *Perceptual and Motor Skills,* 1981, *53* (2), 426.

Johnson, P. A. A comparison of personality traits of superior skilled women athletes in basketball, bowling, field hockey, and golf. *Research Quarterly,* 1972, *43* (4), 409–415.

Johnson, W. O. Marching to euphoria. *Sports Illustrated,* 1980, *53* (3), 72–76, 78–79, 81–82.

Kelly, B. R. Aggression, performance variables, and anger self-report in ice hockey players. *Journal of Psychology,* 1978, *99* (1), 97–101.

King, J. P., and Chi, P. S. Personality and the athletic social structure: A case study. *Human Relations,* 1974, *27* (2), 179–193.

Kirkcaldy, B. D. Personality profiles at various levels of athletic participation. *Personality and Individual Differences,* 1982, *3* (3), 321–326.

Kline, G. M., et al. Estimation of VO_2 max from a one-mile track walk, gender, age, and body weight. *Medicine and Science in Sports and Exercise,* 1987, *19* (3), 253–259.

Kobasa, S. C., Maddi, S. R., and Puccetti, M. C. Personality and exercise as buffers in the stress-illness relationship. *Journal of Behavioral Medicine,* 1982, 5 (4), 391–404.

Konzak, B., and Boudreau, F. Martial arts training and mental health: an exercise in self-help. *Canada's Mental Health,* 1984, 32 (4), 2–8.

Kostrubala, T. *The joy of running.* New York: Lippincott, 1976.

Kostrubala, T. Running and therapy. In M. L. Sachs and G. W. Buffone (Eds.), *Running as therapy.* Lincoln, Neb.: University of Nebraska Press, 1984. Pp. 112–124.

Kraiuhin, C., et al. The Type A behaviour pattern and physique. *Journal of Psychosomatic Research,* 1983, 27 (6), 479–483.

Kretschmer, E. *Physique and character.* (Second Edition, revised). London: Routledge and Kegan Paul, 1945.

Kurz, R., and Prestera, H. *The body reveals: An illustrated guide to the psychology of the body.* New York: Harper and Row, 1976.

Laban, R., and Lawrence, F. C. *Effort.* London: MacDonald and Evans, 1947.

Laban, R. *The mastery of movement.* Boston: Plays, 1971.

Laban, R. *The language of movement.* Boston: Plays, 1974.

Laban, R. *Modern educational dance.* Boston: Plays, 1975.

Lake, B. M., et al. The Type A behavior pattern, physical fitness, and psychophysical reactivity. *Health Psychology,* 1985, 4 (2), 169–187.

Lamb, W. *Body code.* London: Routledge and Kegan Paul, 1979.

LaPorte, R. The relationship of physical activity and physical fitness to cardiovascular disease and health. *Proceedings of the American College of Sports Medicine,* Las Vegas: May 1987.

Leon, A. S. Physical activity levels and coronary heart disease: analysis of epidemiologic and supporting studies. *Medical Clinics of North America,* 1985, 69 (1), 3–20.

Leonard, G. *The ultimate athlete.* New York: Viking Press, 1975.

Leonard, G. (Ed.), Mastery: the secret of ultimate fitness. *Esquire,* 1987, 107 (5), 113–154.

Leunes, A., and Nation, J. R. Saturday's heroes: A psychological portrait of college football players. *Journal of Sport Behavior,* 1982, 5 (3), 139–149.

Levy, R. I., and Feinleib, M. Risk factors for coronary artery disease and their management. In E. Braunwald (Ed.), *Heart disease: a textbook of cardiovascular medicine (volume 2).* Second Edition. Philadelphia: W. B. Saunders, 1984. Pp. 1205–1234.

Lion, L. S. Psychological effects of jogging: a preliminary study. *Perceptual and Motor Skills,* 1978, 47 (3, Pt. 2), 1215–1218.

Lilliefors, J. *The running mind.* Mountain View, Calif.: World Publications, 1978.

Little, J. C. Neurotic illness in fitness fanatics. *Psychiatric Annals,* 1979, 9 (3), 49–56.

Lowen, A. *The language of the body.* New York: Collier Books, 1958.

Lowen, A. *The betrayal of the body.* New York: Collier Books, 1972.

Lowen, A. The body in personality theory: Wilhelm Reich and Alexander

Lowen. In A. Burton (Ed.), *Operational theories of personality.* New York: Brunner/Mazel, 1974.

Lowen, A. *Bioenergetics.* New York: Coward, McCann, and Geoghegan, 1975.

Lucas, J. A., and Smith, R. *The saga of American sports.* Philadelphia: Lea and Febiger, 1978.

Marcenaro, M. Psychometric and psychodynamic investigation of the personality of tennis players. *International Journal of Sport Psychology,* 1979, *10* (4), 217–230.

Markoff, R. A., Ryan, P., and Young, T. Endorphins and mood changes in long distance running. *Medicine and Science in Sports and Exercise,* 1982, *14,* 11–15.

Martens, R. The paradigmatic crisis in American sport personology. *Sportwissenschaft,* 1975, *5,* 9–24.

Martin, J. E., and Dubbert, P. M. Adherence to exercise. In R. L. Terjung (Ed.), *Exercise and sport sciences reviews.* New York: Macmillan, 1985. Pp. 137–167.

Martin, J. E., and Dubbert, P. M. Exercise in hypertension. *Annals of Behavioral Medicine,* 1985, *7,* 13–18.

McCain, G. A. Role of physical fitness training in the fibrositis/fibromyalgia syndrome. *American Journal of Medicine,* 1986, *81* (Supplement 3A), 73–77.

McCarthy, J. F., and Kelly, B. R. Aggression, performance variables, and anger self-report in ice hockey players. *Journal of Psychology,* 1978, *99* (1), 97–101.

McCunny, R. J. Fitness, heart disease, and high-density lipoproteins: a look at the relationships. *The Physician and Sportsmedicine,* 1987, *15* (2), 67–79.

McCutcheon, L. E. Does running make people more creative? *Journal of Sport Behavior,* 1982, *5* (4), 202–206.

McCutcheon, L. E., and Yoakum, M. E. Personality attributes of ultramarathoners. *Journal of Personality Assessment,* 1983, *47* (2), 178–180.

McLeod, B. Field dependence as a factor in sports with a preponderance of open or closed skills. *Perceptual and Motor Skills,* 1985, *60* (2), 369–370.

McMahon, M., and Palmer, R. M. Exercise and hypertension. *Medical Clinics of North America,* 1985, *69* (1), 57–70.

McPhedran, K. Giving yourself a sporting chance. *Verve,* 1986 (October), 22–40.

Mikel, K. V. Extroversion in adult runners. *Perceptual and Motor Skills,* 1983, *57* (1), 143–146.

Miller, P. Forward thinking. *Runner's World,* 1986, *21* (7), 74–75.

Mishra, R. S. *Fundamentals of yoga.* New York: Julian Press, 1959.

Monahan, T. Exercise and depression: Swapping sweat for serenity. *The Physician and Sports Medicine,* 1986, *14* (9), 192–197.

Moore, C. L. *Executives in action.* London: MacDonald and Evans, 1982.

Morgan, W. P. Negative addiction in runners. *The Physician and Sports Medicine,* 1979, *7,* 57–70.

Morgan, W. P. Anxiety reduction following acute physical activity. *Psychiatric Annals,* 1979, *9,* 141–147.

Morgan, W. P. The trait psychology controversy. *Research Quarterly,* 1980, *51* (1), 50–76.

Morgan, W. P., and Roberts, J. Psychological effects of chronic physical activity. *Medicine and Science in Sports and Exercise,* 1970, 2, 213–218.

Morris, D. *The naked ape.* London: Jonathon Cape, 1967.

Morris, D. *Manwatching: a field guide to human behavior.* New York: Harry N. Abrams, 1977.

Morris, D. *Bodywatching: a field guide to the human species.* London: Jonathon Cape, 1985.

Murphy, M., and White, R. *The psychic side of sport.* New York: Addison-Wesley, 1978.

Nideffer, R. M. *The inner athlete.* New York: Thomas Crowell, 1976.

Nideffer, R. M. Concentration and attention control training. In J. M. Williams (Ed.), *Applied sport psychology: Personal growth to peak performance.* Palo Alto, Calif.: Mayfield, 1986.

Nieman, D. C. *The sports medicine fitness course.* Palo Alto, Calif.: Bull Publishing, 1986.

North, M. *Personality assessment through movement.* Boston: Plays, 1972.

Nosanchuk, T. A. The way of the warrior: The effects of traditional martial arts training on aggressiveness. *Human Relations,* 1981, 34 (6), 435–444.

Ogilvie, B. Psychological consistencies within the personalities of high level competitors. *Journal of the American Medical Association,* 1968, 205, 156–202.

Oldridge, N. B. Adherence to adult exercise fitness programs. In J. D. Matarazzo, S. M. Weiss, N. E. Miller, and S. M. Weiss (Eds.). *Behavioral health: a handbook of health enhancement and disease prevention.* New York: Wiley, 1984. Pp. 467–487.

Orwin, A. Treatment of a situational phobia—A case for running. *British Journal of Psychiatry,* 1974, 125, 95–98.

Orwin, A. "The running treatment": a preliminary communication on a new use for an old therapy (physical activity) in the agoraphobia syndrome. In M. H. Sacks and M. L. Sachs (Eds.), *Psychology of running.* Champaign, Ill.: Human Kinetics, 1981. Pp. 32–39.

Paffenbarger, R. A., and Hyde, R. T. Exercise in the prevention of coronary heart disease. *Preventive Medicine,* 1984, 13, 3–22.

Paffenbarger, R. A., et al. A natural history of athleticism and cardiovascular disease. *Journal of the American Medical Association,* 1984, 252, 491–495.

Paffenbarger, R. A. Physical activity, coronary heart disease and longevity. *Proceedings of the American College of Sports Medicine,* Las Vegas: May 1987.

Paffenbarger, R. A. Physical activity and cancer in college alumni. *Proceedings of the American College of Sports Medicine,* Las Vegas: May 1987.

Perkins, K. A., Dubbert, P. M., Martin, J. E., Faulstich, M. E., and Harris, J. K. Cardiovascular reactivity to psychological stress in aerobically trained versus untrained mild hypertensives and normotensives. *Health Psychology,* 1986, 5, 407–421.

Perri, T., and Templer, D. I. The effects of an aerobic exercise program on psychological variables in older adults. *International Journal of Aging and Human Development,* 1985, 20, 167–172.

Perry, S. W., and Sacks, M. H. Psychodynamics of running. In M. H. Sacks and M. L. Sachs (Eds.), *Psychology of running*. Champaign, Ill.: Human Kinetics, 1981. Pp. 69–79.

Pesman, C. Five athletic body types. *Esquire*, 1986, *105* (5), 109–118.

Powell, R. R. Psychological effects of exercise therapy upon institutionalized geriatric mental patients. *Journal of Gerontology*, 1974, *29*, 157–161.

Powell, R. R., and Pohndorf, R. H. Comparison of adult exercisers and nonexercisers on fluid intelligence and selected physiological variables. *Research Quarterly*, 1971, *42* (1), 70–77.

Prestera, H., and Kurz, R. *The body reveals*. New York: Harper and Row, 1976.

Preston, V. *A handbook for modern educational dance*. London: MacDonald and Evans, 1963.

Price, W. A., Dimarzio, and Gardner, P. R. Biopsychosocial approach to premenstrual syndrome. *American Family Physician*, 1986, *33* (6), 117–122.

Pritchard, O. H. Movement and personality: a component analysis and descriptive model. *Momentum*, 1980, *5* (3), 23–32.

Puretz, S. L. Modern dance's effect on the body image. *International Journal of Sport Psychology*, 1982, *13* (3), 176–186.

Pyecha, J. Comparative effects of judo and selected physical education activities on male university freshman personality traits. *Research Quarterly*, 1970, *41* (3), 425–431.

Redfern, H. B. *Concepts in modern educational dance*. London: Henry Kimpton, 1973.

Reich, W. *Character analysis*. New York: Farrar, Strauss, and Giroux, 1949.

Reid, J. G., and Thomson, J. M. *Exercise prescription for fitness*. Englewood Cliffs, N.J.: Prentice-Hall, 1985.

Ribisl, P. M. Developing an exercise prescription for health. In J. D. Matarazzo, S. M. Weiss, N. E. Miller, and S. M. Weiss (Eds.), *Behavioral health: a handbook of health enhancement and disease prevention*. New York: Wiley, 1984. Pp. 448–465.

Rice, P. L. *Stress and health*. Monterey, Calif.: Brooks/Cole, 1987.

Rosenberg, M. *Conceiving the self*. New York: Basic Books, 1979.

Rosenthal, M. M., and Beutell, N. J. Movement and body image: a preliminary study. *Perceptual and Motor Skills*, 1981, *53* (3), 758.

Roth, D. L., and Holmes, D. S. Influence of physical fitness in determining the impact of stressful life events on physical and psychologic health. *Psychosomatic Medicine*, 1985, *47* (2), 164–173.

Rothpearl, A. Personality traits in martial artists: a descriptive approach. *Perceptual and Motor Skills*, 1980, *50* (2), 395–401.

Rummele, E. Sexuality in marathon runners. *Leitungssport*, 1985, *15* (5), 23–26.

Rushall, B. S. Personality profiles and a theory of behavior modification for swimmers. *Swimming Techniques*, 1967, *4*, 66–71.

Sachs, M. L. Running addiction. In M. H. Sacks and M. L. Sachs (Eds.), *Psychology of running*. Champaign, Ill.: Human Kinetics, 1981. Pp. 116–126.

Sachs, M. L. The runner's high. In M. L. Sachs and G. W. Buffone (Eds.),

Running as therapy. Lincoln, Neb.: University of Nebraska Press, 1984. Pp. 273–287.

Sachs, M. L., and Buffone, G. W. (Eds.), *Running as therapy.* Lincoln, Neb.: University of Nebraska Press, 1984.

Sachs, M. L., and Pargman, D. Running addiction. In M. L. Sachs and G. W. Buffone (Eds.), *Running as therapy.* Lincoln, Neb.: University of Nebraska Press, 1984. Pp. 231–252.

Sacks, M. H. Running addiction: a clinical report. In M. H. Sacks and M. L. Sachs (Eds.), *Psychology of running.* Champaign, Ill.: Human Kinetics, 1981. Pp. 127–130.

Sacks, M. H., and Sachs, M. L. *The psychology of running.* Champaign, Ill.: Human Kinetics, 1981.

Schurr, K. T., Ashley, M. A., and Joy, K. L. A multivariate analysis of male athlete personality characteristics: Sport type and success. *Multivariate Experimental Clinical Research,* 1977, *3* (2), 53–58.

Schwartz, G. E., Davidson, R. J., and Goleman, D. J. Patterning of cognitive and somatic processes in the self-regulation of anxiety: effects of medication versus exercise. *Psychosomatic Medicine,* 1978, *40,* 321–328.

Selye, H. *The stress of life.* New York: McGraw Hill, 1956.

Sharkey, B. J. *Physiology of fitness* (second edition). Champaign, Ill.: Human Kinetics, 1984.

Sharp, M. W., and Reilley, R. R. The relationship of aerobic physical fitness to selected personality traits. *Journal of Clinical Psychology,* 1975, *31* (3), 428–430.

Sheehan, G. Body and soul. In M. H. Sacks and M. L. Sachs (Eds.), *Psychology of running.* Champaign, Ill.: Human Kinetics, 1981. Pp. 189–190.

Sheldon, W. H. *The varieties of human temperament.* New York: Harper and Row, 1942.

Sheldon, W. H. *The varieties of human physique.* New York: Harper and Row, 1940.

Shephard, R. J. *Economic benefits of enhanced fitness.* Champaign, Ill.: Human Kinetics, 1986.

Siegel, B. S. *Love, medicine and miracles.* New York: Harper and Row, 1986.

Sime, W. E. Psychological benefits of exercise training in the healthy individual. In J. D. Matarazzo, S. M. Weiss, N. E. Miller, and S. M. Weiss (Eds.), *Behavioral health: a handbook of health enhancement and disease prevention.* New York: Wiley, 1984. Pp. 488–507.

Simons, A. D., Epstein, L. H., McGowan, C. R., and Kupfer, D. J. Exercise as a treatment for depression: an update. *Clinical Psychology Review,* 1985, *5,* 553–568.

Sleet, D. Typecasting: does your body type affect your personality? *Shape,* 1982, *2* (1), 40–42; 90–91.

Slusher, H. Personality and intelligence characteristics of selected high school athletes and non-athletes. *Research Quarterly,* 1964, *35,* 539–543.

Smith, E. W. *The body in psychotherapy.* London: McFarland, 1985.

Solomon, H. A. *The exercise myth.* New York: Harcourt Brace Jovanovich, 1984.

Solomon, E. G., and Bumpus, A. K. The running meditation response: an adjunct to psychotherapy. In M. H. Sacks and M. L. Sachs (Eds.), *Psychology of running*. Champaign, Ill.: Human Kinetics, 1981.

Sonstroem, R. J. Exercise and self-esteem. In R. Terjung (Ed.), *Exercise and sport science reviews*. (volume 12). Lexington, Mass.: D. C. Heath, 1984. Pp. 123–155.

Sours, J. A. Running, anorexia nervosa and perfection. In M. H. Sacks and M. L. Sachs (Eds.), *Psychology of running*. Champaign, Ill.: Human Kinetics, 1981. Pp. 80–91.

Spielberger, C. D. *Anxiety and behavior*. New York: Academic Press, 1966.

Special Report. The great American shape-up. *Life*, 1987, *10* (2), 22–30.

Spence, A. P. *Basic human anatomy*. Menlo Park, Calif.: Benjamin/Cummings, 1982.

Standardized test of fitness: Operations manual. (Second Edition). Ottawa: Fitness and Amateur Sport Canada, 1981.

Stone, M. H., and Wilson, G. D. Resistive training and selected effects. *Medical Clinics of North America*, 1985, *69* (1), 109–122.

Sutton, R. *Body worry*. New York: Viking, 1987.

Swami Rama, Ballentine, R., and Swami Ajaya. *Yoga and psychotherapy: the evolution of consciousness*. Glenview, Ill.: Himalayan Institute, 1976.

Sweigard, L. E. *Human movement potential*. New York: Harper and Row, 1974.

Teshima, H., et al. Psychosomatic aspects of skin diseases from the standpoint of immunology. *Psychotherapy and Psychosomatics*, 1982, 37, 165–175.

Toufexis, A. Getting an F for flabby. *Time*, January 26, 1987. Pp. 54–56.

Thune, J. B. Personality of weight-lifters. *Research Quarterly*, 1949, *20*, 296–306.

Todd, M. E. *The thinking body*. New York: Dance Horizons, 1972.

Tucker, L. A. Weight training experience and psychological well-being. *Perceptual and Motor Skills*, 1982, *55* (2), 553–554.

Tucker, L. A. Muscular strength and mental health. *Journal of Personality and Social Psychology*, 1983, *45* (6), 1355–1360.

USA Today, Walkers outpacing joggers. May 28, 1987.

Valliant, P. M. Personality and injury in competitive runners. *Perceptual and Motor Skills*, 1981, *53* (1), 251–253.

Valliant, P. M., Simpson-Housley, P., and McKelvie, S. J. Personality in athletic and non-athletic college groups. *Perceptual and Motor Skills*, 1981, *52* (3), 963–966.

VanDyke, R. R. Aggression in sport: its implications for character building. *Quest*, 1980, *32* (2), 201–208.

Vanek, M., and Cratty, B. J. *Psychology and the superior athlete*. London: Collier-Macmillan, 1970.

Vaughan, B. L. *Body talk*. Allen, Tex.: Argus Communications, 1982.

Weltman, A. Exercise and diet to optimize body composition. In J. D. Matarazzo, S. M. Weiss, N. E. Miller, and S. M. Weiss (Eds.), *Behavioral health: a handbook of health enhancement and disease prevention*. New York: Wiley, 1984. Pp. 509–523.

Wiggins, D. K. The history of sport psychology in North America. In Silva, J. M., and Weinberg, R. S. (Eds.), *Psychological foundations of sport.* Champaign, Ill.: Human Kinetics, 1984. Pp. 9–34.

Williams, J. M., and Getty, D. Effect of levels of exercise on psychological mood states, physical fitness, and plasma beta-endorphin. *Perceptual and Motor Skills,* 1986, *63* (3), 1099–1105.

World Health Organization. *World Health Organization's Expert Committee on Mental Health.* (Report No. 13). New York: WHO, 1964.

Wrenn, M. Running to extremes. *Life,* 1987, *10* (2), 46–53.

Yates, A., Leehey, K., and Shisslak, C. M. Running—An analogue of anorexia? *New England Journal of Medicine,* 1983, *308* (5), 251–255.

Young, R. J., and Ismail, A. H. Personality differences of adult men before and after a physical fitness program. *Research Quarterly,* 1976, *47* (3), 513–519.

Young, R. J., and Ismail, A. H. Ability of biochemical and personality variables in discriminating between high and low physical fitness levels. *Journal of Psychosomatic Research,* 1978, *22,* 193–199.

Zarski, J. J., West, J. D., and Bubenzer, D. L. Social interest, running, and life adjustment. *Personnel and Guidance Journal,* 1982, *61* (3), 146–149.

Zeitchick, N. Who plays tennis and why. *Tennis,* May 1987, 42–43.

Zillman, D., Katcher, A. H., and Milavsky, B. Excitation transfer from physical exercise to subsequent aggressive behavior. *Journal of Experimental Social Psychology,* 1972, *8* (3), 247–259.

Zuckerman, M. Sensation seeking and sports. *Personality and Individual Differences,* 1983, *52* (2), 511–516.

Index

Aerobics, 12, 14, 209
  aggressive/nonaggressive rating, 207–8
  competitive/noncompetitive rating, 208
  control rating, 211
  disciplined/undisciplined rating, 207
  extension rating, 212
  focused/unfocused rating, 208
  force rating, 211
  linearity rating, 212
  overview of, 13–16, 205–6, 212–13
  risky/safe rating, 208
  social/nonsocial rating, 207
  speed rating, 212
  spontaneous/controlled rating, 207
Aerobics Way, The, 78
Aggressive/nonaggressive, 99, 101–2, 153–54, 156, 158, 162, 164
  aerobics and, 207–8
  body building and, 191–92
  cycling and, 215
  dance and, 237
  golf and, 255
  martial arts and, 229

  racquet sports and, 199–200
  running and, 173
  skiing and, 246
  swimming and, 184
  yoga and, 222
Allport, Gordon, 92
Arnot, R. B., 82–83

Behavior in Public Places, 146–47
Betrayal of the Body, 119
Bioenergetics, 119
Birdwhistell, Ray, 146
Body analysis dimensions (BADs), 129
  of aerobics, 209
  of body building, 193, 195
  of cycling, 216
  of dance, 238, 240
  flexibility, 127
  of golf, 255–56
  of martial arts, 230
  of racquet sports, 201, 203
  of running, 174, 176
  shape, 127